Periodontics and Implants - Contemporary Scientific and Clinical Perspective

Edited by Haim Tal

Published in London, United Kingdom

Periodontics and Implants - Contemporary Scientific and Clinical Perspective
http://dx.doi.org/10.5772/intechopen.1008112
Edited by Haim Tal

Contributors
Alberto Miselli, Alexandra Roi, Alexandre Perez, Ali Khalil, Alyssa Hanel, Benny Barak, Ciprian Ioan Roi, Cristin Coman, Daniele Botticelli, Dan Zhao, Diana-Larisa Ancuța, Dominic Palazzolo, Evgeny Weinberg, Eyal Amar, Gavriel Chaushu, Giancarlo Cuadra, Gregori M. Kurtzman, Haim Tal, Haim Tal, Hari S. Prasad, Houze Li, Itzhak Binderman, Jamil Awad Shibli, Latfiya Al Harthi, Laura-Cristina Rusu, Liat Chaushu, Michal Halperin-Sternfeld, Michel Dard, Mircea Rivis, Nadim Sleman, Nicole Christian, Ofer Moses, Perry Raz, Robert A. Horowitz, Ruxandra Luca, Sara Pecorelli, Shlomo Barak, Simina Boia, Sophie Tomov, Sun Haipeng, Tommaso Lombardi, Vivian Ha, Xiaoxiao Wang, Yaniv Mayer, Yan Wang, Yunyi Xie, Zahra Mustafa Juma Al Lawati, Ziad Albash

First published in London, United Kingdom, 2026 by IntechOpen
IntechOpen is the global imprint of INTECHOPEN LIMITED, registered in England and Wales, registration number: 11086078, 167-169 Great Portland Street, London, W1W 5PF, United Kingdom

For EU product safety concerns: IN TECH d.o.o., Prolaz Marije Krucifikse Kozulić 3, 51000 Rijeka, Croatia, info@intechopen.com or visit our website at intechopen.com.

British Library Cataloguing-in-Publication Data
A catalogue record for this book is available from the British Library

Periodontics and Implants - Contemporary Scientific and Clinical Perspective
Edited by Haim Tal
p. cm.

This title is part of the Dentistry Book Series, Volume 29
Series Editor: Sergio Alexandre Gehrke

Print ISBN 978-1-83635-439-0
Online ISBN 978-1-83635-438-3
eBook (PDF) ISBN 978-1-83635-440-6
ISSN 2631-6218

IntechOpen Book Series
Dentistry
Volume 29

Aims and Scope of the Series

This book series will offer a comprehensive overview of recent research trends as well as clinical applications within different specialties of dentistry. Topics will include overviews of the health of the oral cavity, from prevention and care to different treatments for the rehabilitation of problems that may affect the organs and/or tissues present. The different areas of dentistry will be explored, with the aim of disseminating knowledge and providing readers with new tools for the comprehensive treatment of their patients with greater safety and with current techniques. Ongoing issues, recent advances, and future diagnostic approaches and therapeutic strategies will also be discussed. This series of books will focus on various aspects of the properties and results obtained by the various treatments available, whether preventive or curative.

Meet the Series Editor

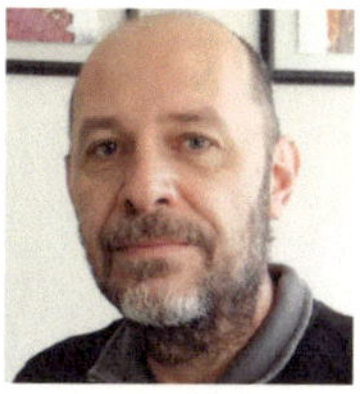

Dr. Sergio Alexandre Gehrke is a doctorate holder in two fields. The first is a Ph.D. in Cellular and Molecular Biology from the Pontificia Catholic University, Porto Alegre, Brazil, in 2010 and the other is an International Ph.D. in Bioengineering from the Universidad Miguel Hernandez, Elche/Alicante, Spain, obtained in 2020. In 2018, he completed a postdoctoral fellowship in Materials Engineering in the NUCLEMAT of the Pontificia Catholic University, Porto Alegre, Brazil. He is currently the Director of the Postgraduate Program in Implantology of the Bioface/UCAM/PgO (Montevideo, Uruguay), Director of the Cathedra of Biotechnology of the Catholic University of Murcia (Murcia, Spain), an Extraordinary Full Professor of the Catholic University of Murcia (Murcia, Spain) as well as the Director of the private center of research Biotecnos – Technology and Science (Montevideo, Uruguay). Applied biomaterials, cellular and molecular biology, and dental implants are among his research interests. He has published several original papers in renowned journals. In addition, he is also a Collaborating Professor in several Postgraduate programs at different universities all over the world.

Meet the Volume Editor

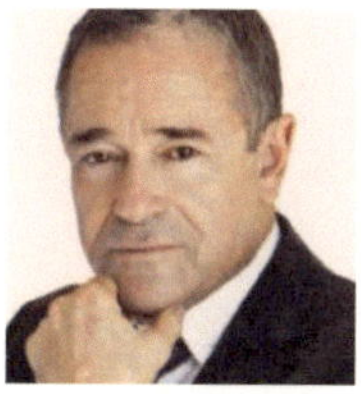

Haim Tal is a Professor (Emeritus) at Tel Aviv University. He served as chairman of the Department of Periodontology and Oral Implants and as Incumbent of the Niznick Chair of Implant Research since 1992. In parallel, he served for 10 years as the Dean of the School of Dental Medicine. Professor Tal graduated (DMD) from Hadassa Faculty of Dental Medicine at the Hebrew University, Jerusalem, and specialized in periodontics and oral medicine at the University of the Witwatersrand, Johannesburg, where he also completed doctoral studies in physical anthropology. He served as an Associate Professor of Periodontology at New York University and held visiting professorships at New York University, the University of Pennsylvania, and the University of Toronto. He served as Chief Clinical Scientist at Tactile Technologies Co., Israel, developers of computer-guided implant systems, and was one of the developers of "OSSIX Collagen membrane of Cobar Co., Israel. Presently, he consults for Core-Bone Co., Israel, developers of a Novel Coral graft for Bone Regeneration and Cartilage Healing.

Contents

Preface

The contemporary era is marked by an exponential expansion of multidisciplinary information encompassing all branches of dentistry. Clinicians are inundated daily with developments from the biological, chemical, technological, and related sciences. Such a continuous influx of information often disrupts professional routines and prompts critical reflection: Are we sufficiently up to date? Have we provided the highest standard of care? Do the techniques in which we are trained and proficient still represent the state of the art? Two domains within restorative dentistry that have witnessed particularly notable advances are periodontology and implant-supported rehabilitation. Periodontal therapy has evolved through innovative regenerative techniques grounded in cutting-edge biological discoveries that parallel advancements in other medical disciplines. Implant therapy, in turn, has benefited from substantial technical, metallurgical, digital, and even electronic innovations.

Printed literature, by its nature, cannot compete with the continuously expanding body of electronic information. The enduring value of scientific literature, in general, and textbooks, in particular, lies in their ability to compile, structure, and critically assess accumulated knowledge in a coherent, logical manner, while emphasizing rigorously selected, evidence-based information that has stood the test of time.

Although natural dentition and dental implants are both anchored within the jaws and surrounded by similar osseous and soft tissues, their biological behaviour differs profoundly. Despite being affected by diseases that appear analogous, and that have even been assigned parallel terminology (periodontitis and peri-implantitis), the only well-established common denominator is the presence of a similar bacterial biofilm accompanied by an acute or chronic inflammatory response in the adjacent tissues. Nevertheless, given that natural teeth and implants serve comparable functional, phonetic, and aesthetic purposes, and share the same anatomical environment within the alveolar ridges, it is both logical and advantageous to address them within a single volume.

This is not a traditional book, nor is it confined to a single topic within periodontology or implantology. Rather, it comprises a curated compendium of chapters, some of which delineate the current state of knowledge, while others explore emerging developments that are still in the process of research and formation.

I believe that these contributions will stimulate curiosity and foster the pursuit of subsequent advancements, clinical, experimental, and philosophical alike.

Haim Tal
Department of Periodontology and Oral Implants,
Tel Aviv University School of Dental Medicine,
Tel Aviv, Israel

Section 1

Innovations

Chapter 1

Cultivated Coral Grafts for Treatment of Bone and Focal Osteochondral Defects: Clinical and Preclinical Observations

Haim Tal and Eyal Amar

Abstract

Bone grafts are an integral component of most oral rehabilitation treatment programs. The similarity between the characteristics of bones and natural coral in terms of composition, structure, strength, and resorption qualities, has led to the widespread use of coral-derived materials in orthopedics and dentistry, particularly for bone augmentation. The use of coral-based xenografts allows circumventing some of the inherent complications associated with the use of autogenous grafts and allografts. Recently, it has been shown that under certain circumstances, coral grafts may also have the potential to induce cartilage growth in some affected sites. This chapter describes the unique qualities of natural cultivated coral skeleton that grows in an optimal artificial environment, making it an ideal biomaterial for bone and cartilage substitutes. This chapter is divided into three parts: *Part I* relates primarily to augmentation of bone following bone loss due to tooth loss, periodontal disease, trauma and other pathological conditions in the oral environment; this part is based on clinical and histological observations. *Part II* presents a multicenter clinical study carried out in three dental centers on 160 participants comparing CoreBone® – a coral bone substitute (experimental) to TCP Curasan AG® (control). *Part III* relates to preliminary results of an ongoing pilot study investigating healing of cartilage defects created by experimental surgical injuries in ovine joints, using a novel coral product, CoreTlage®.

Keywords: periodontitis periimplantitis, bone regeneration, xenograft, coral, cartilage

1. Introduction

1.1 Coral-based bone substitutes

Natural coral skeleton is morphologically and chemically similar to native bone. Porous coralline granules derived from natural corals have several attributes that render them a suitable biomaterial for bone substitution in bone augmentation procedures, while bypassing some of the inherent complications associated with the use of autogenous grafts or allografts. Coral bone substitute (CBS) is an osteoconductive material, designed to serve as a scaffold for bone growth and bone maturation. In addition, CBS does not evoke inflammatory infiltrate or fibrous encapsulation [1, 2].

Since they were first developed in the 1980s, coral (coralline) grafts have been successfully used worldwide to treat a variety of orthopedic, craniofacial and oral bony defects, and to support osseous augmentation procedures. Numerous preclinical and clinical studies, including longitudinal follow-ups have demonstrated successful augmentation using natural coral skeleton, indicating that both natural coral and coralline hydroxyapatite are biocompatible, osteoconductive and resistant to infections [1, 3]. Several studies have shown that calcium carbonate-rich grafts (BioCoral®, France) induced new bone formation after maxillary sinus augmentation [2, 4–6]. A study that compared maxillary sinus augmentation responses to tissue-engineered bone graft obtained by a culture of autogenous osteoblasts seeded on polyglycolicpolylactic scaffolds (Oral Bone®, BioTissue®, Germany) versus calcium carbonate (BioCoral®, France), showed that the mean new bone in the grafted area was 37 and 55%, respectively [5]. A clinical follow-up of socket preservation procedures using CBS in the posterior maxilla and mandible demonstrated successful support of dental implants with no need for additional augmentation procedures. Hence, in successful sites, coral granules can spare residual ridge atrophy and resorption, obviating the need for additional augmentation aids and reducing treatment and costs (**Figure 1**).

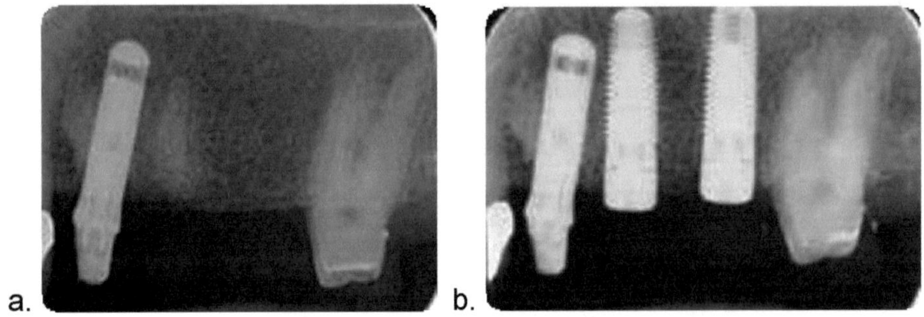

Figure 1.
(a) Radiographic view of an extraction socket site of tooth #25, 4 months after being grafted with CoreBone® 1000. The radio-opaque area shows new bone and graft particles. (b) Radiographic view 5 months after the extraction showing two implants placed at sites #25 and #26.

Histological analyses of core specimens harvested during implant placement in sites that were previously treated with coral grafts, revealed no foreign body reaction to coral grafted particles [1]. Histochemical analysis showed no presence of osteoblasts positive for alkaline phosphatase, and mineralized tissue analysis (von Kossa stain) demonstrated a mature and highly mineralized bone around the grafted particles [7]. **Figure 2** demonstrates a sample of computerized histometric analysis of a typical non-decalcified histological section harvested from a xenograft augmented antral sinus floor.

The fact that almost all grafted particles were in contact with mature bone, supports the claim that this biomaterial is highly osteoconductive. Notably, no fibrous tissue encapsulation was observed [7, 8].

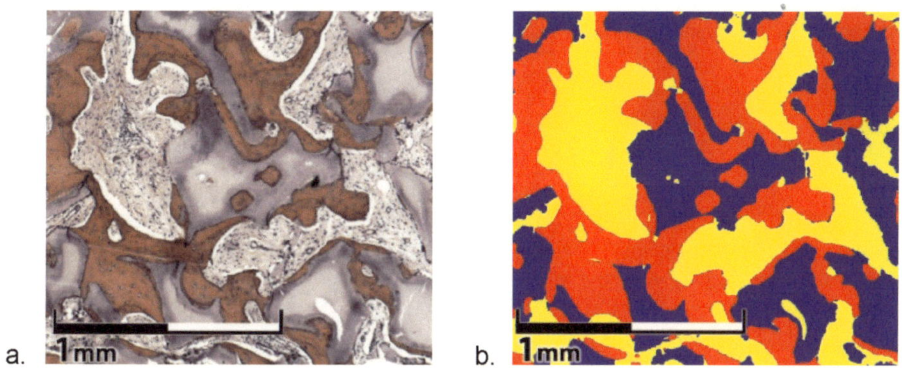

Figure 2.
Histological section of a core harvested from an antral sinus floor augmented with CBS particles. (a) Almost all grafted particles are in contact with new bone. (b) Computerized histometric analysis further supports the microscopic observation.

1.2 Cultivated coral bone substitute: Production and quality

As mentioned above, the bonelike properties of natural coral, in terms of qualities, composition, structure, strength and resorption, have led to their popular use in dental and orthopedic procedures. However, in the last decade, corals have been declared endangered species, and their quality has deteriorated mainly owing to sea pollution. These were among the main reasons to develop CoreBone® as a biomimetic CBS composed of pure coral minerals. This product consists of over 95% calcium carbonate crystals in the form of aragonite, enriched with silicium, strontium, and other non-organic substances. The three main elements – calcium, silicium and strontium – play an important role in bone mineralization and activation of enzymatic reactions in osteogenic cells (**Figure 3**).

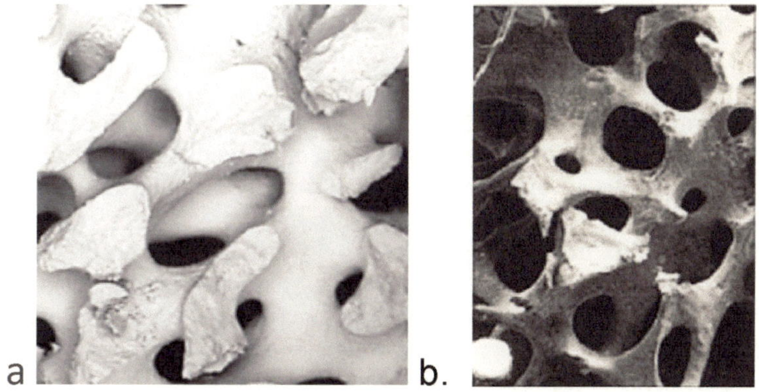

Figure 3.
Scanning electron microscope images showing similarity between (a) CoreBone ® coral porous structure and (b) human bone mineralized tissue.

Table 1 presents the ultimate tensile strength of different bone substitutes. Silicium and strontium contribute to the strength of the CBS, which is up to five times higher than that of synthetic or cancellous bones.

Ultimate tensile strength (MPa, Mega Pascal)	Type of bone substitute
22–17	CoreBone
8–3	Sea corals of different makers
7–3.5	Spongiosa bone
5–2	Synthetic bone

Table 1.
Ultimate tensile strength of different types of bone substitute materials.

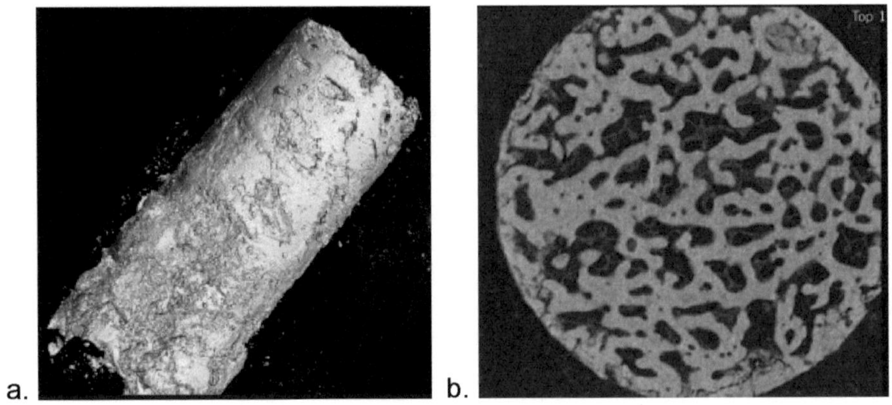

Figure 4.
(a) Micro computed tomography (CT) 3D view of a cylindrical core harvested from a canine extraction socket grafted with core bone®. (b) Cross section at the middle of the core taken 8 weeks after the extraction shows dense, well organized cancellous bone filling the socket.

The CBS comprises a combination of coral types which mimic cortical and cancellous bones and allow optimal bone growth and remodeling using osteoclasts. Its porous structure enables vascular ingrowth and the formation of new bone (**Figure 4**).

Unlike previous products, CoreBone® CBS is produced from corals that are grown in a closed, controlled aquatic system (aquarium) that is fed by proprietary technology laboratory-made sea water enriched with bioactive nutrients. This coral growing technology allows utilizing the bone-like properties of corals while avoiding sea pollution-related risks (**Figure 5**).

Since the structure of corals is affected by its environment (e.g., salinity, minerals, and temperature), the controlled aquatic system enables growing various types of corals, with each type having specific porosity, strength and shape; these may be used for a different indication in dentistry and orthopedics.

Following tooth extraction, various intra-alveolar and extra-alveolar processes – mainly bone resorption – take place in the alveolar ridge and the alveolar process of bone [9, 10]. This pathological bone loss may decrease significantly if graft material is placed in the fresh extraction socket.

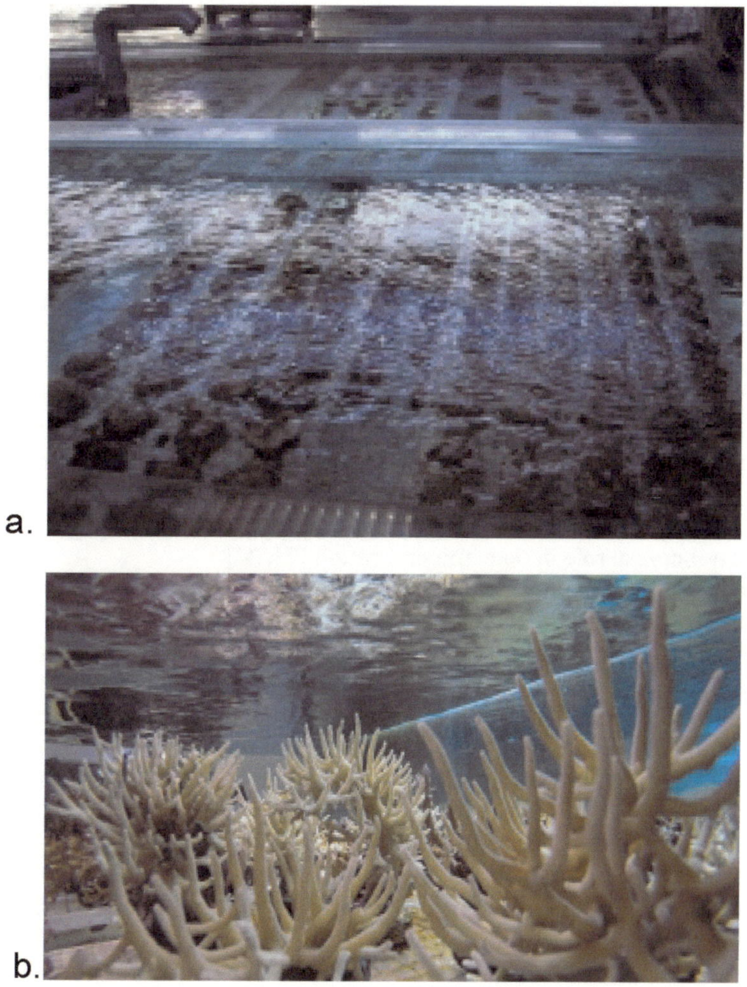

Figure 5.
Cultivated coral aquariums. (a) CoreBone® aquarium provides sea-like water, bioactive enriched with nutrients. (b) Natural growth of cultivated corals in an artificial controlled environment.

The introduction of immediate implant placement, especially at sites in which post-extraction bone resorption is prominent, has made bone augmentation procedures a frequent and integral part of most treatment plans, especially if implant placement is included [11, 12]. Therefore, the use of osseo-integrated oral implants required the establishment of suitable bony contours of the jaw by increasing the bone volume at the implant sites.

The gold-standard treatment for bone defects is bone transplantation, which not only provides physical support to the affected bone but also promotes bone regeneration [13]. There are four types of bone graft materials available, including autologous bone, allogenic bone grafts, artificial bone materials, and xenogeneic bone [14]. Autologous bone is regular bone tissue taken from the patient's body to repair the damaged area. Its main advantage is that it does not cause rejection reactions [15]. However, obtaining the implanted autologous bone requires additional surgery, which can increase patient pain, blood loss, surgical infection rate, and long-term hospitalization costs [16].

Allogeneic demineralized freeze-dried bone cannot fill large bone defects due to the loss of some mechanical properties during the demineralization process [17]. Synthetic materials are better at controlling product quality and can avoid the risk of infection through complete artificial synthesis [18]. However, synthetic materials typically lack the natural porous structure, strength and resorption of autologous or allogeneic bone grafts, leading to slower bone growth [19]. Some materials also have certain toxicity, which can lead to chronic poisoning in patients [20].

Coral exoskeletons are excellent substitutes for bone grafts as they are biocompatible, osteoconductive, and biodegradable [9]. They are derived from marine madreporic corals and have been used for dental applications since 1929 [2]. Coral bone has been available as a medical material since the late 80s [9] and has been used in hundreds of thousands of dental and orthopedic implantations without any reported safety issues [2, 21]. The exoskeletons are rich in calcium carbonate, which allows for cell attachment, growth, spreading and differentiation [22]. Coral exoskeletons are made up of calcium carbonate and various trace elements such as magnesium, strontium, fluorine and phosphorous, all of which play a crucial role in bone mineralization [23, 24].

Coral materials are bioinert and have an affinity for regenerated bone to grow directly on their surface [25]. The pore dimensions and configuration of coral exoskeletons make them ideal for bone ingrowth [26, 27]. The type of bone regenerated in these implants depends on the location of the implant [28]. In humans, implants degrade at different speeds depending on the location and surrounding soft tissue [29]. Coral implants can improve clinical attachment levels, reconstruct defects, and have similar risks compared to bone grafting [30].

Corebone® graft is a type of bone graft substitute derived from the calcium carbonate exoskeleton of coral. Available in various forms and sizes, Corebone® is intended for use in a range of applications. The coral used in the process is sourced from an O.K. coral farm, which employs a closed system with online monitoring. Coral growth is carefully monitored in an aquarium to maintain optimal water quality and growth conditions, minimizing the risk of coral contamination and enhancing product safety.

The following are three clinical examples of cases in which CBS was used for augmentation of different bony defects in the jaws. These will be followed by a prospective double blind, cohort clinical study that relates to augmentation of fresh tooth extraction sockets.

Finally, Part III will deal with an ongoing study using a novel experimental product that is presently being experimented on ovine (sheeps).

2. Part I: Clinical case reports

2.1 Case 1: Socket preservation and immediate implant placement after extraction of the right mandibular first molar (#46) in a 24-year-old woman

Due to a longitudinal crack of the distal root of a right mandibular first molar tooth an atraumatic extraction was performed (**Figure 6**). The extraction socket presented

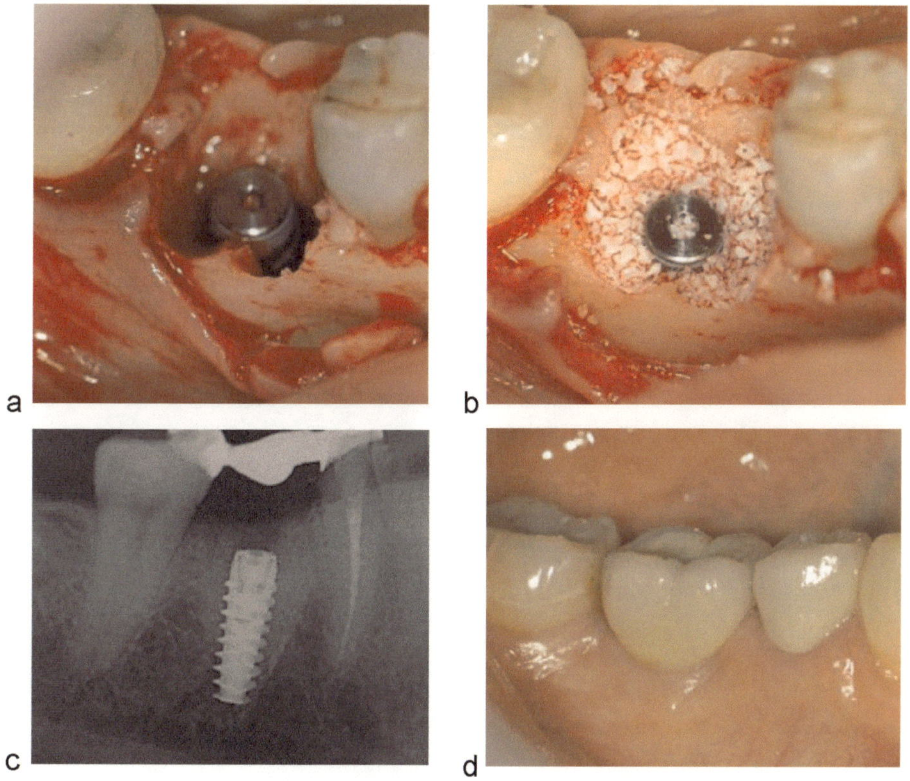

Figure 6.
Immediate implant placement supported by peripheral CBS particles of 600–1000 μm.

bone contours and volume which were suitable for immediate implant placement. An implant, 5 mm in diameter, was placed with the shoulders 1–2 mm below the extraction socket's margins (**Figure 6a**). The space between the alveolar bone proper and the implant surface was filled with CBS particles 600–1000 μm. (**Figure 6b**), and covered with a resorbable collagen membrane. The socket was covered with released coronally positioned gingival flaps. After 6 months, a periapical radiograph presented clinical osseointegration between the newly bone growth and the Implant's surface (**Figure 6c**). The implant was exposed and restored with a zirconia crown (**Figure 6d**).

2.2 Case 2: Augmentation of large bony defect in the right posterior maxilla, following enucleation of a periapical cyst and a sinus floor augmentation procedure

CoreBone 1000® with granule size 600–1000 μm was used (**Figure 7**).

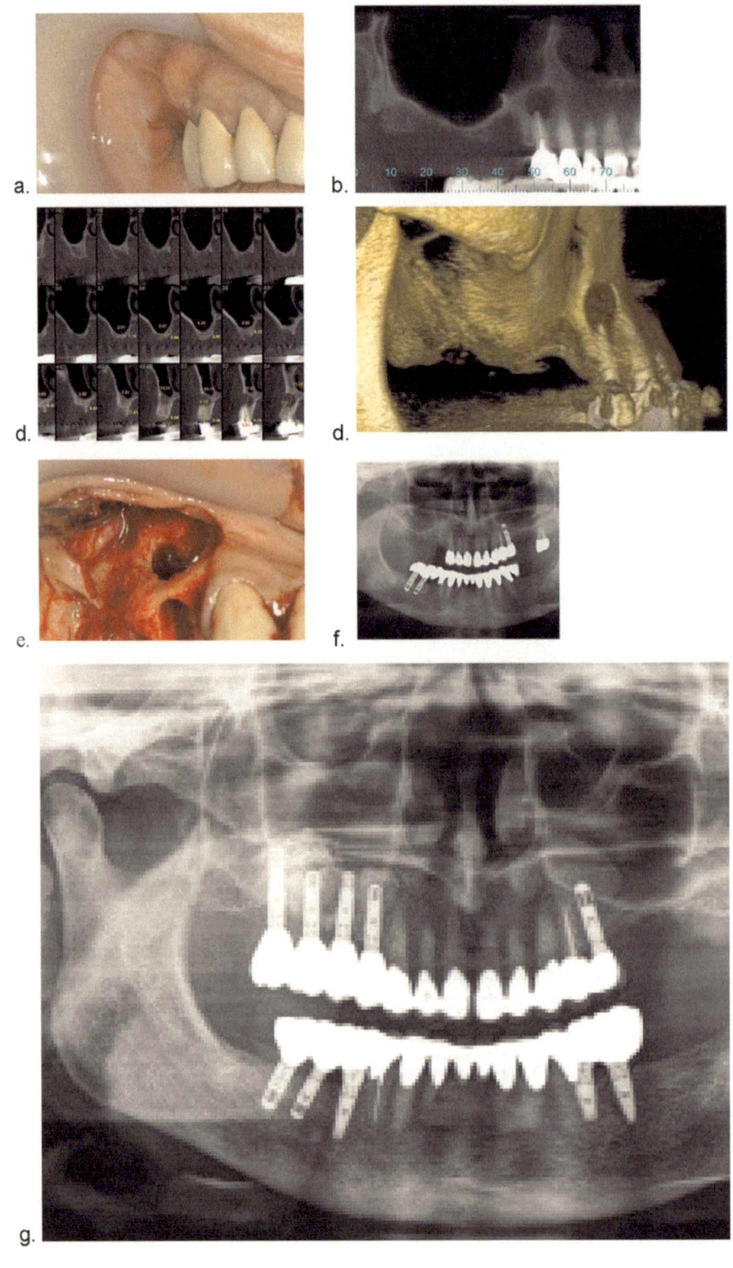

Figure 7.
Case description. Local swelling at the buccal aspect of the upper first right premolar tooth (#14). (b) A longitudinal CT section shows bony defects associated with the first and missing second premolar teeth (#14, #15). (c) Cross CT sections of the upper right posterior maxilla indicate bone loss in the molar region, resulting in a thin (1–2 mm) sinus floor and periapical defect associated with the first premolar. (d) A 3D image of the upper right posterior maxilla showing severe bone loss in the molar region and a periapical defect associated with the first premolar. (e) A surgical view of the upper right posterior maxilla shows severe bone loss in the posterior maxillary crest of bone (molars and second premolar teeth) and an extraction socket and periapical defect associated with the second and first premolars. The bony defects were grafted with CoreBone® 600–1000 um stabilized with collagen membranes. (f) Five months after surgery: a panoramic view shows successful healing of the augmented defects and sinus floor augmentation. (g) Eight months after sinus floor augmentation, the augmented jaw was followed by placement of 4 implants and 5 months after implants placement a panoramic view shows restoration of an implant-supported fixed prosthesis.

2.3 Case 3: Implant placement following extraction sockets preservation procedure in the upper jaw esthetic zone

A 56-year-old woman was scheduled for extractions of the upper central incisors due to a hopeless diagnosis owing to increased mobility (class II+) and surrounding loss of the attachment apparatus with buccal and interproximal probing depth measuring 10–12 mm (**Figure 8a**). Extracted teeth demonstrated soft tissue remnants adherent to the root surfaces leaving wide extraction sockets (**Figure 8b**) with no sufficient apical bone to stabilize immediate implants.

Two dental implants were placed slightly palatal to the original teeth; these were X-rayed after 5 months. Periapical radiograph confirmed successful osseointegration (**Figure 8j**). placement of two dental implants in the grafted region. Final prosthetic restoration at 1 year fulfilled both functional and esthetic criteria (**Figure 8k**).

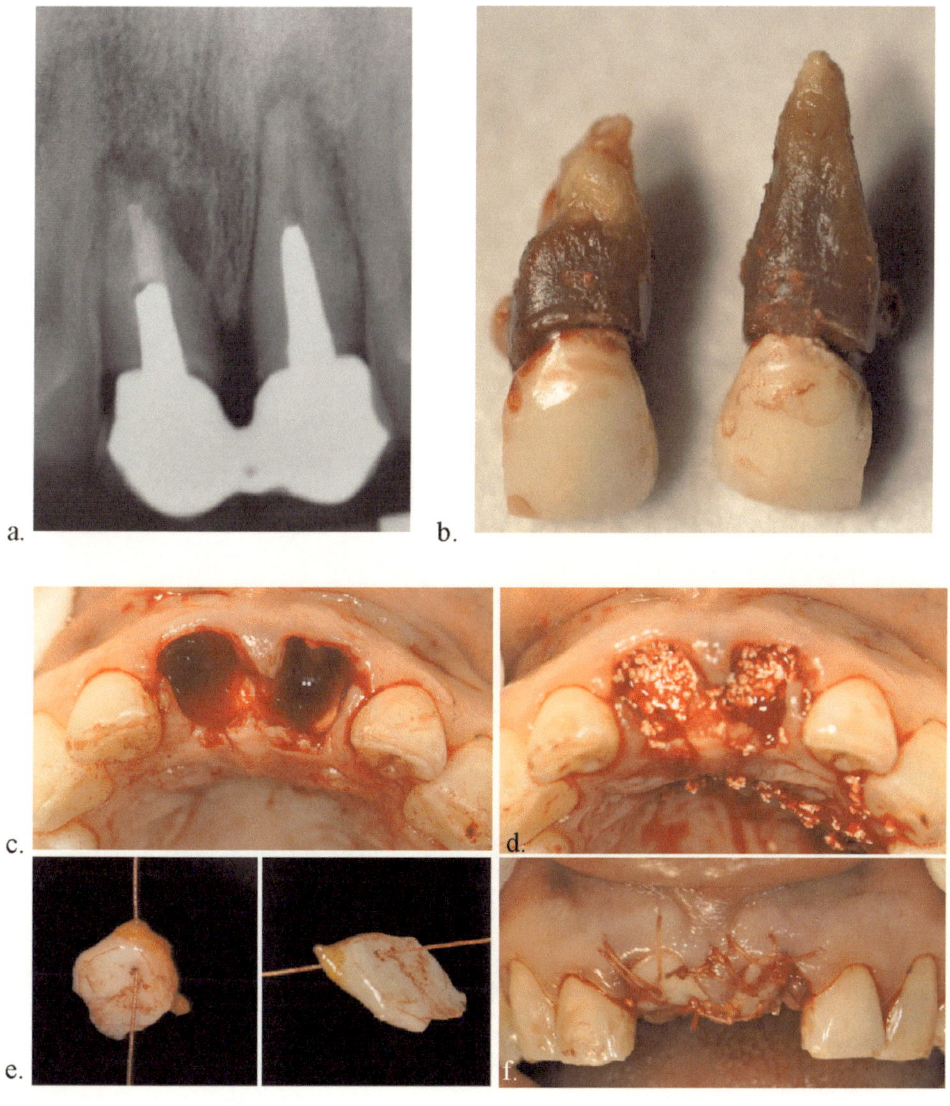

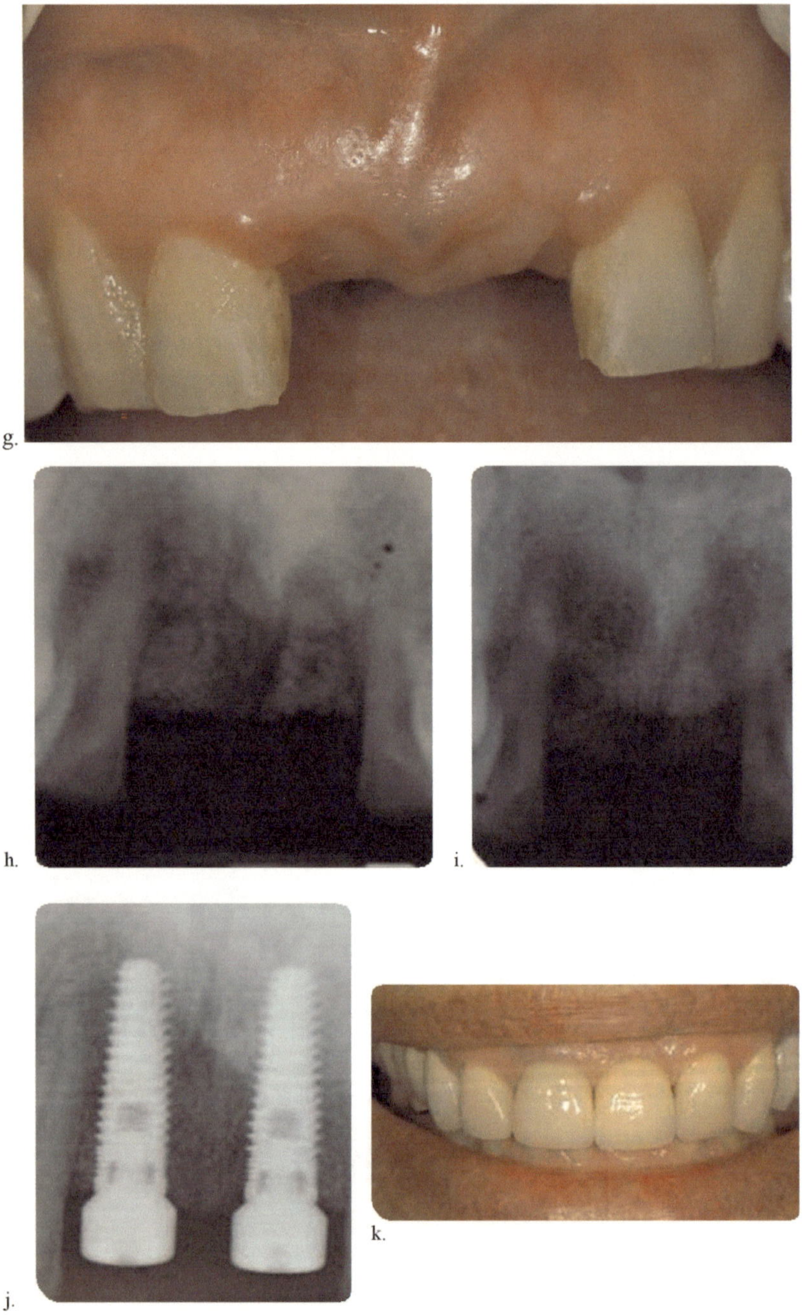

Figure 8.
(a) Preoperative periapical radiograph of the maxillary central incisors reveals increased mobility and surrounding granulation tissue with signs of inflammation. (b) Clinical image of the extracted teeth, demonstrating soft tissue remnants adherent to the root surfaces. Ridge preservation procedure was carried out using (CoreBone®). The grafted sockets (c, d) were sealed with connective tissue grafts (e, f). (c–f) Clinical presentation of the socket preservation procedure. (b) Intraoral view of the post-extraction sockets (upper left) (d) Post-ridge preservation image following grafting with coral-bone 1000 (upper right). (e) Connective tissue grafts taken from the palate designed to seal the socket orifices and stabilize the particulate graft material (lower left). (f) Final sealing of the extraction sites using free gingival grafts, serving both to protect the grafted areas and to augment the keratinized mucosa through autogenous soft tissue augmentation. Satisfactory soft tissue healing was observed at 6 months post-surgery (g). Radiographic follow-up one at 1 m demonstrates successful replacement of the graft material with newly formed native bone (h). This is further confirmed 3 months later (i).

3. Part II: Comparative clinical study analyzing the differences between Corebone® and CTP Curasan AG® as bone substitute materials in socket preservation procedures

Unlike most coral-based products, Corebone® keeps natural form of the coral without any coating or treatments such as HA coating or heat treatment, preserving the pore structure and microscopic rough surface of the coral to better support osteogenesis. This part presents the results of a multicenter, open-label, randomized, parallel-controlled non-inferiority trial aimed at estimating the safety and efficacy of Corebone® compared to the in-market product, **TCP** Curasan AG®. This study is a crucial step in evaluating the potential of Corebone as a bioresorbable bone graft substitute. The trial's primary objective is to demonstrate non-inferiority in safety and efficacy of Corebone® compared to Curasan®. The use of a novel natural coral in the Corebone® product line seeks to maximize the retention of the coral's unique properties, facilitating optimal healing outcomes. The results of this study provide a promising outlook for Corebone® as a safe and effective alternative for bone grafting procedures.

3.1 Study design

The study was carried out as a multicenter, open, randomized, parallel-controlled clinical trial conducted at three medical institutions: Peking University Third Hospital, Peking Union Medical College of the Chinese Academy of Medical Sciences, and Beijing Friendship Hospital affiliated with Capital Medical University. Due to the appearance differences between the test and control products, it was not possible to achieve blinding. Therefore, an open experimental design was used. Random enrollment was conducted to reduce trial bias caused by sampling errors. For random sampling, random letters were assigned to the screened qualified cases. After opening the random letters, each group was given the corresponding treatment, with each random number not indicating the patient's group and treatment. The control product used was dental bone powder produced by Curasan AG (Curasan®). The qualified subjects were randomly divided into experimental and control groups for clinical evaluation.

3.2 Participants

The trial was planned to recruit 168 subjects (1:1 male and female). In this report, participants who had finished follow-up before 28th Feb 2024 were included. The study requires participants between the ages of 18 and 65, who voluntarily provide their consent. Candidates are required to have good oral hygiene habits and require tooth extraction. The surgical wound must be capable of being entirely closed with tight suturing. Prospective participants with a history of osteoporosis and receiving bisphosphonate treatment or those who have undergone radiation therapy and chemotherapy in the maxillofacial, nasopharyngeal, and cervical regions within the past 5 years are prohibited from participating. Individuals with severe degenerative diseases, locally infected areas, and severe systemic diseases are also excluded. Furthermore, individuals with systemic or local bone diseases such as bone cysts, bone tuberculosis, osteoarthritis, and bone tumors, pregnant or lactating women, those with a pregnancy plan within the next 6 months, and people on long-term use of special drugs such as hormones or anticoagulants are not eligible. Prospective participants with mental illness, psychological disorders, and neurological disorders like epilepsy, endocrine and metabolic disorders, hematological disorders, and uncontrolled cardiovascular diseases are also prohibited from participating. Additionally, individuals who smoke more than 10 cigarettes per day, have poor oral hygiene habits, severe bone defects, or diabetes, and those with a severe allergic constitution are also excluded. Researchers believe that other factors may also render an individual unsuitable for participation in the study. All participants are required to provide written informed consent. Additional details regarding inclusion/exclusion criteria are available in the supplementary information section.

3.3 Randomization

This clinical trial was executed utilizing a randomized enrollment approach to mitigate the potential bias introduced by sampling errors. The statistical department provided random numbers for each subject, which were generated through the PLAN process of SAS 9.2 on an electronic computer. The subjects were then assigned to either the test or control groups in a 1:1 ratio, following predetermined rules. It is noteworthy that this randomization process is reproducible and that the parameters utilized in the process, such as the length of the block group and the initial seed parameter of the random number, are recorded in the randomization table.

The specific method employed for randomizing the subjects entails the assignment of random letters in sequential order to the screened cases. These random letters are subsequently revealed to determine the group to which the subject belongs, and the appropriate treatment is dispensed accordingly. It is pertinent to note that each random number, in isolation, does not suggest the patient's group or treatment.

3.4 Procedures

The purpose of this study was to perform minimally invasive socket preservation using local anesthesia (ativanacaine) after tooth extraction in eligible patients. After the extraction, granulation tissue present within the socket was removed, whereas the alveolar socket was filled with Corebone bone graft in the test group or β-tricalcium phosphate artificial bone from Corusan AG in the control group. Following this, both groups were covered with Geistlich Bio-Gide, a resorbable biofilm (membrance) from Geistlich Pharmaceuticals AG, Switzerland, and the extraction wounds were tightly closed with silk sutures. Postoperative antibiotics were administered to prevent infection.

A cone-beam computed tomography (CBCT) was conducted immediately after the procedure to determine the height and width of the alveolar ridge bone. The vertical height is the distance from the top of the alveolar ridge to the lowest horizontal plane of the jawbone.

Width reference point, the horizontal width of the alveolar bone 5 mm along the vertical direction toward the root from point e is width. Adverse events and corresponding clinical responses were noted, along with any instrumentation defects and the documentation of medication combinations. However, anesthetics and hemostatic drugs used during surgery were not considered as combined medications.

CBCT was utilized to record the bone morphology of the implant area 180 days after surgery to determine the alveolar ridge bone height and width at 6 months postoperatively, as well as to calculate the change in alveolar ridge bone height and width. Any adverse events and corresponding clinical responses were recorded, along with the presence of instrumentation defects and the documentation of medication combinations.

3.5 Outcomes

The primary outcome is the change in alveolar ridge bone height immediately after surgery and at 6 months post-op.

3.6 Patient and public involvement

In order to prevent trial bias and data sampling, it is imperative that researchers adhere strictly to the inclusion and exclusion criteria. Moreover, it is recommended that they undertake the following measures: carefully review the instruction manual before employing the product, attend a CoreBone product training session or watch a demonstration video, meticulously inspect the product before use, and prepare supplementary products. These procedures should be carried out solely by trained and qualified physicians, and the assessment of outcomes must be consistent throughout testing and evaluation by trial outcome assessors.

3.7 Statistical analysis

The evaluation methods for the trial to determine non-inferiority are based on the Guidelines for clinical trials of bone substitute materials for repairing alveolar bone defects in China. To be considered non-inferior, the lower limit of the 95% confidence interval difference of ΔHFBT (ΔHFBT (Corebone group) - ΔHFBT (Curasan group)) at 6 months after surgery should be greater than −0.35 mm [31]. A non-parametric test was used to compare the alveolar bone height and alveolar bone horizontal width between Corebone and Curasan on day 2 after surgery and 6 months after surgery [31].

3.8 Results

3.8.1 Participants

A total of 168 subjects were involved in this study (84 subjects treated with Corebone, and 84 subjects treated with Curasan). By now, 160 of them have completed the final examinations. The participant's profile is summarized below. There was no significant different in age or gender between Corebone and Curasan group (**Figure 9**).

3.8.2 Primary outcome

On the first day following the surgical procedure, a cone beam computed tomography (CBCT) scan was performed to evaluate the surgical outcomes of the Corebone and Curasan groups. The primary objective was to determine whether any dissimilarities existed between the two groups and to assess the reliability of the baseline. Findings from the initial postoperative CBCT results revealed no significant differences between the Corebone and Curasan groups (**Figure 2**). Similarly, no significant variance was observed in the postoperative alveolar bone height and horizontal alveolar bone width among the groups, which indicated the dependability of the baseline for both groups (**Figure 10**).

The height and width of alveolar bone after implant bone graft (Corebone or Curasan). All the patients used bio-membrane to cover the wound after implant bone graft. There was no difference between Corebone and Curasan after 1 day of surgery. An unpaired nonparametric test was used for the statistics analyzed. $P < 0.05$ was considered a significant difference. V2:1 day after surgery (**Figure 10**).

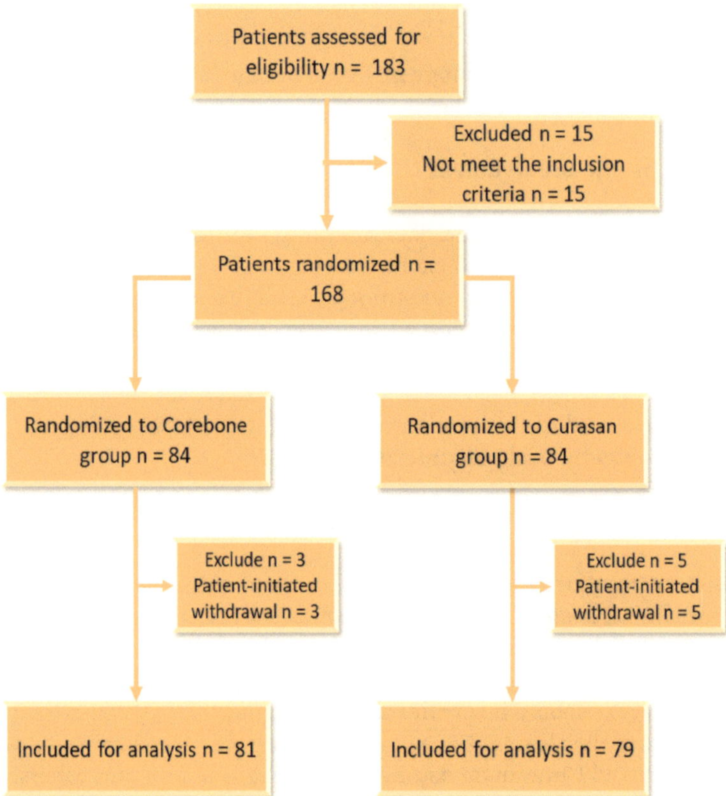

Figure 9.
Subject involvement and exclude situation of the trial.

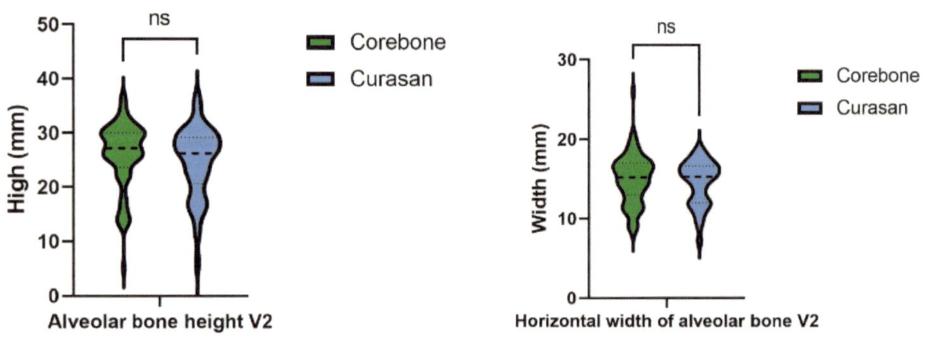

Figure 10.
The height and width of alveolar bone 1 day after surgery of Corebone and Curasan treatment.

A secondary cone beam computed tomography (CBCT) scan was performed 180 days post-surgery to evaluate the stability and efficacy of Corebone, in comparison to Curasan, a well-established market product renowned for its efficacy and stability. The results of the study indicated that Corebone was not inferior to Curasan in terms of stability and efficacy. The majority of subjects who underwent surgery with Corebone and Curasan experienced no changes in alveolar bone height and alveolar bone horizontal width after 6 months. The alveolar bone dimensions did not differ significantly between Corebone and Curasan (**Figure 3**). These findings demonstrate that Corebone is a robust and effective long-term solution. As per the "Guidelines for Clinical Trials of Bone Substitute Materials for Repairing Alveolar Bone Defects" in China, Corebone has an IC 95% lower limit of 0.0368 mm, which is higher than the non-inferior requirement of −0.035 mm (**Tables 2** and **3**). These results confirm that Corebone is non-inferior to Curasan's product (**Figures 11** and **12**).

Group		Corebone	Curasan	p value
Subjects involved		81	79	
Gender	Female	52 (64%)	51 (55%)	0.914
	Male	29 (36%)	28 (45%)	
Age	Average	29.05 (year)	27.89 (year)	
	20 ~ 30	73 (90%)	66 (86%)	0.439
	31 ~ 40	5 (7%)	9 (12%)	
	41 ~ 50	1 (1%)	2 (1%)	
	51 ~ 60	1 (1%)	0 (0%)	
	61 ~ 70	1 (1%)	2 (1%)	

Table 2.
Brief summary of enrollment subjects' distribution.

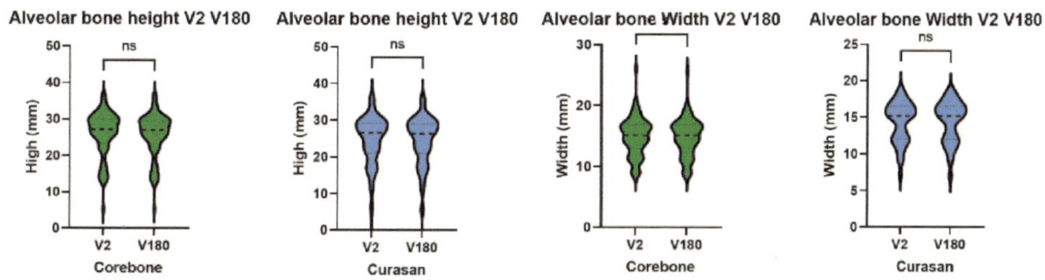

Figure 11.
Comparison of alveolar bone height and width at 1 day after surgery and 180 days after surgery. Comparison of alveolar bone height and width at 1 day after surgery and 180 days after surgery. There is no significant difference between V2 and V180 after surgery in Corebone or Curasan group. Unpaired nonparametric test was used for the statistic analyzed. P < 0.05 was considered significant difference. V2: 1 day after surgery. V180: 180 days after surgery.

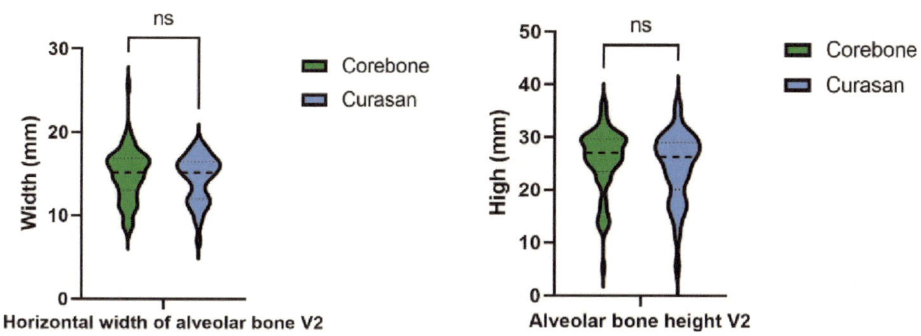

Figure 12.
Comparison of alveolar bone height and width at 180 days after surgery.

4. Part III: Evaluation of cultivated coral implants for regeneration of focal osteochondral defects in ovine model

4.1 Cartilage injuries and healing

Cartilage injuries present a significant clinical challenge. Lesions involving the femoral condyles or patellofemoral articular cartilage may result from overuse, direct trauma, malalignment, or malrotation. Such chondral defects are frequently encountered during knee arthroscopy, with studies reporting their presence in up to 36% of cases [32, 33]. Due to its avascular nature and limited chondrocyte population, articular cartilage has a poor intrinsic regenerative capacity. However, fibrocartilage formation and symptom stabilization may occur.

The most widely used surgical intervention remains microfracture surgery (marrow stimulation), which offers only a $\sim$ 30% improvement rate [33].

Without treatment, even minor lesions can grow in size to more substantial lesions and may progress to widespread joint degeneration and osteoarthritis. Current treatments (microfracture, chondroplasty, autograft/allograft transplantation, ACI, etc.) are often staged, require cell harvesting/expansion, or yield mechanically inferior repair tissue.

4.2 Preclinical study overview

An ovine (sheep) study was conducted to evaluate the safety and effectiveness of the CoreTlage® implant in repairing critical-size osteochondral defects.

CoreTlage is made from cultured coral, specifically cultivated for this indication, and includes a patented central channel to enhance cells migration toward the cartilage layer (**Figure 13**).

In each sheep knee, cylindrical defects (6 mm $\times$ 8 mm) were surgically drilled into the load-bearing medial femoral condyle. Each defect was immediately treated in a single-stage procedure by press-fitting a CoreTlage® implant flush with the surrounding bone (**Figure 14**).

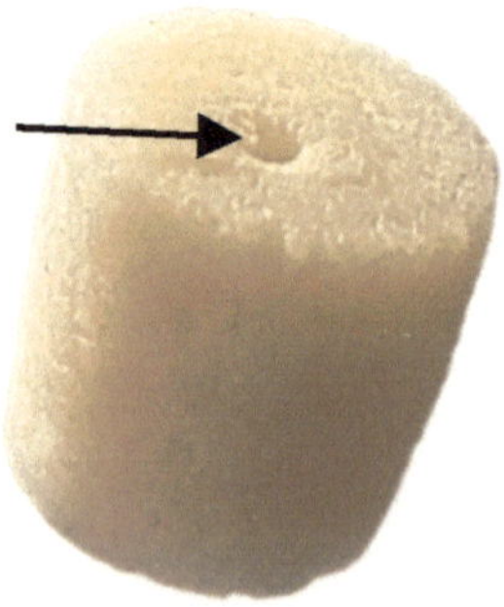

Figure 13.
Coral plug with through vertical channel.

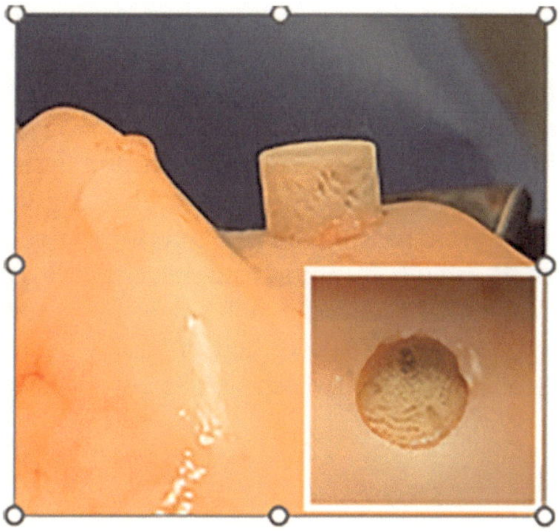

Figure 14.
Scaffold flush with the subchondral bone.

The study consisted of eight animals in total:

- Two animals were followed for 4.5 months post-operatively for preliminary evaluation.
- Six animals were followed for 6 months post-operatively,

Postoperative care and monitoring were conducted according to standard protocols for large-animal cartilage studies, including unrestricted weight-bearing, analgesia, and daily welfare observations. At the designated endpoints, animals were humanely sacrificed and the knees harvested for gross, micro–CT, and histological analyses.

Outcomes included clinical monitoring, gross/macro scoring (e.g., ICRS criteria), high-resolution micro-computed tomography (micro-CT) of the explanted joints, and comprehensive histology (hematoxylin-eosin, Masson's trichrome and safranin-O/fast green staining) of the repair sites. Histological slides were semi-quantitatively graded for tissue reaction (0 = normal to 4 = severe) and cartilage morphology by board-certified pathologists.

4.2.1 Safety and biocompatibility results

Throughout the study, animals showed normal recovery with no adverse reactions. At explant, no signs of joint irritation. Most importantly, no chronic inflammation or foreign-body response was observed in any CoreTlage®-treated joint. Histopathology consistently noted "very clean" tissue fields. Bone and cartilage around the implants were free of inflammatory infiltrates or necrosis.

Natural bone was observed growing directly onto and into the coral-based material. No signs of thick fibrous encapsulation or giant cells were seen around any implant. In all samples, no residual coral fragments were found. These findings suggest that the coral matrix is well-tolerated in the joint environment.

4.2.2 Macroscopic and imaging outcomes

4.2.2.1 Gross morphology

At the post-procedure analysis, all CoreTlage®-treated defects appeared well-healed. The repair sites were flat or slightly convex, blending with surrounding cartilage. According to blinded gross scoring, all implants evaluated at 6 months achieved Grade I-II (nearly normal) in texture, color, and defect fill (**Figure 15**). In plain view, the cartilage covering the implant looked continuous and smooth. As noted in the study report, the treated defects were described as "smoothly contoured, well-filled, and flush with the adjacent cartilage," which we see as encouraging preliminary outcomes.

4.2.3 Micro-CT analysis

High-resolution micro-CT scans performed at 4.5 months post implantation (**Figure 16**). The coral scaffold was completely encased by new bone, restoring an anatomically normal subchondral bone structure. In cross-section images, the implant (light gray) was interspersed with dark-gray newly formed trabeculae, yielding a uniform appearance. Importantly, no radiolucency or implant displacements were observed, underscoring excellent osseointegration.

4.2.4 Bone regeneration efficacy

Micro-CT at sacrifice demonstrated that all defects had become densely filled with new trabecular bone, seamlessly integrating the implant. In cross-section, the coral (high X-ray attenuation) was indistinguishable from host bone, with continuous bony trabeculae spanning the former defect boundary. No gaps were observed between implant and host. By 6 months, the repaired subchondral region was essentially remodeled into normal-appearing bone.

Histological analysis revealed that new bone tissue had filled nearly the entire defect area beneath the joint surface. Masson's trichrome staining showed thick, mineralized bone trabeculae (red) interdigitating with the coral matrix as shown in

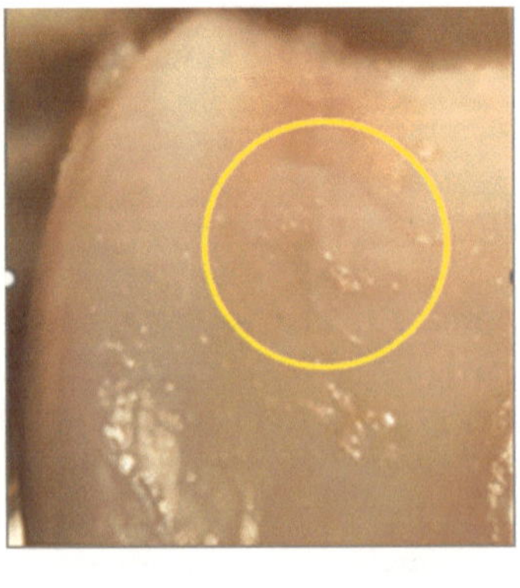

Figure 15.
Gross appearance of a treated osteochondral defect at 18 weeks post-implantation. The yellow circle highlights the defect region, which is completely filled with cartilage-like repair tissue that is smooth and level with the surrounding native cartilage.

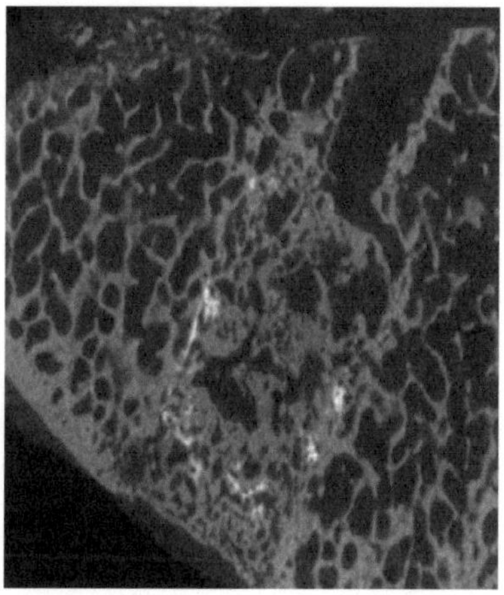

Figure 16.
Micro-CT cross-sectional image of an explanted femoral condyle treated with a CoreTlage® implant (center of image). The coral scaffold (lighter gray) is fully integrated with the surrounding host bone. New trabecular bone formation is evident within and around the implanted scaffold, restoring the subchondral bone structure beneath the defect.

Figure 17. As the evaluating pathologist noted: "the area of implantation is filled with new bone trabeculae that are wide and massive including mineralization."

Across samples, the subchondral plate and trabecular architecture were rebuilt to near-normal geometry. Bone bridges often thickened across the defect. Histology noted a thickened trabecular network underlying the new cartilage. Grossly, the articular surface was supported by a solid bony foundation: all CoreTlage® defects were described as "well-filled" and flush with the native subchondral plate. In sum, CoreTlage® proved highly osteoconductive, guiding new bone formation to reestablish the subchondral bone stock.

4.2.5 Cartilage regeneration efficacy

4.2.5.1 Hyaline-like cartilage formation

A hallmark finding was the regeneration of cartilage at the defect surface. By 6 months, histology consistently revealed a continuous cartilage layer covering the CoreTlage®. Staining with Safranin-O/Fast Green revealed rich proteoglycan content within the new matrix—shown by bright red staining—suggesting the presence of glycosaminoglycans similar to those found in healthy natural cartilage (**Figures 14** and **15**). The superficial cartilage surface was smooth and unbroken, and chondrocytes were organized in columns similar to native tissue in the deeper zones. In top-performing implants, the tidemark (interface) between new cartilage and underlying bone was clear, mimicking a normal osteochondral junction. It was also encouraging to see that cartilage formation was localized to the defect area, with seamless integration into surrounding host tissue and no signs of osteophytes or ectopic cartilage formation.

4.2.5.2 Matrix quality

Overall, the repair cartilage tended toward hyaline character. Immunostains showed predominantly type II collagen, and the semi-quantitative scores for proteoglycan staining were high. However, pathologists did note that the new cartilage was not always perfectly hyaline. In some cases the matrix was somewhat more fibrous than native cartilage (**Figures 17–19**). Overall, CoreTlage® supported the formation of hyaline-like cartilage that was structurally and functionally superior to untreated healing, and no adverse degeneration of adjacent cartilage was seen in any sample.

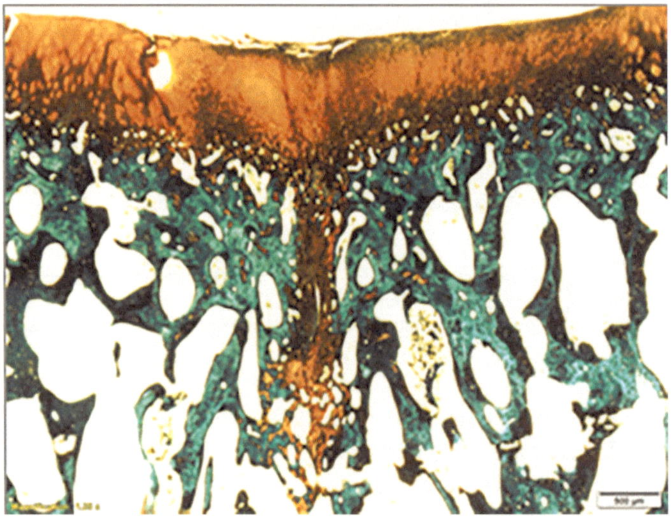

Figure 17.
Safranin-O/Fast Green–stained section of a treated defect at 6 months post-implantation. A layer of hyaline-like cartilage (red staining at top) has regenerated over the defect, with proteoglycan-rich matrix and a smooth articular surface. Underneath, the fast green stain highlights the regenerated subchondral bone (green), demonstrating reconstitution of the bone-cartilage interface. No notable gaps or inflammatory tissue are present at the implant site.

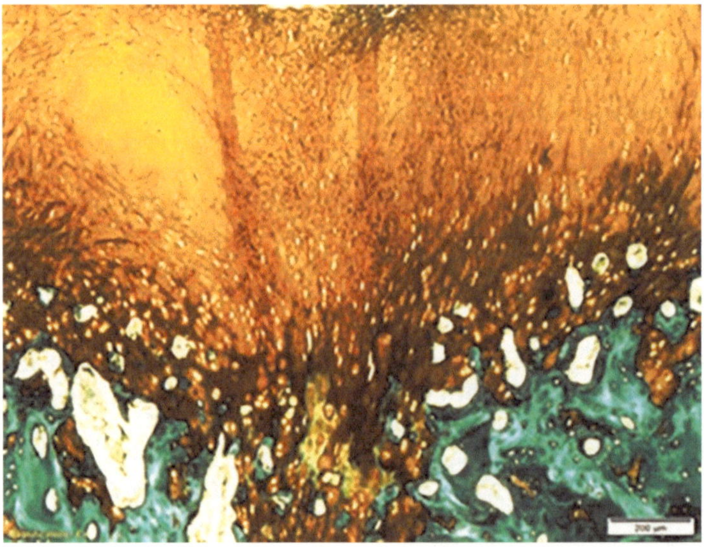

Figure 18.
Safranin-O/fast green-stained section 6 months after implantation reveals formation of hyaline-like cartilage at the articular surface with appropriate proteoglycan content. No significant inflammatory response at the implant interface. (4x magnification).

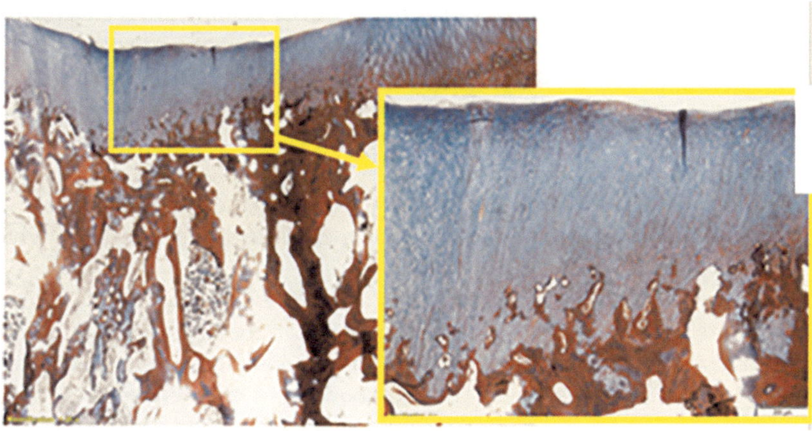

Figure 19.
Histological section of a CoreTlage®-treated defect ~6 months post-surgery (Masson's Trichrome stain). The defect space is being filled with regenerated tissues: new bone (red-stained trabeculae, bottom) is present within the coral scaffold, and a layer of nascent cartilaginous matrix (blue staining) is extending over the surface of the new bone (see inset). This indicates progressive osteochondral healing, with cartilage formation emerging from the underlying bone.

ΔHFBT 95% confidence interval			Statistic	Standard Error
ΔHFBT	Mean value		.1381	0.04105
	95% confidence interval of the average value	Lower limit	.0368	
		Upper limit	.2114	
	5% mean after clipping		.1141	
	Median		.0000	
	Variance		.151	
	Standard deviation		.37204	
	Minimum		−.50	
	Maximum		1.80	
	Range		2.30	
	Quartile distance		.25	

No product-related adverse events were reported during the trial.

Table 3.
Adverse events.

5. Discussion

Coral has been used as a bone substitute graft material for many years. Several FDA and CE approved products for dental and orthopedic indications have shown good ability in promoting bone regeneration in the treatment of bone defects. However, most coral-based products on the market are made from marine harvested coral, which is at risk of contamination from the sea and its environment. To address this issue, high-temperature calcination is used, which can cause changes in the microstructure of the coral and create a dense surface of the pores. These changes may reduce the effectiveness of bone regeneration.

Corebone graft is a type of bone substitute material made from the calcium carbonate exoskeleton of coral. It is available in different forms and sizes for various application scenarios and is bioresorbable, meaning it is absorbed by the body over time. The coral used is grown in the company Coral farm, which is a closed system with online monitoring to ensure water quality and growth conditions are continuously monitored. This reduces the possibility of coral contamination and improves product safety. Corebone process ensures the retention of the pore structure and microscopic rough surface of the coral, which better supports osteogenesis.

The results of the multicenter, open-label, randomized, parallel-controlled non-inferiority trial to estimate the safety and efficacy of Corebone compared to Curasan have shown no significant difference between the two products after surgery or after finishing the follow-up. This suggests that Corebone has similar effect as Curasan in promoting bone growth in repairing bone defects in the jaw. The trial involved three medical institutions, Peking University Third Hospital, Peking Union Medical College of the Chinese Academy of Medical Sciences, and Beijing Friendship Hospital affiliated with Capital Medical University, and included a significant number of participants.

An important limitation of the present study lies the relatively short follow-up time (12 months); after 12 months, we do not know if the radiographic and clinical parameters remain stable.

Based on these findings, it may be concluded that Corebone is as effective as Curasan in repairing bone defects in the jaw. This is significant as it provides an alternative option for patients who require bone grafting. The use of Corebone can potentially reduce the need for additional surgeries to obtain autologous bone, which may increase patient pain, blood loss, surgical infection rate, and long-term hospitalization costs. Additionally, being produced from corals grown in a safe and monitored environment, the use of Corebone avoids the risk of infection. Overall, the results of this trial demonstrate that Corebone is a safe and effective option for promoting bone regeneration in the repair of bone defects in the jaw.

Orthopedics: Coral grafts designed for treating focal osteochondral defects - CoreTlage have shown promising healing including chondral growth within the injury sites. The key findings of the present study demonstrate that the CoreTlage implant provides a highly effective environment for the repair of critical-size osteochondral defects in a large weight-bearing ovine model. At the 6-month follow-up, the treated defects achieved near-normal macroscopic appearances, consistently reaching high macroscopic scores. Histological analysis revealed the formation of hyaline-like cartilage characterized by a smooth articular surface, rich proteoglycan content as evidenced by intense Safranin-O staining, and the presence of predominantly Type II collagen. Crucially, the subchondral bone was fully restored, with the biphasic scaffold facilitating a seamless transition between the regenerated bone and the overlying cartilaginous layer.

The biocompatibility and safety of the CoreTlage implant were evidenced by the total absence of chronic inflammation, foreign-body giant cell reactions, or joint irritability across all subjects. This observation is particularly significant given the dynamic, load-bearing environment of the ovine stifle joint. The direct integration of host bone with the implant interface, without intervening fibrous tissue, confirms the high osteoconductivity of the cultivated coral material. These findings are supported by Pountos & Giannoudis [26] who identified coral-derived substitutes as highly biocompatible and effective in bone repair. Furthermore, the long-term safety and bone-forming capacity of coral-derived materials are well-established, with studies by

Piattelli et al. [1] and Demers et al. [2] highlighting successful bone augmentation and resorption characteristics in both orthopedic and dental applications.

When compared to current clinical standards, CoreTlage offers several distinct advantages. As noted by Liao et al. [34], many current treatments remain palliative and fail to restore the native structure and function of the joint. Traditional marrow-stimulation techniques, such as microfracture, frequently result in the formation of mechanically inferior fibrocartilage (Type I collagen), which lacks durability and often leads to clinical decline. While autografts provide healthy tissue, they are limited by supply and a high risk of donor-site morbidity—reported in up to 50% of cases. Cell therapies like ACI address some of these issues but are hindered by high costs, staged surgeries, and the risk of chondrocyte dedifferentiation. CoreTlage addresses these deficiencies as a single-stage, off-the-shelf solution. A notable performance benchmark is the multilayer collagen scaffold described by Levingstone et al. [35]; while that scaffold required 12 months for maturation in a caprine model, CoreTlage achieved robust bone fill and cartilage maturation within only 6 months. Overall, CoreTlage demonstrated a significantly accelerated rate of tissue maturation and superior structural integration compared to existing biphasic constructs.

The success of this biphasic implant provides further mechanistic support for coral-derived aragonite in joint preservation. These results align with the biological rationale behind established platforms like Agili-C. CoreTlage incorporates a full-length central canal, extending the concept of mechanical modification described by Kon et al. [36]. In that study, 1–2 mm deep drilled channels were shown to be essential for facilitating nutrient supply and the recruitment of Mesenchymal Stem Cells (MSCs) from the subchondral bone marrow. Our findings demonstrate that the regenerative outcomes of the CoreTlage system measure up to these established benchmarks, achieving comparable hyaline-like cartilage formation and robust bone fill within a similar timeframe. This suggests that the biphasic aragonite structure, particularly when modified with a central canal to enhance biological access, serves as an effective "homing device" for osteochondral regeneration. Furthermore, our findings extend this evidence to a large weight-bearing model, confirming that the specific porosity and mineral composition of the cultivated coral scaffold are suited for simultaneous bone and cartilage regeneration.

Despite of these promising results, several limitations must be acknowledged. This study utilized a relatively small sample size (n = 8), and the 6-month follow-up period may not fully capture the long-term durability of the regenerated tissue under years of physiological loading. Additionally, human clinical translation involves complexities such as varying age, activity levels, and potential degenerative changes in the joint.

The preclinical evidence presented suggests that cultivated coral-derived CoreTlage scaffolds can support coordinated regeneration of subchondral bone and hyaline-like cartilage in a large animal model without eliciting adverse inflammatory responses. Future research should focus on longer-term studies and randomized clinical trials to confirm the efficacy and durability of CoreTlage in treating focal osteochondral lesions in human patients.

6. Conclusions

1. Coral has been used as a bone graft material for many years with several FDA and CE approval as a bone graft substitute for oreal and orthopedic indications.

2. The results of this trial demonstrate that cultivated Corebone products are safe and effective option for promoting bone regeneration in the repair of bone defects in the jaw.

3. Corebone process ensures the retention of the pore structure and microscopic rough surface of the coral, which better supports osteogenesis.

4. A clinical multicenter, open-label, randomized, parallel-controlled has shown similar safety and efficacy of Corebone compared to Curasan.

5. Evaluation of cultivated coral implants for regeneration of focal osteochondral defects in an ovine model have shown promising healing including chondral growth within the injury sites; these findings need further animal and human trials.

6. While further in human validation is required, this strategy represents a promising paradigm shift toward single-stage, acellular osteochondral regeneration driven by biomimetic scaffold design.

7. CoreTlage implant provides a highly effective environment for the repair of critical-size osteochondral defects in a large weight-bearing ovine model.

Author details

Haim Tal[1*] and Eyal Amar[2]

1 Department of Periodontology and Oral Implants, School of Dental Medicine, Gerald A Niznick Chair of Implant Research at the Tel Aviv University, Gray Faculty of Medicine, Israel

2 Tel Aviv University, Gray Faculty of Medicine, Head of Minimally Invasive Orthopedic Unit and Sports Injuries Service, Tel Aviv Medical Centre, Israel

*Address all correspondence to: talhaim@tauex.tau.ac.il

References

[1] Piattelli A, Podda G, Scarano A. Clinical and histological results in alveolar ridge enlargement using coralline calcium carbonate. Biomaterials. 1997;**18**:623-627

[2] Demers C, Hamdy CR, Corsi K, et al. Natural coral exoskeleton as a bone graft substitute: A review. Bio-medical Materials and Engineering. 2002;**12**: 15-35

[3] Begley CT, Doherty MJ, Mollan RA, et al. Comparative study of the osteoinductive properties of bioceramic, coral and processed bone graft substitutes. Biomaterials. 1995;**16**:1181-1185

[4] Figueiredo M, Henriques J, Martins G, et al. Physicochemical characterization of biomaterials commonly used in dentistry as bone substitutes - Comparison with human bone. Journal of Biomedical Materials Research. Part B, Applied Biomaterials. 2010;**92**:409-419

[5] Mangano C, Piattelli A, Mangano A, et al. Combining scaffolds and osteogenic cells in regenerative bone surgery: A preliminary histological report in human maxillary sinus augmentation. Clinical Implant Dentistry and Related Research. 2009;**11**: e92-e102

[6] Sàndor GK, Kainulainen VT, Queiroz JO, et al. Preservation of ridge dimensions following grafting with coral granules of 48 post-traumatic and post-extraction dento-alveolar defects. Dental Traumatology. 2003;**19**:221-227

[7] Magan A, Ripamonti U. Geometry of porous hydroxyapatite implants influences osteogenesis in baboons (Papio ursinus). The Journal of Craniofacial Surgery. 1996;**7**:71-78

[8] Walsh WR, Chapman-Sheath PJ, Cain S, et al. A resorbable porous ceramic composite bone graft substitute in a rabbit metaphyseal defect model. Journal of Orthopaedic Research. 2003;**21**:655-661

[9] Amler MH. The time sequence of tissue regeneration in human extraction wounds. Oral Surgery, Oral Medicine, and Oral Pathology. 1969;**27**:309-318

[10] Auraújo MG, Lindhe J. Dimensional ridge alterations following tooth extraction: An experimental study in the dog. Journal of Clinical Periodontology. 2005;**32**:212-218

[11] Souyris F, Pellequer C, Payrot C, Servera C. Coral, a new biomedical material. Experimental and first clinical investigations on Madreporaria. Journal of Maxillofacial Surgery. 1985;**13**:64-69

[12] Molly L, Vandromme H, Quirynen M, et al. Bone formation following implantation of bone biomaterials into extraction sites. Journal of Periodontology. 2008;**79**(6):1108-1115

[13] Xue N et al. Bone tissue engineering in the treatment of bone defects. Pharmaceuticals (Basel). 2022;**15**(7)

[14] Kim YK et al. Tooth-derived bone graft material. Journal of the Korean Association of Oral and Maxillofacial Surgeons. 2013;**39**(3):103-111

[15] Ferraz MP. Bone grafts in dental medicine: An overview of autografts, allografts and synthetic materials. Materials (Basel). 2023;**16**(11)

[16] Migliorini F et al. Autologous bone grafting in trauma and orthopaedic surgery: An evidence-based narrative review. Journal of Clinical Medicine. 2021;**10**(19)

[17] Sethi AK et al. Use of plasma-enriched demineralized freeze-dried bone matrix in postsurgical jaw defects. National Journal of Maxillofacial Surgery. 2018;**9**(2):174-183

[18] Steijvers E, Ghei A, Xia Z. Manufacturing artificial bone allografts: A perspective. Biomaterials Translational. 2022;**3**(1):65-80

[19] Roberts TT, Rosenbaum AJ. Bone grafts, bone substitutes and orthobiologics: The bridge between basic science and clinical advancements in fracture healing. Organogenesis. 2012;**8**(4):114-124

[20] Prikrylova J, Prochazkova J, Podzimek S. Side effects of dental metal implants: Impact on human health (metal as a risk factor of implantologic treatment). BioMed Research International. 2019;**2019**:2519205

[21] Zhao R et al. Bone grafts and substitutes in dentistry: A review of current trends and developments. Molecules. 2021;**26**(10)

[22] Krishani M et al. Development of scaffolds from bio-based natural materials for tissue regeneration applications: A review. Gels. 2023;**9**(2)

[23] Levy S, Mass T. The skeleton and biomineralization mechanism as part of the innate immune system of stony corals. Frontiers in Immunology. 2022;**13**:850338

[24] Neto AS, Ferreira JMF. Synthetic and marine-derived porous scaffolds for bone tissue engineering. Materials (Basel). 2018;**11**(9)

[25] Macha IJ, Ben-Nissan B. Marine skeletons: Towards hard tissue repair and regeneration. Marine Drugs. 2018;**16**(7)

[26] Pountos I, Giannoudis PV. Is there a role of coral bone substitutes in bone repair? Injury. 2016;**47**(12):2606-2613

[27] Gorna K, Gogolewski S. Preparation, degradation, and calcification of biodegradable polyurethane foams for bone graft substitutes. Journal of Biomedical Materials Research. Part A. 2003;**67**(3):813-827

[28] Patat JL, Guillemin G. Natural coral used as a replacement biomaterial in bone grafts. Annales de Chirurgie Plastique et Esthétique. 1989;**34**(3):221-225

[29] Nuss KM, von Rechenberg B. Biocompatibility issues with modern implants in bone - a review for clinical orthopedics. The Open Orthopaedics Journal. 2008;**2**:66-78

[30] Yamada M, Egusa H. Current bone substitutes for implant dentistry. Journal of Prosthodontic Research. 2018;**62**(2):152-161

[31] Suyoung K, Seong-Gon K. Advancements in alveolar bone grafting and ridge preservation: A narrative review on materials, techniques, and clinical outcomes. Maxillofacial Plastic and Reconstructive Surgery. 2024;**46**(1):14-21

[32] Chahla J, Sweet MC, Okoroha KR, et al. Osteochondral allograft transplantation in the patellofemoral joint: A systematic review. The American Journal of Sports Medicine. 2019;**47**(12):3009-3018

[33] Flanigan DC, Harris JD, Trinh TQ, Siston RA, Brophy RH. Prevalence of chondral defects in athletes' knees: A systematic review. Medicine and Science in Sports and Exercise. 2010;**42**(10):1795-1801

[34] Liao XY, Xue Y, Zheng XN, et al. Expert consensus on clinical randomized

controlled trial design and evaluation methods for bone grafting or substitute materials in alveolar bone defects[J]. West China Journal of Stomatology, 2025;**43**(5):613-619

[35] Levingstone TJ et al. Cell-free multi-layered collagen-based scaffolds demonstrate layer specific regeneration of functional osteochondral tissue in caprine joints. Biomaterials. 2016;**87**:69-81

[36] Kon E et al. Osteochondral regeneration using a novel aragonite-hyaluronate bi-phasic scaffold in a goat model. Knee Surgery, Sports Traumatology, Arthroscopy. 2014;**22**:1452-1464

Chapter 2

Pulsed Electromagnetic Fields in Medicine and Dentistry: Mechanisms, Applications, and Clinical Advances

Shlomo Barak, Yaniv Mayer, Michel Dard, Benny Barak and Jamil Awad Shibli

Abstract

Pulsed electromagnetic fields (PEMFs) represent a revolutionary non-invasive therapeutic modality that has gained significant recognition across medical and dental disciplines. This technology utilizes precisely controlled electromagnetic pulses to interact with biological systems at the cellular and molecular levels, influencing fundamental processes including DNA synthesis, gene expression, cell migration, and tissue regeneration. The therapeutic applications of PEMFs span from pain management and inflammation reduction to enhanced bone healing and antimicrobial effects. In dentistry, PEMFs have demonstrated remarkable potential in improving dental implant stability, promoting osseointegration, and managing peri-implant diseases. The introduction of miniaturized electromagnetic devices represents an innovation in implant dentistry, offering targeted therapy that may improve treatment outcomes and reduce complications. This chapter provides a comprehensive examination of PEMF technology, exploring its underlying mechanisms, clinical applications across medical fields, basic research foundations, and specialized dental applications, with particular emphasis on recent advances in implant therapy and antimicrobial effects.

Keywords: pulsed electromagnetic fields, PEMF therapy, dental implants, osseointegration, tissue regeneration, antimicrobial effects, non-invasive treatment, microbiome modulation

1. Introduction

The intersection of physics and medicine has yielded numerous therapeutic innovations, with pulsed electromagnetic fields (PEMFs) emerging as one of the most promising non-invasive treatment modalities of the modern era. PEMF technology harnesses the fundamental properties of electromagnetic radiation to influence biological systems. Evidence indicates it may promote healing, reduce inflammation, and enhance cellular function under certain conditions. The growing body of evidence supporting PEMF applications has led to its integration into diverse medical specialties, with particularly notable advances in orthopedics and dentistry [1–3].

The therapeutic potential of electromagnetic fields was first recognized in the nineteenth century, building upon the foundational work of Michael Faraday and James Clerk Maxwell in electromagnetism.1 However, it was not until the mid-twentieth century that systematic investigation into the biological effects of electromagnetic fields began to reveal their therapeutic applications. The discovery of the piezoelectric effect in bones by Yasuda in 1957 marked a pivotal moment, demonstrating that bone tissue could respond to electromagnetic stimulation by generating electrical potentials that influence bone formation and repair processes [2].

Modern PEMF therapy represents a sophisticated evolution of these early discoveries, incorporating precise control over field parameters including frequency, intensity, pulse duration, and treatment protocols. The technology's non-invasive nature, combined with its proven safety profile and broad therapeutic applications, has positioned it as an attractive alternative to pharmacological interventions for numerous conditions. The development of miniaturized electromagnetic devices has further expanded the clinical utility of PEMF therapy, particularly in dental applications where targeted, localized treatment can significantly enhance outcomes (**Figure 1**) [3].

2. Technology overview: Principles and mechanisms

2.1 Fundamental principles

Pulsed electromagnetic fields comprise synchronized magnetic and electric field components that interact with biological tissues through well-defined physical principles. Unlike static magnetic fields, PEMFs are characterized by their time-varying nature, which enables them to induce electrical currents within biological tissues

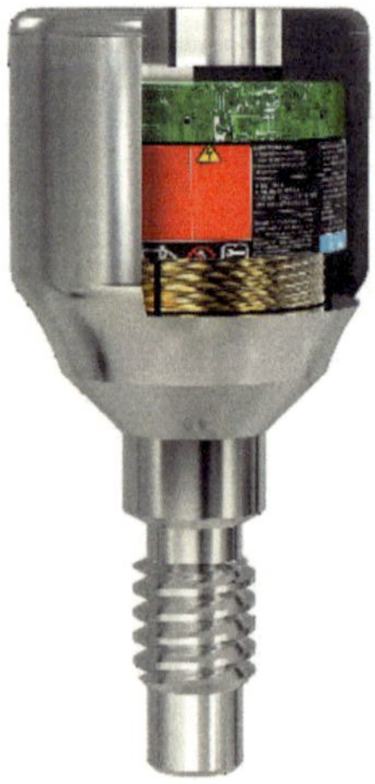

Figure 1.
A cross-sectional view of the Miniaturized Electromagnetic Device (MED) healing abutment (Courtesy of Magdent Ltd.).

according to Faraday's law of electromagnetic induction. This property allows PEMFs to penetrate deeply into tissues, making them particularly effective for treating conditions affecting deeper structures that are difficult to access with other non-invasive modalities [1, 2].

The therapeutic effectiveness of PEMF therapy depends on several critical parameters. Frequency selection typically ranges from extremely low frequencies (1–300 Hz) to higher frequencies approaching the radio frequency spectrum, with different frequency ranges demonstrating optimal efficacy for specific therapeutic applications. Low frequencies (1–10 Hz) are commonly employed for pain management and sleep enhancement, while medium frequencies (10–100 Hz) show effectiveness in anti-inflammatory applications. Higher frequencies (100–1000 Hz) are frequently utilized for bone healing and tissue regeneration applications [4].

Field intensity represents another crucial parameter, typically measured in Gauss or Tesla units. Low-intensity fields (1–10 Gauss) are effective for chronic pain and inflammatory conditions, while medium-intensity fields (15–30 Gauss) demonstrate optimal results for bone healing applications. The pulse characteristics, including pulse width, rise time, and duty cycle, further influence the biological response, with shorter pulses often providing more targeted cellular effects [2, 5].

2.2 Cellular and molecular mechanisms

The biological effects of PEMF therapy result from complex interactions at multiple levels of biological organization, from molecular to systemic. At the cellular level, PEMFs exert their primary effects through the modulation of ion channel activity and membrane potential. The oscillating electromagnetic fields cause forced vibration of free ions on cell membrane surfaces, potentially leading to alterations in ion channel gating and disruption of transmembrane protein equilibrium [5].

These membrane-level changes trigger cascades of intracellular signaling events that ultimately influence cellular behavior. PEMF exposure affects the entire signal transduction pathway, altering both cell surface receptor expression and downstream signaling cascades. Key signaling pathways influenced by PEMF therapy include the mitogen-activated protein kinase (MAPK) pathway, cyclic adenosine monophosphate (cAMP)/protein kinase A (PKA) pathway, and the Wnt/beta-catenin signaling system [5, 6].

The MAPK pathway, including ERK, JNK, and p38 components, plays a crucial role in mediating PEMF effects on cell proliferation, differentiation, and apoptosis. PEMF stimulation can activate these pathways, leading to both pro-survival and pro-differentiation responses depending on the cellular context and field parameters. The modulation of nuclear factor-kappa B (NF-kappaB) activity by PEMFs contributes to their anti-inflammatory effects by reducing the expression of pro-inflammatory cytokines [2].

Calcium signaling represents another fundamental mechanism through which PEMFs influence cellular function. PEMF exposure enhances Ca^{2+} influx through voltage-gated calcium channels and affects intracellular calcium release from stores. This calcium signaling modulation is particularly important for osteoblast function, where calcium plays essential roles in bone matrix synthesis and mineralization processes [7].

Adenosine-related signaling intersects with osteogenesis; A2A receptor activation triggers Akt signaling and enhances nuclear localization of beta-catenin in osteoblasts, supporting a mechanistic rationale relevant to PEMF-responsive pathways [8, 9].

3. Medical applications and clinical evidence

3.1 Orthopedic applications

The orthopedic applications of PEMF therapy represent some of the most extensively studied and clinically validated uses of this technology. The FDA approval of PEMF devices for bone healing in the 1970s provided official recognition of their therapeutic value and paved the way for broader clinical adoption. PEMF therapy has demonstrated clinically meaningful results in treating fracture non-unions, with success rates often exceeding those of conventional treatments [1, 2].

Osteoporosis management represents another significant application area where PEMF therapy has shown considerable promise. The technology's ability to stimulate osteoblast activity while inhibiting osteoclast function makes it particularly well-suited for addressing the bone density loss characteristic of osteoporotic conditions. Clinical studies have demonstrated that regular PEMF treatment can improve bone mineral density and reduce fracture risk in osteoporotic patients [4].

The treatment of osteoarthritis with PEMF therapy has gained substantial clinical support, with numerous controlled studies demonstrating significant improvements in pain levels, joint function, and quality of life measures. The anti-inflammatory effects of PEMF therapy contribute to reduced joint inflammation and improved cartilage health, making it an attractive non-pharmacological option for arthritis management [10].

3.2 Pain management and inflammation

PEMF therapy has established itself as a valuable tool in pain management across various clinical contexts. The analgesic effects of PEMF treatment appear to involve multiple mechanisms, including modulation of pain signaling pathways, reduction of inflammatory mediators, and enhancement of endogenous pain control systems. Clinical applications range from acute post-operative pain management to chronic pain conditions [11].

Interstitial cystitis/bladder pain syndrome represents a specific pain condition where PEMF therapy has demonstrated particular efficacy. Both full-body and targeted treatment protocols have shown promising results in reducing pain intensity and improving bladder function in affected patients. The non-invasive nature of PEMF therapy makes it particularly attractive for conditions where conventional treatments may have limited effectiveness or significant side effects [12].

The anti-inflammatory properties of PEMF therapy extend beyond pain management to encompass broader inflammatory conditions. PEMF treatment can promote the production of anti-inflammatory mediators while reducing pro-inflammatory cytokine expression. This dual anti-inflammatory action contributes to improved tissue healing and reduced chronic inflammation [2].

3.3 Wound healing and tissue regeneration

The wound healing applications of PEMF therapy have shown remarkable clinical potential, particularly in challenging cases such as diabetic ulcers and chronic wounds. PEMF treatment enhances multiple aspects of the wound healing process, including angiogenesis promotion, collagen synthesis enhancement, and acceleration of epithelialization. The technology's ability to improve circulation and reduce tissue hypoxia contributes to its effectiveness in wound healing applications [2, 13].

Diabetic wound healing represents a particularly challenging clinical scenario where PEMF therapy has demonstrated significant benefits. The impaired healing response characteristic of diabetic patients can be substantially improved through PEMF treatment, which enhances myofibroblast activity and collagen fiber production, leading to accelerated wound closure and improved healing quality [14].

Neurological applications of PEMF therapy have shown promise in conditions such as stroke recovery, Parkinson's disease, and multiple sclerosis. The neuroprotective effects of PEMF treatment, including reduction of neuronal necrosis and enhancement of neuroplasticity, contribute to improved functional outcomes in neurological conditions [15].

3.4 Comparative effectiveness

The comparative effectiveness of PEMF therapy versus other treatment modalities has been extensively studied across various applications. When compared to low-level laser therapy (LLLT) for conditions such as diabetic foot ulcers and myofascial pain, PEMF therapy has demonstrated superior outcomes in several clinical parameters. The dual heating and molecular resonance effects of PEMF treatment have been suggested to contribute to muscle relaxation and improved circulation compared to laser therapy, although further validation is required [16].

However, the optimal approach often involves understanding the unique advantages of each modality and potentially combining treatments for synergistic effects. Laser therapy demonstrates particular strengths in wound regeneration through photobiomodulation mechanisms, while PEMF therapy excels in deeper tissue penetration and broader systemic effects. The combination of PEMF and laser therapy has shown potential for enhanced therapeutic outcomes in certain clinical scenarios [17].

The long-term effects of PEMF therapy require careful consideration in clinical practice. While most applications demonstrate excellent safety profiles, prolonged exposure to high-intensity fields may produce oxidative stress effects in some biological systems. However, clinical studies of long-term PEMF use have generally shown positive outcomes with minimal adverse effects when appropriate treatment protocols are followed [18].

4. Basic research: In vitro and in vivo studies

4.1 Cellular response mechanisms

The foundation of PEMF therapy's clinical effectiveness lies in its profound effects on cellular function demonstrated through extensive in vitro research. Cell cycle regulation represents one of the most fundamental areas where PEMF treatment exerts significant influence. Exposure to precisely controlled electromagnetic fields can modulate cell cycle progression, with specific parameters promoting proliferation in regenerative contexts while potentially inducing apoptosis in pathological conditions [5].

The osteogenic differentiation of mesenchymal stem cells under PEMF stimulation has been extensively studied, revealing the involvement of multiple signaling pathways including transforming growth factor-beta (TGF-beta), bone morphogenetic proteins (BMPs), and the mechanistic target of rapamycin (mTOR) pathway. These pathways collectively contribute to enhanced osteoblast differentiation and bone matrix synthesis, providing the mechanistic basis for PEMF therapy's effectiveness in bone healing applications [19].

4.2 Molecular pathway modulation

The molecular mechanisms underlying PEMF therapy effects involve complex interactions among multiple signaling pathways. The Wnt/beta-catenin signaling system plays a central role in mediating PEMF effects on bone formation, with electromagnetic field exposure leading to beta-catenin accumulation and nuclear translocation. This pathway activation results in enhanced expression of genes involved in osteoblast differentiation and bone matrix synthesis [6].

Adenosine-related signaling represents another crucial axis influenced by PEMF-related biology. PEMF-relevant studies indicate that activation of A2A receptors can trigger Akt signaling and enhance nuclear localization of beta-catenin in osteoblasts. This intersects with broader osteoanabolic pathways relevant to bone repair and regeneration [8, 9].

The interaction between PEMF therapy and growth factor expression extends beyond IGF to include other critical factors such as BMP and TGF-beta. These growth factors work synergistically to promote tissue regeneration and repair, with PEMF treatment enhancing their synthesis and biological activity. The coordinated regulation of multiple growth factor systems contributes to the broad therapeutic effectiveness of PEMF therapy [2, 19].

4.3 Antimicrobial effects and biofilm modulation

Recent research has revealed significant antimicrobial properties of PEMF therapy, particularly relevant for preventing and treating biofilm-associated infections. In vitro studies using polymicrobial biofilm models demonstrated that PEMF treatment can significantly alter bacterial colonization patterns and reduce total bacterial loads. These effects are particularly pronounced for problematic species commonly associated with implant-related infections (**Figures 2** and **3**) [20].

The antimicrobial mechanism of PEMF therapy appears to involve multiple pathways, including direct effects on bacterial cell membrane integrity and indirect effects through enhancement of host immune responses. PEMF treatment can reduce the colonization of pathogenic species such as *Streptococcus anginosus*, *Fusobacterium nucleatum*, and *Streptococcus mutans*, while promoting more favorable microbial environments [21].

The ability of PEMF therapy to modulate biofilm formation represents a significant advantage in clinical applications, particularly in implant dentistry where biofilm-associated infections pose substantial challenges. The technology's capacity to reduce initial bacterial colonization while promoting healing responses makes it an attractive adjunctive treatment for implant-related infections [21].

4.4 In vivo validation studies

In vivo studies have provided crucial validation for the cellular and molecular mechanisms identified through in vitro research. Animal studies using rat models have demonstrated that PEMF treatment can significantly improve tissue perfusion through enhanced arteriolar dilation and improved capillary blood flow. These vascular effects contribute to reduced tissue hypoxia and enhanced healing responses [22].

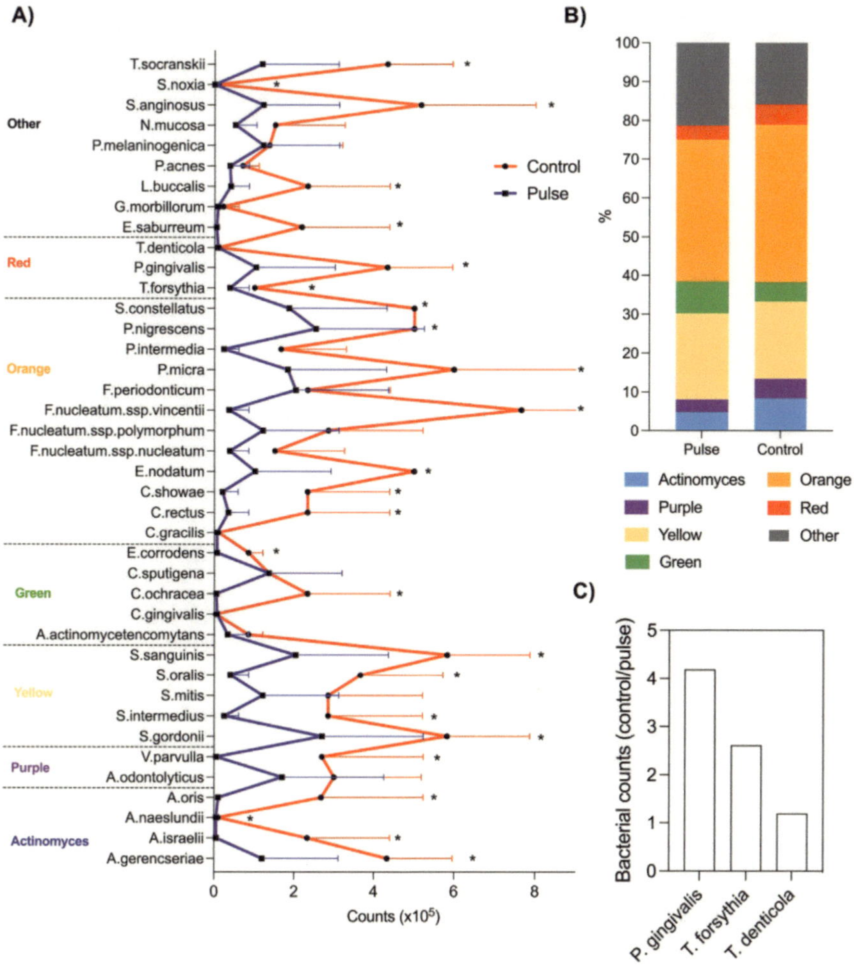

Figure 2.

In vitro polymicrobial biofilm formation under pulsed electromagnetic field (PEMF) exposure, assessed by checkerboard DNA–DNA hybridization for 40 bacterial species linked to implant-related infections. (A) Mean ± SD bacterial counts (×10^5) in pulse (activated PEMF) vs. control (non-activated) groups. (B) Bacterial proportions by periodontal microbial complexes (Actinomyces -blue, yellow, green, purple; secondary colonizers - orange; late colonizers - red). (C) Fold change (control/pulse) for key pathogenic species associated with tissue damage. Indicates significant difference ($p < 0.05$, t-test).

The translation of PEMF effects from cellular studies to whole organism responses has been particularly well demonstrated in bone healing applications. Studies using rabbit tibia models with titanium implants have shown that PEMF treatment enhances the expression of osteogenesis-related genes at the implant-bone interface, leading to improved osseointegration outcomes. Micro-computed tomography and histomorphometric analysis have confirmed the superior bone formation achieved with PEMF treatment [23].

Neurological applications of PEMF therapy have shown promising results in animal models of stroke and neurodegenerative conditions. The neuroprotective effects of PEMF treatment, including reduced inflammation and enhanced neuroplasticity, translate into improved functional outcomes in animal studies [24].

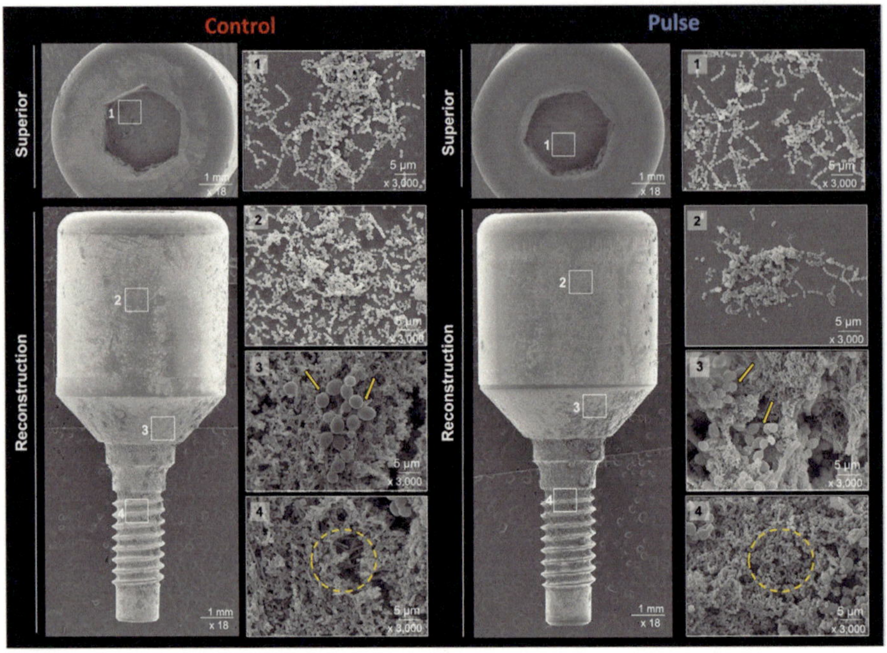

Figure 3.
*Scanning electron microscopy micrographs of both groups after 72 h of biofilm formation. The circles and yellow lines represent microbial (streptococcal) aggregates or mixed-species aggregation on the surface. * Indicates statistical difference ($p < 0.05$) by t-test.*

5. Dental applications: Revolutionizing oral healthcare

5.1 Dental implant stability and osseointegration

The application of PEMF therapy in dental implantology represents one of the most significant advances in implant treatment protocols. The primary challenge in implant dentistry involves achieving reliable osseointegration, particularly in patients with compromised bone quality or systemic conditions that impair healing. PEMF therapy addresses these challenges by enhancing the biological processes that govern implant-bone integration (**Figure 4**) [23].

The miniaturized electromagnetic device (MED) represents a breakthrough innovation in implant therapy, providing targeted PEMF treatment directly at the implant site. This device, constructed from titanium alloy and incorporating sophisticated electromagnetic field generation capabilities, can be screwed directly into the implant in place of conventional healing abutments (**Figure 1**). The localized delivery of PEMF therapy maximizes treatment effectiveness while minimizing systemic exposure [3].

Clinical studies evaluating the effectiveness of MED therapy have demonstrated significant improvements in implant stability quotient (ISQ) measurements, particularly during the critical early healing period. Resonance frequency analysis has shown that PEMF-treated implants achieve superior stability values compared to conventional healing protocols, with benefits becoming apparent as early as two weeks post-implantation and continuing throughout the osseointegration period [25].

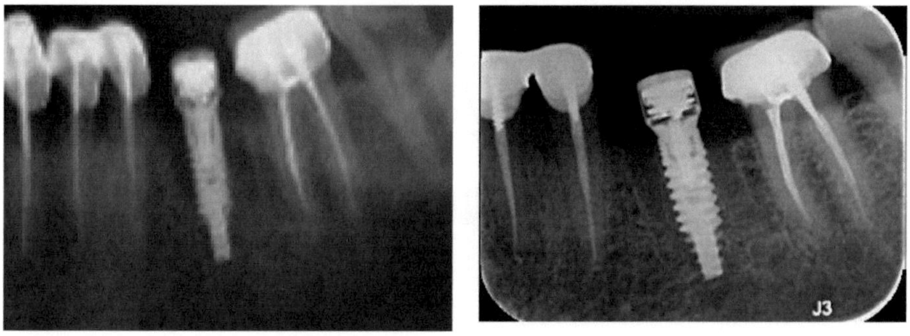

Figure 4.
Increased bone volume density after 30 days of pulsed electromagnetic field at implant site.

The radiographic evidence supporting PEMF therapy in implant treatment includes improved bone density around implant surfaces and enhanced bone-to-implant contact ratios. These improvements are particularly pronounced in challenging cases involving type IV bone or patients with systemic conditions that compromise healing. The enhanced bone formation achieved with PEMF therapy can significantly reduce the time required for implant loading, improving treatment efficiency and patient satisfaction (**Figure 4**) [23].

5.2 Histological and molecular evidence

Histological analysis of implants treated with PEMF therapy reveals enhanced osseointegration characterized by increased direct bone-to-implant contact and improved bone quality around the implant surface. Ground sections of retrieved implants show evidence of enhanced osteogenesis, with more rapid and complete bone formation compared to conventional healing protocols. These histological improvements are particularly evident in challenging bone types where conventional osseointegration may be compromised [23].

The molecular mechanisms underlying improved osseointegration with PEMF therapy involve the upregulation of key osteogenic genes and proteins. Enhanced expression of Runx2, osterix, and collagen type I contributes to accelerated osteoblast differentiation and bone matrix synthesis. The activation of the Wnt/beta-catenin signaling pathway further supports osteogenesis, leading to improved bone formation around implant surfaces [6].

Growth factor expression is significantly enhanced by PEMF therapy, with increased levels of bone morphogenetic proteins (BMPs), transforming growth factor-beta (TGF-beta), and insulin-like growth factors (IGFs). These growth factors work synergistically to promote osteoblast recruitment, proliferation, and differentiation, ultimately leading to enhanced bone formation and implant integration [19].

5.3 Peri-implantitis management

Peri-implantitis represents one of the most challenging complications in implant dentistry, with conventional treatment approaches often providing limited long-term success [26–28].

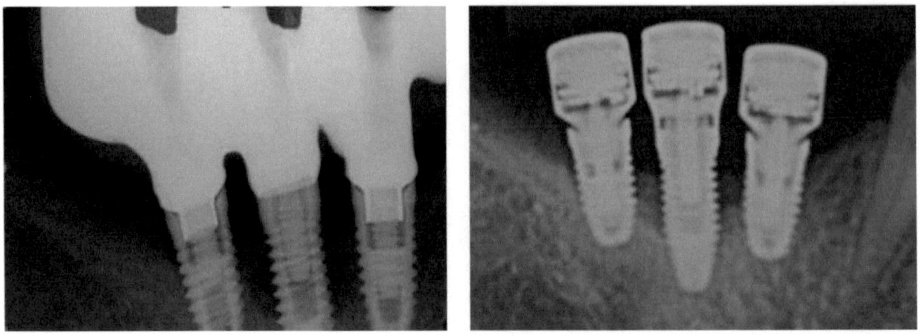

Figure 5.
Clinical and radiographic outcomes of MED treatment in advanced peri-implantitis.

PEMF therapy offers a novel nonsurgical approach to peri-implantitis management that addresses both the infectious and regenerative aspects of the condition (**Figure 5**) [21]. Clinical studies of PEMF therapy for peri-implantitis have demonstrated significant improvements in clinical parameters including probing depth reduction, bleeding on probing improvement, and crestal bone preservation. A randomized controlled trial testing the effectiveness of nonsurgical treatment for peri-implantitis management using PEMFs as an adjunctive measure for 30 days recorded greater bone defect fill at 3 months and a decrease in the levels of interleukin-1beta at 2 weeks following mechanical debridement [29].

The long-term follow-up data for PEMF therapy in peri-implantitis management shows sustained improvements in clinical parameters over 12–26 month observation periods. Extended follow-up studies have demonstrated that PEMF therapy maintains clinical benefits over time, with patients showing continued improvements in probing depth reduction and bone level maintenance [30].

The mechanism of action in peri-implantitis treatment involves multiple pathways, including direct antimicrobial effects, enhanced immune system function, and promotion of tissue regeneration. PEMF therapy has been shown to increase the expression of anti-inflammatory cytokine IL-10 while reducing the expression of pro-inflammatory cytokine IL-1, contributing to improved tissue health and reduced disease progression. The modulation of inflammatory mediators creates an environment more conducive to healing and tissue regeneration around affected implants (**Figure 6**) [21, 29].

5.4 Antimicrobial and microbiome effects

Recent advances in understanding the oral microbiome have revealed the complex bacterial communities associated with implant health and disease. PEMF therapy has demonstrated remarkable ability to modulate these microbial communities, promoting more favorable bacterial populations while reducing pathogenic species. This microbiome modulation represents a significant advancement in implant therapy, addressing one of the fundamental challenges in long-term implant success (**Figures 2** and **3**) [21].

The antimicrobial effects of PEMF therapy extend beyond simple bacterial reduction to include sophisticated modulation of biofilm formation and maturation. Studies have shown that PEMF treatment can significantly alter the composition of multispecies biofilms, with reductions in pathogenic species such as *Porphyromonas*

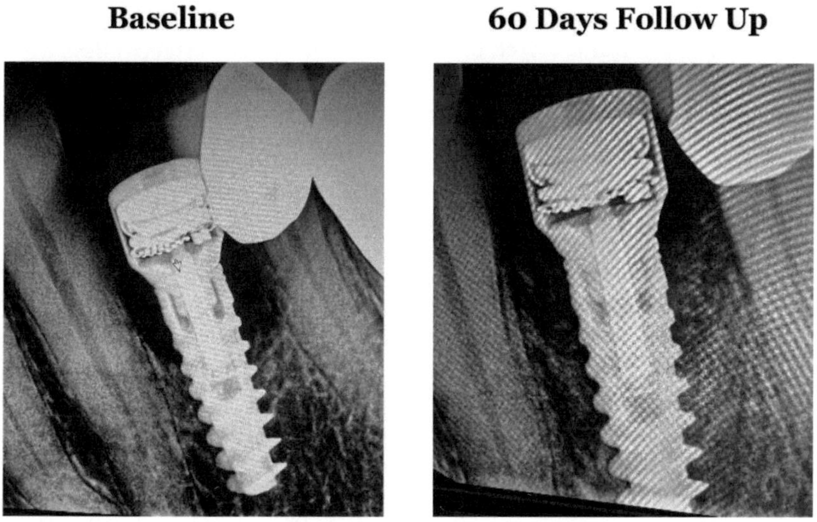

Figure 6.
A 54-year-old systemically healthy patient presented 1.5 years after placement of the definitive prosthetic crown, reporting pain and localized swelling around the implant site. Clinical examination revealed probing depths of 6 mm circumferentially, with bleeding on probing. A periapical radiograph demonstrated crestal bone loss involving the coronal third of the implant. The prosthetic crown was removed, and mechanical debridement with deep curettage of the affected peri-implant tissues was performed. Subsequently, a Magdent MED healing abutment generating Pulsed Electromagnetic Field (PEMF) was applied for a period of 60 days as a non-surgical therapeutic intervention. At the 60-day follow-up, radiographic evaluation showed new bone apposition at the previously resorbed coronal region, accompanied by complete resolution of inflammation and pocket reduction to physiological levels. The outcome demonstrates a favorable peri-implant bone regeneration and soft tissue healing response following adjunctive PEMF therapy.

gingivalis, *Tannerella forsythia*, and *Prevotella intermedia*. These changes in biofilm composition contribute to improved implant health and reduced risk of peri-implant disease [20, 31].

The emerging understanding of biofilm resistance mechanisms has highlighted the importance of treatments that can effectively penetrate established biofilms and disrupt bacterial communication systems. PEMF therapy appears to affect bacterial quorum sensing and biofilm matrix integrity, making it particularly effective against mature biofilms that are resistant to conventional antimicrobial treatments [32].

5.5 Clinical applications and treatment protocols

The integration of PEMF therapy into clinical dental practice requires careful consideration of treatment protocols and patient selection criteria. The miniaturized electromagnetic device has been specifically designed to integrate seamlessly into existing implant workflows, requiring minimal changes to established surgical and prosthetic procedures. The device activation and monitoring protocols ensure consistent treatment delivery while maintaining patient safety [3].

Patient selection for PEMF therapy should consider factors such as bone quality, systemic health status, smoking history, and diabetes status. Patients with compromised healing capacity may derive particular benefit from PEMF therapy, as the treatment can partially compensate for impaired biological responses. The therapy has shown effectiveness across diverse patient populations, including elderly patients and those with systemic conditions that complicate healing [29].

The treatment duration and field parameters for dental applications have been optimized through clinical research to maximize therapeutic effectiveness while ensuring patient safety. Typical treatment protocols involve continuous or intermittent field application over periods ranging from several weeks to several months, depending on the specific clinical indication and patient response [2, 33].

5.6 Future directions and emerging applications

The rapid advancement of PEMF technology in dentistry has opened new avenues for clinical application and research. Emerging applications include the treatment of temporomandibular joint disorders, acceleration of orthodontic tooth movement, and enhancement of oral wound healing. These expanding applications demonstrate the broad therapeutic potential of PEMF technology in oral healthcare [33, 34].

The development of next-generation PEMF devices with enhanced precision and control capabilities promises to further expand the clinical utility of this technology. Advanced field shaping and targeting capabilities may enable more sophisticated treatment protocols tailored to specific anatomical and pathological conditions [34].

The integration of PEMF therapy with other advanced treatments represents an exciting frontier in dental medicine. Combination approaches involving PEMF therapy with regenerative techniques such as growth factor therapy, stem cell treatments, and advanced biomaterials may provide synergistic benefits that exceed the effectiveness of individual treatments [32, 33, 35, 36].

6. Conclusions

Pulsed electromagnetic field (PEMF) therapy is increasingly recognized as a non-invasive modality with relevance across medicine and dentistry. Experimental and clinical data indicate that PEMF can modulate key cellular processes, including proliferation, differentiation, and tissue repair. These properties make it particularly relevant in conditions where healing is compromised or inflammation plays a central role. The body of research, extending from basic laboratory studies to controlled clinical trials, provides a scientific basis for further clinical application.

In dental medicine, PEMF has gained attention primarily in the field of implant therapy. Here, it has been investigated as a means to enhance osseointegration and improve implant stability. The development of miniaturized devices adapted for intraoral use represents an important step, enabling direct clinical translation. Current evidence points to dual benefits, namely, stimulation of bone formation and modulation of the peri-implant microbiota, both of which are critical determinants of implant success.

The reported safety profile of PEMF is favorable. Adverse events are uncommon, and patients generally tolerate the therapy well. Its non-invasive nature provides an alternative to pharmacological or surgical interventions, which is of practical importance for patients who cannot undergo more aggressive treatment.

Beyond clinical outcomes, potential economic implications have been discussed. If PEMF contributes to reduced complication rates, lower medication use, or improved implant survival, it may yield meaningful savings at both patient and healthcare system levels. These aspects are particularly relevant in light of the shift toward value-based models of care.

Looking ahead, there is growing interest in tailoring PEMF parameters to individual patient characteristics. Advances in diagnostic technologies and biomarker discovery may allow for more precise treatment adaptation. In parallel, computational approaches such as artificial intelligence and machine learning are being explored as tools to refine treatment protocols and monitor patient response.

Finally, while the primary focus remains on bone healing and implantology, ongoing research is expanding into other domains, including neurodegenerative and autoimmune conditions, as well as regenerative medicine more broadly. Although many of these applications remain preliminary, they underscore the potential versatility of PEMF as a therapeutic tool.

In conclusion, PEMF has progressed from an experimental concept to a modality with demonstrated clinical utility in selected areas. For implant dentistry, in particular, it offers a scientifically supported approach to improve outcomes by addressing both biological integration and microbial challenges. Continued clinical research, especially long-term and multicenter studies, will be essential to establish its role more firmly within evidence-based dental practice.

Author details

Shlomo Barak[1], Yaniv Mayer[2,3], Michel Dard[4,5], Benny Barak[6]* and Jamil Awad Shibli[1,4,7,8]

1 Department of Periodontology, Dental Research Division, Guarulhos University, Guarulhos, SP, Brazil

2 Department of Periodontology, Rambam Health Care Campus, Haifa, Israel

3 Rappaport Faculty of Medicine, Technion Israel Institute of Technology, Haifa, Israel

4 Columbia University, College of Dental Medicine, New York, USA

5 Department of Mechanical Engineering, University of Washington, Seattle, USA

6 Independent Researcher, Tel Aviv, Israel

7 School of Dental Medicine, Albert Einstein Israelite Hospital, São Paulo, SP, Brazil

8 Department of Oral Medicine, Infection, and Immunity, Harvard School of Dental Medicine, Boston, Massachusetts, USA

*Address all correspondence to: barakbenny8@gmail.com

References

[1] Markov MS. Pulsed electromagnetic field therapy history, state of the art and future. Environmentalist. 2007;**27**:465-475

[2] Cadossi R, Massari L, Racine-Avila J, Aaron RK. Pulsed electromagnetic field stimulation of bone healing and joint preservation: Cellular mechanisms of skeletal response. Journal of the American Academy of Orthopaedic Surgeons. Global research & reviews. 2020;**4**(5):e1900155

[3] Barak S, Matalon S, Dolkart O, Zaban B, Mortellaro C, Piatelli A, et al. A miniaturized electromagnetic device abutment improves stability of the dental implants. The Journal of Craniofacial Surgery. 2019;**30**(4):1055-1057

[4] Caliogna L, Medetti M, Bina V, Brancato AM, Castelli A, Jannelli E, et al. Pulsed electromagnetic fields in bone healing: Molecular pathways and clinical applications. International Journal of Molecular Sciences. 2021;**22**(14):7403

[5] Maziarz A, Kocan B, Bester M, Budzik S, Cholewa M, Ochiya T, et al. How electromagnetic fields can influence adult stem cells: Positive and negative impacts. Stem Cell Research & Therapy. 2016;**7**(1):54

[6] Jing D, Zhai M, Tong S, Xu F, Cai J, Shen G, et al. Pulsed electromagnetic fields promote osteogenesis and osseointegration of porous titanium implants in bone defect repair through a Wnt/beta-catenin signaling-associated mechanism. Scientific Reports. 2016;**6**:32045

[7] Wang J, An Y, Li F, Li D, Jing D, Guo T, et al. The effects of pulsed electromagnetic field on the functions of osteoblasts on implant surfaces with different topographies. Acta Biomaterialia. 2014;**10**(2):975-985

[8] Ham J, Evans BA. An emerging role for adenosine and its receptors in bone homeostasis. Frontiers in Endocrinology. 2012;**3**:113

[9] Borhani S, Corciulo C, Larranaga-Vera A, Cronstein BN. Adenosine A2A receptor activation triggers Akt signaling and enhances nuclear localization of beta-catenin in osteoblasts. The FASEB Journal. 2019;**33**(6):7555-7562

[10] Markov MS. Expanding use of pulsed electromagnetic field therapies. Electromagnetic Biology and Medicine. 2007;**26**(3):257-274

[11] Ross CL, Teli T, Harrison BS. Electromagnetic field devices and their effects on nociception and peripheral inflammatory pain mechanisms. Alternative Therapies in Health and Medicine. 2016;**22**(3):52-64

[12] Ross C, Overholt T, Xu R, Badlani G, Evans RJ, Matthews CA, et al. Pulsed electromagnetic field (PEMF) as an adjunct therapy for pain management in interstitial cystitis/bladder pain syndrome. International Urogynecology Journal. 2022;**33**(3):487-491

[13] Strauch B, Herman C, Dabb R, Ignarro LJ, Pilla AA. Evidence-based use of pulsed electromagnetic field therapy in clinical plastic surgery. Aesthetic Surgery Journal. 2009;**29**(2):135-143

[14] Choi MC, Cheung KK, Li X, Cheing GL. Pulsed electromagnetic field (PEMF) promotes collagen fibre deposition associated with increased myofibroblast population in the early

healing phase of diabetic wound. Archives of Dermatological Research. 2016;**308**(1):21-29

[15] Park HJ, Choi JH, Nam MH, Seo YK. Induced neurodifferentiation of hBM-MSCs through activation of the ERK/CREB pathway via pulsed electromagnetic fields and physical stimulation promotes neurogenesis in cerebral ischemic models. International Journal of Molecular Sciences. 2022;**23**(3):1177

[16] Emes Y, Akca K, Aybar B, Yalcin S, Cavusoglu Y, Baysal U, et al. Low-level laser therapy vs. pulsed electromagnetic field on neonatal rat calvarial osteoblast-like cells. Lasers in Medical Science. 2013;**28**(3):901-909

[17] Shanb AA, Youssef EF, Al Baker WI, Al-Khamis FA, Hassan A, Jatoi NA. The efficacy of adding electromagnetic therapy or laser therapy to medications in patients with diabetic peripheral neuropathy. Journal of Lasers in Medical Sciences. 2020;**11**(1):20-28

[18] Li B, Li W, Bi JQ, Zhao J, Qu Z, Lin C, et al. Effect of long-term pulsed electromagnetic field exposure on hepatic and immunologic functions of rats. Wiener Klinische Wochenschrift. 2015;**127**(9-10):959-962

[19] Ferroni L, Gardin C, Dolkart O, Salai M, Barak S, Piattelli A, et al. Pulsed electromagnetic fields increase osteogenetic commitment of MSCs via the mTOR pathway in TNF-alpha mediated inflammatory conditions: An in-vitro study. Scientific Reports. 2018;**8**:5108

[20] Faveri M, Miquelleto DEC, Bueno-Silva B, Pingueiro JMS, Figueiredo LC, Dolkart O, et al. Antimicrobial effects of a pulsed electromagnetic field: An in vitro polymicrobial periodontal subgingival biofilm model. Biofouling. 2020;**36**(7):862-869

[21] Souza JGS, Nagay BE, Martins R, Bertolini M, Shibli JA, Aparicio C, et al. Microbiome modulation of implant-related infection by a novel miniaturized pulsed electromagnetic field device. npj Biofilms and Microbiomes. 2025;**11**:36

[22] Bragin DE, Bragina OA, Hagberg S, Nemoto EM. Pulsed electromagnetic field (PEMF) mitigates high intracranial pressure (ICP) induced microvascular shunting (MVS) in rats. Acta Neurochirurgica. Supplement. 2018;**126**:93-95

[23] Barak S, Dolkart O, Chechik O, Kinarty A, Amir A, Galoyan N, et al. A new device for improving dental implants anchorage: A histological and micro-computed tomography study in the rabbit. Clinical Oral Implants Research. 2016;**27**(8):935-942

[24] Premi E, Benussi A, La Gatta A, Visconti S, Costa A, Gilberti N, et al. Modulation of long-term potentiation-like cortical plasticity in the healthy brain with low frequency-pulsed electromagnetic fields. BMC Neuroscience. 2018;**19**:34

[25] Nayak BP, Dolkart O, Satwalekar P, Kumar YP, Chandrasekar A, Fromovich O, et al. Effect of the pulsed electromagnetic field (PEMF) on dental implants stability: A randomized controlled clinical trial. Materials. 2020;**13**(7):1667

[26] Rakic M, Galindo-Moreno P, Monje A, Radovanovic S, Wang HL, Cochran D, et al. How frequent does peri-implantitis occur? A systematic review and meta-analysis. Clinical Oral Investigations. 2018;**22**(4):1805-1816

[27] Cosgarea R, Sculean A, Shibli JA, Salvi GE. Prevalence of peri-implant diseases - a critical review on the current evidence. Brazilian Oral Research. 2019;**33**(Suppl. 1):e063

[28] Esposito M, Grusovin MG, Worthington HV. Treatment of peri-implantitis: What interventions are effective? A Cochrane systematic review. European Journal of Oral Implantology. 2012;**5**(Suppl.):S21-S41

[29] Mayer Y, Khoury J, Horwitz J, Ginesin O, Canullo L, Gabay E, et al. A novel nonsurgical therapy for peri-implantitis using focused pulsed electromagnetic field: A pilot randomized double-blind controlled clinical trial. Bioelectromagnetics. 2023;**44**(7-8):144-155

[30] Mayer Y, Gabay E, Younis A, Ginesin O, Siroma RS, Barak S, et al. Pulsed electromagnetic field therapy on nonsurgical treatment of peri-implantitis: 12-26 months follow-up. Journal of periodontology. 2025. DOI: 10.1002/jper.11384. Advance online publication

[31] Ceccarelli G, Bloise N, Mantelli M, Gastaldi G, Fassina L, De Angelis MGC, et al. A comparative analysis of the in vitro effects of pulsed electromagnetic field treatment on osteogenic differentiation of two different mesenchymal cell lineages. Bioresearch Open Access. 2013;**2**(4):283-294

[32] Monje A, Amerio E, Mallor I, Aparicio C. Emerging locally delivered antimicrobial and immunomodulatory approaches for the prevention/treatment of peri-implant diseases. Periodontology 2000. 2025. DOI: 10.1111/prd.12638. Advance online publication

[33] da Silveira LE, Canullo L, Murillo GDC, Garcia IL, Berberi A, Munoz FA, et al. Pulsed electromagnetic therapy: Literature review and current update. Brazilian Dental Journal. 2024;**35**:e24-e6109

[34] Flatscher J, Pavez Lorie E, Mittermayr R, Meznik P, Slezak P, Redl H, et al. Pulsed electromagnetic fields (PEMF)-physiological response and its potential in trauma treatment. International Journal of Molecular Sciences. 2023;**24**(14):11239

[35] Canullo L, Genova T, Wang HL, Carossa S, Mussano F. Plasma of argon increases cell attachment and bacterial decontamination on different implant surfaces. The International Journal of Oral & Maxillofacial Implants. 2017;**32**:1315-1323

[36] Alsahhaf A, Alrabiah M, Ali K, Vohra F, Abduljabbar T. Implant abutment disinfection using plasma of argon and 0.2% chlorhexidine gel applications immediately before prosthesis delivery: Clinical and radiographic status at 5-years of follow-up. European Review for Medical and Pharmacological Sciences. 2023;**27**:116-121

Chapter 3

Peri-Implantitis Therapy: From Conventional Methods to Innovative Solutions

Liat Chaushu, Gavriel Chaushu and Haim Tal

Abstract

Peri-implantitis is one of the most challenging biological complications in contemporary implant dentistry. It is characterized by peri-implant mucosal inflammation and progressive bone loss that may ultimately lead to implant failure. The condition represents a multifactorial breakdown of host-implant homeostasis, influenced by microbial biofilms, host immune dysregulation, and biomechanical factors. Despite significant progress in preventive strategies and surface decontamination techniques, achieving a long-term resolution of peri-implantitis and predictable re-osseointegration remains challenging. This chapter provides a comprehensive overview of the current understanding of peri-implantitis, spanning its pathophysiology, diagnostic principles, and therapeutic approaches. It critically evaluates both conventional treatment modalities—mechanical and chemical debridement, antimicrobial protocols, laser and photodynamic therapy, and regenerative interventions. Particular attention is given to novel implant-surface renewal strategies, which may enable minimally invasive, prosthesis-preserving management of advanced peri-implantitis. In addition, the chapter examines the evolving role of systemic and molecular biomarkers in disease monitoring and precision risk assessment. By integrating current clinical evidence with experimental advances, this chapter outlines the transition of peri-implantitis management from conventional decontamination toward regenerative, biomarker-guided, and implant-design-driven paradigms, offering a forward-looking perspective on the future of personalized peri-implant therapy.

Keywords: peri-implantitis, biomarkers, implant design, re-osseointegration, systemic inflammation, regenerative therapy

1. Introduction

The advent of dental implants has redefined restorative dentistry, achieving exceptional success rates and offering durable functional and esthetic rehabilitation of edentulous sites. However, with increasing implant use, peri-implant diseases, particularly peri-implantitis, have emerged as significant biological complications. Peri-implantitis is characterized by inflammation of peri-implant mucosa and progressive bone loss, which may ultimately lead to implant failure [1]. The disease shares features with periodontitis but presents unique clinical and histopathological dynamics [2–4]. Peri-implantitis is a multifactorial inflammatory condition typically initiated by a dysbiotic biofilm at the implant–mucosa interface. Its onset and progression depend on host susceptibility and modifying factors, as well as implant/prosthetic design and biomechanical loading. Risk factors include poor oral hygiene, history of periodontitis, smoking, systemic diseases (e.g., diabetes), and genetic predisposition [5, 6]. The disease typically begins as peri-implant mucositis, progressing to peri-implantitis if left untreated. Clinical signs include redness, swelling, bleeding on probing, suppuration, and increased probing depths. Radiographically, the disease is characterized by vertical or crater-like bone loss around the implant. Histologically, peri-implantitis lesions exhibit a dense inflammatory infiltrate, osteoclastic bone resorption, and disorganization of the collagen matrix [7].

This chapter outlines the current understanding of peri-implantitis etiology, diagnosis, and treatment, with a focus on recent evidence and novel modalities. The discussed innovations include systemic biomarker assessment and a newly designed two-piece implant system with a replaceable titanium sleeve, which holds potential for advancing peri-implantitis management.

2. Pathogenesis and diagnosis of peri-implantitis

Recent diagnostic studies [1, 8] have included the use of biomarkers in gingival crevicular fluid (GCF) and peri-implant sulcular fluid (PISF), providing non-invasive options for disease detection and monitoring. Biomarkers such as interleukin-1β (IL-1β), tumor necrosis factor-α (TNF-α), and matrix metalloproteinases (MMPs) have shown elevated levels in peri-implant disease and may provide early warning signs.

In particular, IL-1β is a pivotal pro-inflammatory cytokine that orchestrates leukocyte recruitment and stimulates osteoclast differentiation through the RANK/RANKL/OPG pathway, thereby promoting bone resorption and connective-tissue degradation. Its concentration rises significantly in both peri-implant mucositis and peri-implantitis, correlating positively with disease severity and marginal bone loss [9]. Following successful therapy, whether mechanical, surgical, or regenerative, IL-1β levels typically decrease, reflecting resolution of inflammation and stabilization of bone metabolism. This bidirectional change makes IL-1β a valuable biomarker not only for diagnosis but also for monitoring treatment response [10].

The use of multiplex assays and high-throughput analysis has enhanced the capacity to detect multiple biomarkers simultaneously, increasing diagnostic sensitivity. Multiplex platforms allow simultaneous measurement of key inflammatory mediators (e.g., IL-1β, RANKL, MMP-8, TNF-α, and specific miRNAs), which are strongly correlated with early peri-implant tissue breakdown and bone loss. These biomarkers form a self-amplifying inflammatory–destructive cycle in peri-implant tissues. The bacterial biofilm induces the release of IL-1β and TNF-α, which promote RANKL expression and osteoclast activation, leading to bone resorption. Simultaneously, MMP-8 degrades collagen and soft tissue, exposing further bacterial and host antigens that sustain cytokine production and chronic inflammation. Dysregulated miRNAs modulate this cascade, preventing resolution and favoring continuous tissue destruction. Together, these mediators explain the strong correlation between their elevated levels and early peri-implant tissue breakdown [9].

High-throughput proteomic and molecular analyses further enhance diagnostic precision by identifying complex biomarker profiles associated with disease activity and progression. For instance, diagnostic kits, such as aMMP-8 point-of-care tests, provide immediate results during the clinical visit, facilitating real-time assessment of tissue-destructive activity. This enables clinicians to detect subclinical inflammation before irreversible loss occurs [11]. Moreover, the development of chairside diagnostic kits now enables the rapid and cost-effective identification of peri-implant inflammation, allowing for timely and minimally invasive intervention before bone loss occurs [12].

Beyond biochemical markers, advances in imaging technologies, such as cone-beam computed tomography (CBCT) and fluorescence-based probes, provide additional insights into disease progression and the extent of bone destruction [13, 14]. These tools, when integrated with clinical and biomarker data, contribute to a more comprehensive and individualized diagnostic approach. However, their clinical utility in peri-implantitis is still under investigation and not yet standard practice [15].

Collectively, these diagnostic tools underscore the transition toward precision medicine in implant dentistry, where early detection, risk profiling, and personalized treatment plans have become standard components of peri-implant disease management.

3. Conventional treatment approaches

Current therapeutic modalities aim to reduce bacterial load and halt disease progression. These include mechanical debridement, chemical disinfection, systemic and local antibiotics, and surgical intervention, such as open flap debridement. These approaches are essential for reducing the initial bacterial load but are often insufficient alone for advanced disease [16].

Mechanical debridement methods include curettes, ultrasonic devices, and air-polishing. However, the complex microtopography of rough surfaces harbors bacteria deep within microgrooves and pits, making it difficult for mechanical methods. As a result, complete decontamination of the rough implant surface remains challenging, and long-term success is unpredictable [17].

Clinical and microbiological evidence indicate that when mechanical debridement is used alone in peri-implant sites, microbial recolonization may begin as early as 2 to 3 weeks post-treatment. As a result, more virulent pathogenic species can repopulate the niche rapidly [18]. This rapid recolonization highlights the limited durability of mechanical therapy when used alone and underscores the need for adjunctive modalities, such as antimicrobial agents, laser-assisted decontamination, or photodynamic therapy, to achieve more sustained suppression of the peri-implant biofilm [19]. Implant surface decontamination using adjunctive chemical agents (e.g., chlorhexidine and local antibiotics) as well as physico-chemical methods, such as photodynamic therapy, has also been investigated [20, 21].

However, their clinical efficiency was not superior. Systemic antibiotic regimens, including metronidazole and amoxicillin, have been used in conjunction with mechanical treatment. The combination of amoxicillin and metronidazole is commonly employed. Systemic antibiotics can provide additional short-term clinical improvements, especially in terms of probing depth and bleeding on probing; however, concerns about compliance, together with concerns about resistance and limited long-term benefits, restrict their routine use [15]. Meta-analyses indicate greater odds of treatment success and reduced bleeding and suppuration on probing in the first 1–2 years post-surgery [22]. However, no substantial long-term benefits (≥3 years) have been demonstrated, and the need for additional surgical intervention is not significantly reduced by adjunctive antibiotics [23]. The Academy of Osseointegration and American Academy of Periodontology consensus states that adjunctive systemic antibiotics do not consistently improve surgical outcomes [24].

Laser therapy, particularly Er:YAG and diode lasers, has been proposed as a less invasive method with promising results in reducing bacterial loads on implant surfaces. Even though laser therapy has been found to be, in some studies, effective and a less invasive treatment for peri-implantitis [25], current evidence indicates that these modalities do not consistently outperform conventional mechanical debridement in terms of clinical outcomes or long-term disease control. Clinical trials and meta-analyses confirm that Er:YAG laser therapy can reduce inflammation and bacterial load. However, the improvements in clinical parameters are comparable to those achieved with mechanical debridement alone. Moreover, there is no significant advantage in preventing crestal bone loss or achieving long-term disease resolution [26].

In the management of advanced peri-implantitis [27], regenerative surgical techniques using bone grafts and barrier membranes are well-documented procedures. Clinical improvements, such as reduction in probing depth, bleeding on probing, and radiographic bone fill, were achieved. However, in terms of re-osseointegration, the results remain elusive. Most studies report only partial bone regeneration, with long-term success rates for disease resolution and implant survival. Other studies have also documented cases requiring retreatment due to disease recurrence or progression over time. The extent of bone fill and clinical improvement is influenced by defect morphology, implant surface characteristics, and the disease severity at baseline. No specific biomaterial or protocol has demonstrated clear superiority. The addition of reconstructive procedures to access flap surgery does not consistently yield better outcomes in terms of probing depth or bleeding on probing at long-term follow-up [1, 28].

4. Systemic biomarker response and disease monitoring

Recent studies have highlighted the systemic impact of peri-implant infections [29, 30]. An experimental peri-implantitis was induced in a dog model. Mechanical debridement was performed using titanium implant curettes (HU-FRIEDY, Chicago, IL, USA). No clinically apparent macroscopic damage to the implant surface was observed during the procedure; however, microscopic surface alterations cannot be excluded.

Blood count was assessed before and after treatment. The authors found altered complete blood count (CBC) values, including increases in WBC, RBC, hemoglobin, MCHC, and platelets, prior to treatment. These changes returned to baseline following surgical debridement, suggesting a reversible systemic inflammatory response linked to local peri-implant pathology (**Figure 1**) [29].

Complementing this, biochemical analyses revealed elevated serum inflammatory and hepatic markers (total protein, albumin, ALT, AST), which normalized post-treatment (**Figure 2**) [30].

These findings underscore the bidirectional relationship between peri-implant health and systemic status, supporting the concept of peri-implantitis as not solely a local but a systemic disease.

Therefore, monitoring hematological and biochemical parameters before and after therapy may provide valuable insights into disease activity, severity, and treatment response.

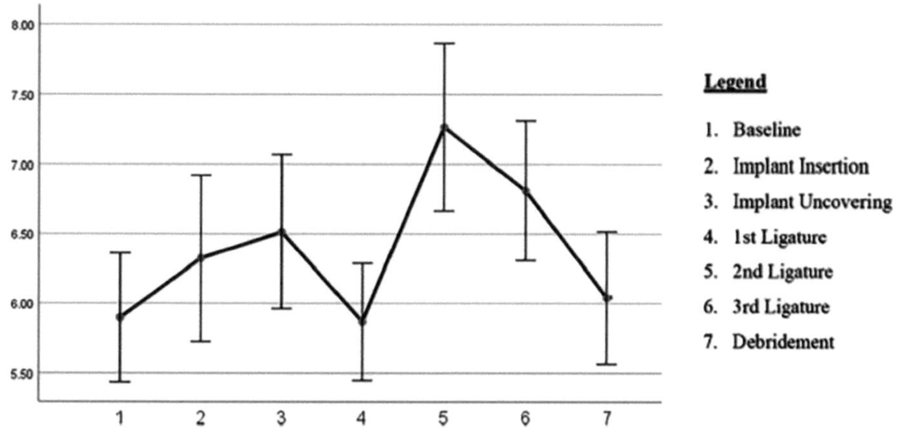

Figure 1.
RBC dynamics (cells per microliter of blood × 1000).

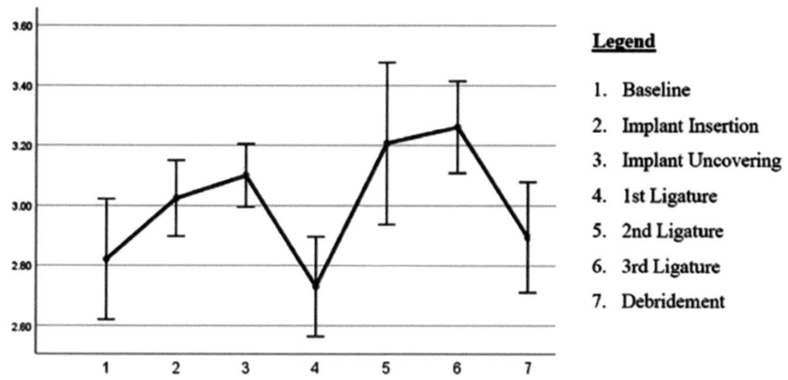

Figure 2.
Albumin concentration (g/dL) dynamics.

5. A novel implant design: Two-piece implant with replaceable sleeve

Traditional implants have a single-body or two-part configuration with fixed surfaces, which complicates decontamination once peri-implantitis sets in. A novel two-piece implant system (NGI100; Implant B, NGT, Israel) addresses this issue with a detachable coronal titanium sleeve (4.2 mm height, 0.2 mm thick), allowing for the mechanical removal and replacement of the contaminated surface (**Figure 3**).

This pre-assembled design facilitates the surgical procedure while preserving prosthetic components. During peri-implantitis treatment, the sleeve can be removed using a specialized trephine and replaced with a sterile one, restoring a pristine surface conducive to re-osseointegration. By replacing only the outer sleeve, removal of the entire implant is avoided, preserving osseointegration at the apical portion and minimizing patient morbidity.

Moreover, this approach provides a practical and cost-effective solution for both clinicians and patients, as it minimizes surgical invasiveness, preserves existing prosthetic structures, and allows for chairside intervention. The procedure could potentially be integrated into regular peri-implant maintenance programs.

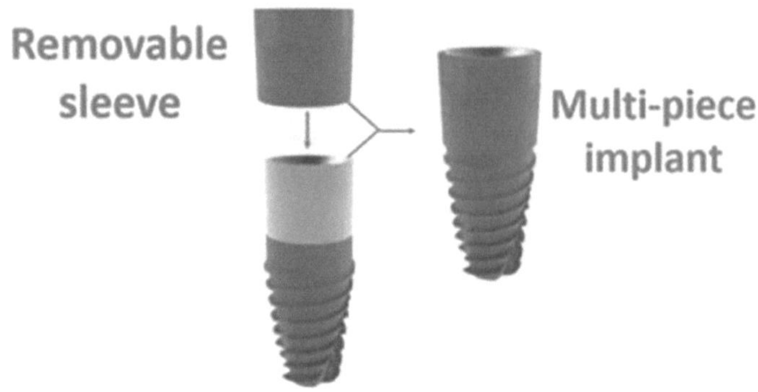

Figure 3.
A two-piece dental implant comprising a replaceable thin titanium sleeve.

In a controlled dog study [31], seven dogs were included. Each received both a conventional rough surface implants and a two-piece with a replaceable sleeve implants. Experimental peri-implantitis was induced using a ligature-based model. After the establishment of peri-implantitis, during peri-implantitis treatment, mechanical debridement was carried out using titanium implant curettes (HU-FRIEDY, Chicago, IL, USA), which are preferred over stainless-steel instruments due to their reduced risk of implant surface alteration. No obvious macroscopic surface damage was observed following debridement.

The implants were treated according to the assigned decontamination and resurfacing protocol in the four study groups:

- E1: Sleeve removed, implant decontaminated, new sleeve inserted
- E2: Sleeve removed, implant decontaminated, no sleeve replacement
- C1: Sleeve not removed, only decontamination
- C2: Standard implant, decontaminated

Histological analysis revealed the lowest inflammatory infiltrate in Group E2, followed by E1, C2, and C1. These findings suggest that removing the contaminated sleeve, with or without replacement, is more effective than decontamination alone. Moreover, turned surfaces (Group E2) were associated with better outcomes than roughened ones (Group C1) (**Figure 4**).

Additional findings indicated that the mesio-distal regions of the implants demonstrated more severe inflammation than the bucco-lingual aspects, possibly due to reduced access for decontamination tools. These anatomical insights could guide clinical strategies for flap design and debridement techniques.

Another important conclusion showed that conventional dental implants complicate the decontamination process in peri-implantitis primarily due to their surface roughness, thread geometry, and microstructural features. Biofilm adheres more tenaciously to the roughened surfaces, and even advanced decontamination protocols often fail to achieve complete removal, leaving residual bacteria and organic debris [17].

Future studies should focus on slow-release materials on the implant surface that may enhance osseointegration on one hand and reduce the risk for peri-implantitis.

DOI: http://dx.doi.org/10.5772/intechopen.1014443

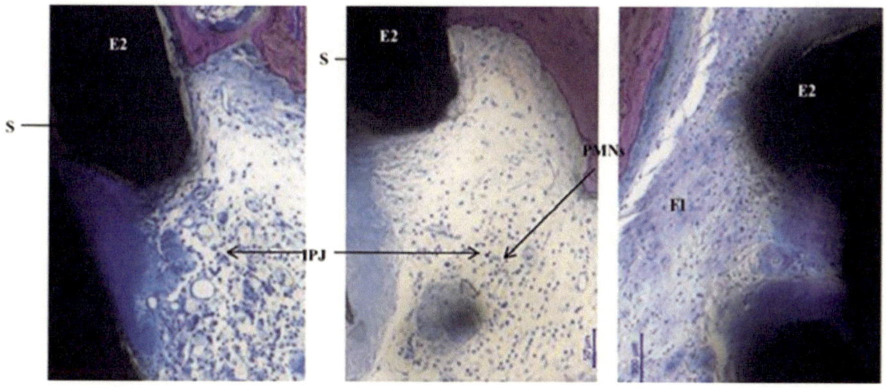

Figure 4.
The area apical to the sleeve implant junction in group E2 showed rare signs of residual inflammatory reaction. BT-bone tissue; IPJ-inflammatory pocket epithelium at sleeve to implant junctions; PMNS-polymorphonuclear cells (predominant); S-sleeve FI-Fibrosis.

6. Re-osseointegration potential

Re-osseointegration refers to the re-establishment of a direct, functional connection between bone and the previously contaminated implant surface, following disease resolution and surgical intervention. Achieving true re-osseointegration after peri-implantitis has long been a challenge in implant dentistry due to persistent bacterial contamination, altered surface topography, and chronic inflammation.

While many studies report bone fill or radiographic stability after treatment [32], only a limited number have demonstrated histological evidence of re-osseointegration characterized by intimate bone-to-implant contact on a previously diseased surface. These cases are rare, and the regenerative outcomes have often been partial or unpredictable, particularly on rough implant surfaces that are more susceptible to bacterial colonization and more difficult to decontaminate effectively [33–34].

These findings suggest that, unlike traditional one-piece implants, the novel two-piece system may suggest a more predictable and minimally invasive solution for the management of peri-implantitis. It is particularly in cases where preserving the implant and its prosthetic restoration is critical [31].

7. Clinical implications and future directions

These findings propose a paradigm shift in peri-implantitis treatment: instead of merely attempting to decontaminate, clinicians may now consider physically removing the infected surface. Two-piece implant with a removable sleeve system enables a minimally invasive, prosthetic-preserving intervention with the potential to improve long-term outcomes.

Additionally, systemic monitoring via CBC and serum biomarkers could be integrated into diagnostic and follow-up protocols, offering insights into disease severity and therapeutic efficacy.

Future clinical trials are warranted to confirm these preclinical findings and assess the long-term stability, cost-effectiveness, and patient satisfaction associated with the novel implant system. Furthermore, the development of adjunctive agents that enhance the decontamination and re-osseointegration process, such as antimicrobial peptides, growth factors, or nanocoating, may further improve outcomes.

8. Conclusion

Peri-implantitis presents a significant challenge in implant dentistry. Current treatment modalities often fall short in achieving complete disease resolution. Recent innovations, including systemic biomarker analysis and a replaceable sleeve implant design, offer promising avenues for both diagnosis and therapy. By combining localized treatment with systemic monitoring and regenerative strategies, peri-implant disease management may enter a new era of precision and predictability.

Author details

Liat Chaushu*, Gavriel Chaushu and Haim Tal
Tel Aviv University, Tel Aviv, Israel

*Address all correspondence to: liat.natanel@gmail.com

References

[1] Hirooka H, Renvert S. Diagnosis of periimplant disease. Implant Dentistry. 2019;**28**(2):144-149. DOI: 10.1097/ID.0000000000000868

[2] Berglundh T, Zitzmann NU, Donati M. Are peri-implantitis lesions different from periodontitis lesions? Journal of Clinical Periodontology. 2011;**38**(Suppl. 11):188-202. DOI: 10.1111/j.1600-051X.2010.01672.x

[3] Robitaille N, Reed DN, Walters JD, Kumar PS. Periodontal and peri-implant diseases: Identical or fraternal infections? Molecular Oral Microbiology. 2016;**31**(4):285-301. DOI: 10.1111/omi.12124. Epub 2015 Sep 15

[4] Heitz-Mayfield LJ, Lang NP. Comparative biology of chronic and aggressive periodontitis vs. peri-implantitis. Periodontology 2000. 2010;**53**:167-181. DOI: 10.1111/j.1600-0757.2010.00348.x

[5] Berglundh T, Armitage G, Araujo MG, Avila-Ortiz G, Blanco J, Camargo PM, et al. Peri-implant diseases and conditions: Consensus report of workgroup 4 of the 2017 world workshop on the classification of periodontal and peri-implant diseases and conditions. Journal of Periodontology. 2018;**89**(Suppl. 1):S313-S318. DOI: 10.1002/JPER.17-0739

[6] Schwarz F, Sculean A, Engebretson SP, Becker J, Sager M. Animal models for peri-implant mucositis and peri-implantitis. Periodontology 2000. 2015;**68**(1): 168-181. DOI: 10.1111/prd.12064

[7] Lindhe J, Meyle J, Group D of European Workshop on Periodontology. Peri-implant diseases: Consensus report of the sixth European workshop on periodontology. Journal of Clinical Periodontology. 2008;**35**(8 Suppl.):282-285. DOI: 10.1111/j.1600-051X.2008.01283.x

[8] La Monaca G, Pranno N, Patini R, Polimeni A, Cordaro M, Cristalli MP. Biomarkers in peri-implant crevicular fluid of healthy implants and those with peri-implant diseases: A systematic review and meta-analysis. Journal of Oral Pathology & Medicine. 2025;**54**(5):267-282. DOI: 10.1111/jop.13612. Epub 2025 Mar 18

[9] Hentenaar DFM, De Waal YCM, Vissink A, Van Winkelhoff AJ, Meijer HJA, Liefers SC, et al. Biomarker levels in peri-implant crevicular fluid of healthy implants, untreated and non-surgically treated implants with peri-implantitis. Journal of Clinical Periodontology. 2021;**48**(4):590-601. DOI: 10.1111/jcpe.13423. Epub 2021 Feb 16

[10] Moaven H, Giacaman A, Beltrán V, Sam YH, Betancur D, Mainas G, et al. Biomarker expression of peri-implantitis lesions before and after treatment: A systematic review. International Journal of Environmental Research and Public Health. 2022;**19**(21):14085. DOI: 10.3390/ijerph192114085

[11] Lähteenmäki H, Pätilä T, Pärnänen CP, Räisänen I, Tervahartiala T, Gupta S, et al. aMMP-8 point-of-care - Diagnostic methods and treatment modalities in periodontitis and peri-implantitis. Expert Opinion on Therapeutic Targets. 2023;**27**(7):627-637. DOI: 10.1080/14728222.2023.2240014. Epub 2023 Jul 31

[12] Carinci F, Romanos GE, Scapoli L. Molecular tools for preventing and

improving diagnosis of peri-implant diseases. Periodontology 2000. 2019;**81**(1):41-47. DOI: 10.1111/prd.12281

[13] Tzortzakis NG, Damaskos S, Dimakopoulou K, Chatzipetros E, Angelopoulos C. Periapical radiographs vs cone beam CT imaging for the evaluation of peri-implant bone defects: An ex vivo study. Medicina Oral, Patología Oral y Cirugía Bucal. 2025;**30**(3):e322-e332. DOI: 10.4317/medoral.26777

[14] Sahrmann P, Kühl S, Dagassan-Berndt D, Bornstein MM, Zitzmann NU. Radiographic assessment of the peri-implant site. Periodontology 2000. 2024;**95**(1):70-86. DOI: 10.1111/prd.12577. Epub 2024 Jul 1

[15] Hakkers J, Vangsted TE, van Winkelhoff AJ, de Waal YCM. Do systemic amoxicillin and metronidazole during the non-surgical peri-implantitis treatment phase prevent the need for future surgical treatment? A retrospective long-term cohort study. Journal of Clinical Periodontology. 2024;**51**(8):997-1004. DOI: 10.1111/jcpe.14024. Epub 2024 Jun 4

[16] Baima G, Citterio F, Romandini M, Romano F, Mariani GM, Buduneli N, et al. Surface decontamination protocols for surgical treatment of peri-implantitis: A systematic review with meta-analysis. Clinical Oral Implants Research. 2022;**33**(11):1069-1086. DOI: 10.1111/clr.13992. Epub 2022 Sep 7

[17] Ravidà A, Dias DR, Lemke R, Rosen PS, Bertolini MM. Efficacy of decontamination methods for biofilm removal from dental implant surfaces and Reosseointegration: An AAP/AO systematic review on Peri-implant diseases and conditions. The International Journal of Oral & Maxillofacial Implants. 2025;**4**:91-160

[18] Di Spirito F, Pisano M, Di Palo MP, Franci G, Rupe A, Fiorino A, et al. Peri-implantitis-associated microbiota before and after peri-implantitis treatment, the biofilm "competitive balancing" effect: A systematic review of randomized controlled trials. Microorganisms. 2024;**12**(10):1965. DOI: 10.3390/microorganisms12101965

[19] Feng Z, Zhu J, Zhang L, Li C, Su D, Wang H, et al. Microbiological and functional traits of peri-implant mucositis and correlation with disease severity. mSphere. 2024;**9**(7):e0005924. DOI: 10.1128/msphere.00059-24. Epub 2024 Jul 9

[20] Wilensky A, Shapira L, Limones A, Martin C. The efficacy of implant surface decontamination using chemicals during surgical treatment of peri-implantitis: A systematic review and meta-analysis. Journal of Clinical Periodontology. 2023;**50**(Suppl. 26):336-358. DOI: 10.1111/jcpe.13794. Epub 2023 Mar 12

[21] Rakasevic D, Gabrić D. The effect of implant surface design and their decontamination methods in peri-implantitis treatment. In: Current Concepts in Dental Implantology – From Science to Clinical Research. London, UK: IntechOpen; 2022. DOI: 10.5772/intechopen.99753

[22] Ramanauskaite A, Fretwurst T, Schwarz F. Efficacy of alternative or adjunctive measures to conventional non-surgical and surgical treatment of peri-implant mucositis and peri-implantitis: A systematic review and meta-analysis. International Journal of Implant Dentistry. 2021;**7**(1):112. DOI: 10.1186/s40729-021-00388-x

[23] Antonoglou GN, Papageorgiou SN, Carrillo de Albornoz A, Payer M, Stavropoulos A. Do systemic antibiotics

offer benefits to the surgical treatment of peri-implantitis? A systematic review with meta-analyses. Journal of Clinical Periodontology. 2025;**52**(12):1746-1759. DOI: 10.1111/jcpe.70021. Epub 2025 Aug 27

[24] Wang HL, Avila-Ortiz G, Monje A, Kumar P, Calatrava J, Aghaloo T, et al. AO/AAP consensus on prevention and management of peri-implant diseases and conditions: Summary report. Journal of Periodontology. 2025;**96**(6):519-541. DOI: 10.1002/JPER.25-0270. Epub 2025 Jun 12

[25] Romanos GE, Estrin NE. Laser applications in peri-implantitis therapy: A narrative review. Journal of Dentistry. 2025;**162**:106081. DOI: 10.1016/j.jdent.2025.106081. Epub 2025 Sep 1

[26] Di Gianfilippo R, Wang CW, Xie Y, Kinney J, Sugai J, Giannobile WV, et al. Effect of laser-assisted reconstructive surgical therapy of peri-implantitis on protein biomarkers and bacterial load. Clinical Oral Implants Research. 2023;**34**(4):393-403. DOI: 10.1111/clr.14059. Epub 2023 Mar 16

[27] Froum SJ, Rosen PS. A proposed classification for peri-implantitis. The International Journal of Periodontics & Restorative Dentistry. 2012;**32**(5):533-540

[28] Schwarz F, Jepsen S, Obreja K, Galarraga-Vinueza ME, Ramanauskaite A. Surgical therapy of peri-implantitis. Periodontology 2000. 2022;**88**(1):145-181. DOI: 10.1111/prd.12417

[29] Chaushu L, Tal H, Sculean A, Fernández-Tomé B, Chaushu G. Peri-implant disease affects systemic complete blood count values-an experimental in vivo study. Clinical Oral Investigations. 2020;**24**(12):4531-4539. DOI: 10.1007/s00784-020-03318-0. Epub 2020 May 16

[30] Chaushu L, Tal H, Sculean A, Fernández-Tomé B, Chaushu G. Effects of peri-implant infection on serum biochemical analysis. Journal of Periodontology. 2021;**92**(3):436-445. DOI: 10.1002/JPER.20-0048. Epub 2020 Aug 26

[31] Chaushu L, Tal H. Long-term inflammatory outcome after placement of a novel two-piece dental implant in a dog model experimental peri-implantitis. Clinical Oral Investigations. 2024;**28**(10):519. DOI: 10.1007/s00784-024-05907-9

[32] Madi M, Htet M, Zakaria O, Alagl A, Kasugai S. Re-osseointegration of dental implants after Periimplantitis treatments: A systematic review. Implant Dentistry. 2018;**27**(1):101-110. DOI: 10.1097/ID.0000000000000712

[33] Heitz-Mayfield LJA, Salvi GE, Mombelli A, Faddy M, Lang NP. Anti-infective surgical therapy of peri-implantitis. A 12-month prospective clinical study. Clinical Oral Implants Research. 2012;**23**(2):205-210. DOI: 10.1111/j.1600-0501.2011.02276.x. Epub 2011 Aug 9

[34] Monje A, Pons R, Ramanauskaite A, Castro A, Schwarz F, Chambrone L. Long-term surgical treatment outcomes of peri-implantitis. Periodontology 2000. 2025. DOI: 10.1111/prd.12643. Epub ahead of print

Chapter 4

Effectiveness of Health Belief Model on the Compliance of Periodontal Patients with Plaque Control: A Randomized Control Trial

Zahra Mustafa Juma Al Lawati and Latfiya Al Harthi

Abstract

The study aims to evaluate the effectiveness of the Health Belief Model (HBM) on patients' plaque control and periodontal condition compared with generic counseling and oral hygiene instructions. This Randomized Control Trial was tested in the "Periodontal Department of the Military Dental Center of the Armed Forces Medical Services", Oman. The control and experimental groups were the subjects referred to the Department of Periodontology from the Outpatient Dental Department [OPD]. They were examined and recruited from September 2020 to September 2021. At 12 months of follow-up, Bleeding on Probing (BOP) was substantially reduced in the experimental group in contrast to the non-experimental group ($p < 0.001$). At 12 months of monitoring, a substantial change was found in the plaque percentage between the two groups ($p < 0.001$). Both groups showed nearly no change in Clinical Attachment Level (CAL) at the 12-month evaluation, with the experimental group scoring CAL at 1.85 mm, while the CAL for the control group was 1.93 mm ($p = 0.095$). The study provided valuable knowledge on the impact of HBM on patients with periodontal diseases and their adherence to oral hygiene practices. Furthermore, this study found that self-efficacy plays an important role in improving compliance behavior.

Keywords: periodontitis, clinical attachment loss, health belief model, dental plaque, health belief model

1. Introduction

The two most common diseases related to oral health are "dental caries" and "periodontal diseases", which both can be prevented in early stages [1]. According to the World Workshop on the Classification of Periodontal Diseases and Conditions in 2017, periodontal diseases were classified into gingival and periodontal health, periodontitis, and other conditions affecting the periodontium [2, 3]. Periodontitis is a chronic inflammatory disease that leads to gingival inflammation and loss of bone

 IntechOpen

caused by the bacteria in the dental plaque. The composition of the dental plaque consists of 80% water and 20% solids, and according to the area of the location, it is classified into supragingival and subgingival plaque. It is the sixth most predominant disease globally, and it is linked with affecting the quality of life, masticatory dysfunction, and an increase in the cost of dental health treatment [4]. In addition to its effect on the health of the oral tissue, periodontitis has a direct impact on multiple general diseases such as diabetes mellitus (DM) [5, 6], cardiovascular disease (CVD) [5, 6], and preterm low birth weight [6, 7]. Globally, the burden of severe periodontitis is approximately 11% [4]. In Oman, the burden of severe periodontitis was estimated to be about 36% of the study population [8], which is higher than the reported prevalence globally.

Oral hygiene maintenance is the key to controlling plaque accumulation [9]. Establishing success after non-surgical periodontal therapy can be a challenge. Individuals with periodontitis require a high standard of oral hygiene to maintain periodontal health. This needs effective methods to encourage adherence to the oral hygiene instructions, as it is a chronic disease [3]. A study by Axelsson et al. has shown that patients who clean their teeth well have less dental caries and periodontitis compared with those who do not perform well cleaning [10]. Different studies reported on compliance with plaque control in the periodontitis group. These studies have noted that compliance is one of the challenging parts of the treatment of patients with periodontitis [1, 3].

Successful treatment of periodontitis involves the quality of the debridement, patients' compliance with plaque control, and their dental visits [11]. This is challenging if quality debridement is not achieved and the compliance of the patient toward plaque control through proper brushing and the use of interdental aids is not optimal [12]. Moreover, a study by Tonetti et al. reported that patients' compliance with long-term maintenance is fundamental to this success [12]. Many reasons have been reported in the literature for the lack of compliance. Some studies have found a positive relationship between socio-economic status and self-efficacy and brushing or flossing behaviors [13, 14]. Further studies have shown that multiple psychological constructs related to self-efficacy, attitudes, and dental coping beliefs are positively related to self-reported oral health behavior [15, 16]. Therefore, different methods should be used to improve the patient's compliance. However, these studies did not clarify which methods were used to improve patient compliance.

There are many psychological theories and models explaining how to change behaviors in improving own beliefs, aiming for better and more successful treatment. The most used are the Health Belief Model (HBM) [17], Self-Efficacy Model (SEM) [18], and Social Learning Theory (SLT) [18].

HBM is one of the most elaborate models. It was introduced in the 1950s to explore why some individuals are more interested in healthcare services while others neglect them. The primary variables of HBM include perceived susceptibility, benefits, severity, challenges, cues to action, and self-efficacy [19]. The susceptibility factor of the HBM indicates that when a patient is literate enough to know the severity of the disease, they willingly follow the suggested oral hygiene practices [20]. One of the most important applications of HBM is behavioral guidance, which assesses and recognizes health-related attitudes and includes preventive dental habits. Early diagnosis of the oral disease helps prevent future progression of the illness [21].

Current advancements have been included in preventive dentistry, focusing on behavioral models to recognize patients' psychology and enhance self-care and compliance with suggested dental treatments [22]. Dental fear is one of the most important causes of the progression of the disease. Several factors, including past dental trauma, specific personality traits, and depression in adults, lead to the development of dental anxiety in adults. The prevalence rate of dental phobia in adults is 9.4–19% [23]. According to HBM, the combined effect of perceived seriousness, susceptibility, advantages, barriers, cues to action, and self-efficacy helps to identify whether an individual takes preventive measures to stop the disease progression, go for screening, or improve health-related behavior. HBM significantly promotes self-care and healthy habits, and as per different studies, perceived behavior and self-efficacy were dominant parameters in oral health behavior [24, 25].

Few studies have explained if they used the full cycle of HBM in assessing the compliance of periodontal patients with plaque control [26, 27]. Newton et al. in a meta-analysis study found that two studies [26, 27], concluded that HBM has a small effect in predicting the related behavior to the oral hygiene of individuals with periodontitis [28]. In Kuhner's and Retzek's study, they used HBM to assess the compliance of patients with periodontitis during the treatment phase by measuring the bleeding index. From baseline to reevaluation appointments, the mean score of BOP decreased, and the average improvement was 51.2%. They assumed that health beliefs play a significant role in the determination of health-related behavior. Therefore, this chapter aims to evaluate the effectiveness of the HBM on patients' plaque control and periodontal condition compared with generic counseling and oral hygiene instructions.

2. Methodology

2.1 Research design and methods

This is a randomized controlled trial [RCT], single-blinded with two arms. RCT is a scientific study used to test a specific intervention or treatment. The subjects are divided into two groups: A control group receiving a standard treatment and an experimental group receiving an investigational intervention. In a single-blinded RCT, subjects are unaware of their group division, but the researchers are aware of it.

2.2 Study population

This RCT study was tested in the "Periodontal Department of the Military Dental Center of the Armed Forces Medical Services", Oman. The control and experimental groups were the subjects referred to the Department of Periodontology from the Outpatient Dental Department [OPD]. The subjects were recruited from the same medical center's OPD. OPD is when a patient undergoes treatment without any surgical procedure. They were examined and recruited from September 2020 to September 2021. RCT usually follows fixed recruiting periods to ensure data is gathered within a specific timeframe.

2.3 Eligibility criteria

The following criteria were considered to determine the subjects' eligibility.
Inclusion Criteria

- The inclusion criteria for the RCT were:
- Both genders included from 18 years to 70 years.
- Patients are referred to the periodontal department.
- Patients capable of traveling and attending all the study visits.
- Patients with stage I to III Periodontitis.
- A minimum of 20 teeth must be present in the oral cavity.

Exclusion Criteria:

- The exclusion criteria for the RCT were:
- Advanced Periodontal Disease (stage IV).
- Uncontrolled chronic systemic diseases (diabetes and immunocompromised) [29–33].
- Patients having an increased risk of tuberculosis.
- Patients with a history of bleeding disorders.
- Pregnant or lactating females.
- Subjects showing unavailability issues.
- Need antibiotic cover.
- Patients who took antibiotics 1 month before the start of the process.
- Specialist periodontal treatment in the previous 6 months.

Study Outcome Measures:
The following key indicators of progression of periodontal disease were evaluated,

- Changes in plaque index and bleeding on probing [BOP].
- Clinical attachment level [CAL].

Changes in plaque index and [BOP] were included in the study measures to assess the subjects' oral hygiene and gingival health status. Dental plaque biofilm indicates the oral hygiene status and the risk of developing gum disease or carious lesions. BOP occurs when there is an underlying inflammation of the soft tissues, indicating gingivitis or periodontal disease [34]. CAL was evaluated to test the severity of the periodontal disease and the treatment outcome. CAL is the area between the periodontal pocket base and the exact point on the tooth, which shows the attachment loss between the gingiva and the teeth. A deeper pocket indicates extensive attachment loss between the gums and the teeth. Examining the changes in these measurements over time gives beneficial information about the successful outcomes of periodontal treatments. Therefore, in assessing these outcome measures, the study intended to completely evaluate the intervention's impact on periodontal health.

2.4 Randomization

Patients referred to the periodontal department were randomized to one of two groups using a simple randomization method. The randomization was performed using sealed envelopes. Concealment of allocation was achieved using a sealed envelope containing the allocated intervention arm for the patient. An equal number of labels were divided into Letter A, which referred to the control group, and Letter B, which referred to the experimental group. This was opened immediately before ZAL conducted the clinical examination.

Figure 1 shows the randomization process and how the patients referred to the OPD were allocated into two groups. An equal quantity of labels was used, with "A"

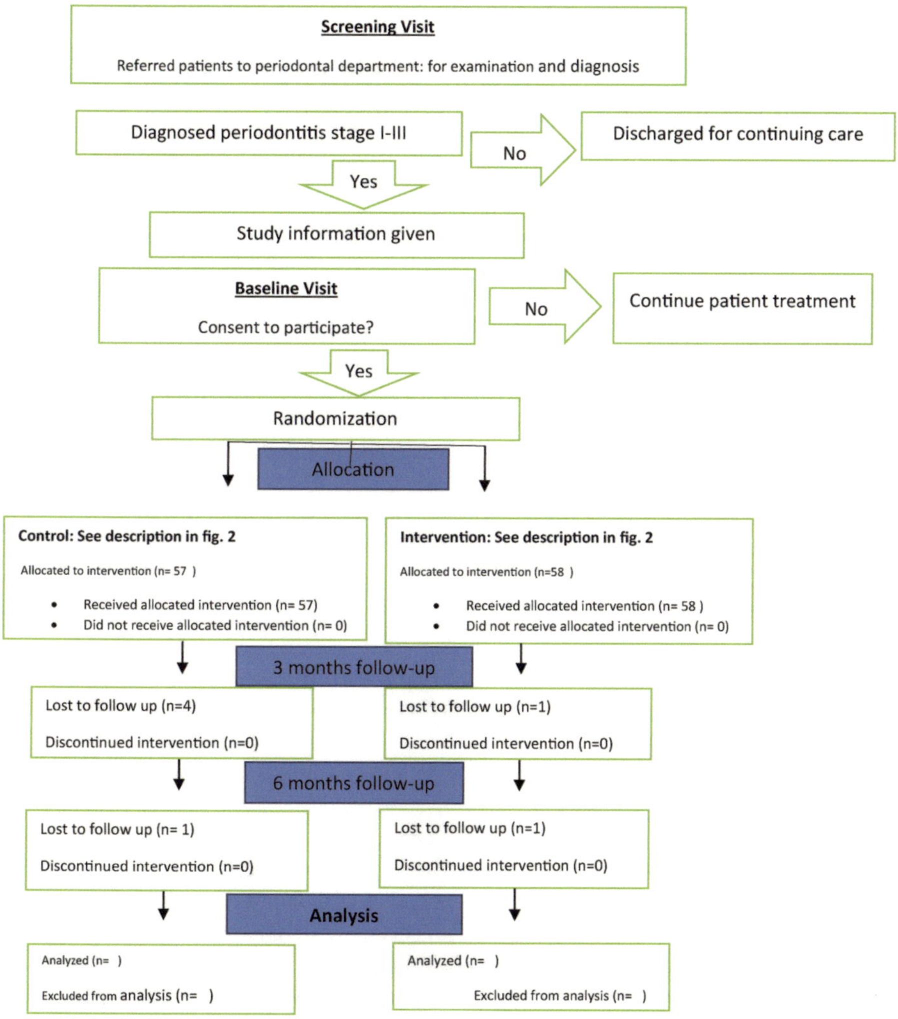

Figure 1.
CONSORT flow diagram for a randomized controlled trial.

indicating the control group and "B" indicating the experimental group, promoting equal allocation. The envelopes were opened right before the clinical evaluation, ensuring that the allocation remained hidden until the last minute, protecting against potential biases and preserving the integrity of the study's conclusions.

2.5 Masking

Masking, or blinding, is a strategy used in the study to prevent bias by keeping the participants ignorant of the important aspects of the study. In this study, participants were unaware of the intervention provided under investigation and the allocation of the groups. The researcher gathered and analyzed the clinical data and masked it into group divisions using anonymized coded samples. Data entry was performed by ZAL, who was the only one who had access to all the stored data. The masked researcher analyzing the data was ignorant about the group allocation throughout the data entry.

Masking is a crucial technique used in the study to reduce bias and improve the authenticity of the study outcomes. It prevents any influence of the subject's knowledge on their behavior or reactions by keeping them unaware of essential characteristics of the research, such as the intervention under investigation and group allocation. This strategy eliminates any possibility that their expectations would impact the findings.

2.6 Participant dropout

Dropout criteria were followed based on the non-availability of the participants. Suppose the participant became ineligible, possibly due to an alteration or improvement in their overall periodontal health. Some participants withdraw their consent to participate. Therefore, they were removed from the study. This indicates that the involvement of the patients in the study was voluntary, and participants could leave the study whenever they wanted.

The participants' willingness was included in the ethical guidelines of the research because it ensures the rights of the participants in decision-making regarding whether to continue with the study or leave without their treatment being affected.

3. Study procedure

Study Schedule: The study's timeframe begins with the screening of the patients, recording baseline data, and providing treatment. Subsequently, participants were followed up at 3, 6, and 12 months.

3.1 Screening visit

Patients were referred from the OPD to the periodontal department. It was based on the basic periodontal treatment [BPE] scores. A BPE score of 3 or 4 warranted a referral for assessment and management. Zal screened all the participants using routine clinical procedures, including medical history, and examined them to see if they fit the study's eligibility criteria. ZAL explained the study to the eligible participants, and the participants who decided to be part of the study filled out a written consent form. After that, they were asked to complete a validated questionnaire.

3.2 Baseline visit

It refers to the initial evaluation of the patients before the start of intervention or recommendation of ant treatment. It offers the baseline characteristics and health status of the participants. Clinical assessment of the patients was performed by LAH, including plaque score, bleeding from the gingiva, gingival pocket depth, and gingival recession. The plaque score was measured according to O'Leary et al. [35]. A disclosing agent was applied to the teeth' surfaces to assess the plaque's presence. A periodontal probe was used to run circumferentially around each tooth within the gingival sulcus or pocket depth to evaluate the bleeding from the gingiva. The following sites of the tooth were used to check the gingival bleeding score: MB, B, DB, MP, P, and DP. The pocket depth and recession of the gingiva were measured at six sites on all erupted teeth, excluding wisdom teeth, and performed using a mirror and a periodontal probe (CC Williams Probe 10 mm). OPG was taken for all the patients to assess the level of bone resorption. ZAL did the counseling according to the randomization. After completing the examination, the hygienist NAM completed periodontal treatment according to the prescription given by LAH.

4. Treatment visits

4.1 Initial visit

Control Group: Generic counseling and oral hygiene instructions that include brushing and flossing techniques were delivered to participants with the aid of models while the participants were sitting on the dental chair without using the Health Belief Model [HBM]. NAM carries out the periodontal treatment if needed. Incentives such as toothbrushes and interdental brushes were distributed to participants.

Experimental group: Participants received specific counseling according to the HBM and tailored oral hygiene instructions. Tailored oral hygiene was done by showing them the correct technique of tooth brushing in front of the mirror using a toothbrush with soft bristles (Swedish brand TePe, Malmo, Sweden), which was done in three steps. First, I will watch them systematically or randomly. After that, they evaluated which technique they were using while brushing their teeth. Finally, they were assessed to see if they looked at the mirror while brushing. Then, ZAL repeated all the steps with an explanation of the correct brushing technique in front of the mirror. If the patient had interdental spaces, the proper size of the interdental brush(Tepe brushes) with the correct diameter was given.

Moreover, dental floss (dentotape, Johnson & Johnson, Sollentuna, Sweden) was recommended for patients with narrow interdental spaces. A leaflet was distributed to the patients with all the information given, and the action plan agreed upon. Then, NAM completed the periodontal treatment, which was done based on the guided biofilm therapy that encompasses the use of air polishing devices, followed by selective scaling using the EMS system. Incentives such as toothbrushes, interdental brushes, and dental floss were also distributed. All patients were given a manual toothbrush (Tepe brushes) to standardize self-performed plaque control at home.

Three- and six-month follow-up:

Control group: LAH re-examined the participant's oral health, and NAM performed the regular maintenance procedures previously performed.

Experimental group: LAH re-examined the participant's overall periodontal health. ZAL re-counseled the patients according to HBM, and NAM performed the periodontal maintenance.

Twelve-month follow-up:

Both groups were asked to complete a second questionnaire similar to the one done at baseline. LAH re-examined both groups. ZAL counseled all of them according to the HBM and tailored oral hygiene instructions. Treatment was provided if required. Incentives such as toothbrushes and interdental brushes were distributed to them. Then, they were given review appointments in the dental hygiene department.

Figure 2 is a graphic illustration of the study process, which provides the outline of the methods followed during the patients' initial visits, followed by 3, 6, and 12 months follow-up for both the control and experimental groups. During the initial

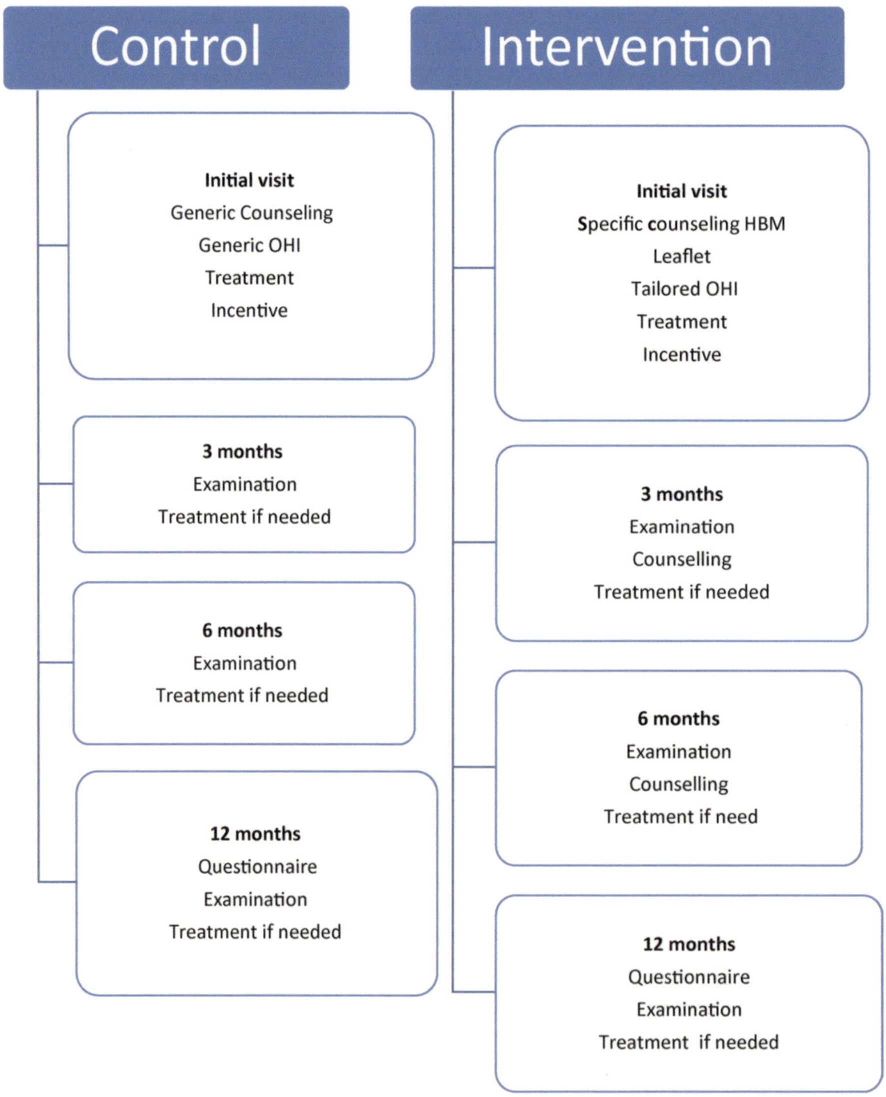

Figure 2.
Control and intervention plan.

visit, participants were given counseling based on HBM. The goal was to improve the participant's attitude toward oral health. On 3- and 6-month follow-ups, re-examination and treatment were performed in the control group, and counseling and therapy were conducted in the experimental group. On the 12-month follow-up, a questionnaire was filled out along with examination and treatment if required.

5. Data collection and analysis

5.1 Sample size calculation

Sample size calculation determines the number of participants to evaluate the significant effect of the study. The calculated sample size is 128 (64 in each group). The estimate was based on the anticipated effect size of 0.50 (medium), alpha error of 5%, and power of 80%. The effect size represents the degree of difference between the two groups. The allocation ratio considered is 1:1 to reduce the bias and maintain the balance between the two groups. To overcome the attrition bias (anticipating 15%), the sample size increased to 148 (74 in each group). Attrition refers to the dropping out of participants. G*Power version 3.1.9.2 was used to calculate the sample size.

5.2 Statistical analysis

Continuous elements were summarized using mean and standard deviation. Frequency and percentages were reported for categorical elements. Pearson's correlation coefficient was applied to determine the relationship between two continuous variables. An unpaired t-test is used to compare the means of two individual groups. A paired test was performed to compare the pre-post mean score. A chi-square test (Fisher's exact/likelihood ratio) was applied to determine the relationship between two categorical variables. A two-way mixed ANOVA was used to evaluate the main and interaction effects of the type of intervention and time on the outcome variables. A p-value of 0.05 was considered statistically significant. All the analyses were done using IBM SPSS version 28.0.

6. Results

6.1 Patient baseline characteristics

The 115 participants received individual standard treatment, with 58 individuals in the intervention and 57 in the non-intervention group. **Table 1** shows the independent t-test to assess the mean ages between the control and the experimental groups, represented as Group A and Group B, respectively. The mean age of group A is 29.81 years, with a standard deviation of 8.808. Group B shows a mean age of 29.95 with a standard deviation of 7.473. The p-value is 0.926, greater than 0.05, indicating no statistically significant difference in the mean ages between Group A and Group B. Additionally, no significant difference between the genders was observed between the groups ($p = 0.85$). This result is analyzed using Fisher's exact test, which identifies whether two categorical variables are related, as illustrated in **Table 1**.

Table 2 compares control and experimental groups at initial evaluation and 12 months across different variables: susceptibility, severity, benefits, barriers, and

Variable	Group		P-value
	Experimental	Control	
	n (%)	n (%)	
Age, mean ± SD	29.95 ± 7.47	29.81 ± 8.81	0.926
Sex			
Male	29 (50.0)	27 (47.4)	0.853
Female	29 (50.0)	30 (52.6)	

Test: Independent samples t-test, Fisher's exact test.

Table 1.
Baseline characteristics of the study participants.

Group Statistics					
	Group	N	Mean	Std. Deviation	P-value
Susceptibility – initial	Control	57	7.16	1.461	0.955
	Experimental	58	7.17	1.313	
Susceptibility – 12 months	Control	57	8.02	1.541	0.744
	Experimental	58	8.10	1.266	
Severity – initial	Control	57	11.16	2.548	0.948
	Experimental	58	11.19	2.685	
Severity – 12 months	Control	57	12.33	2.107	0.712
	Experimental	58	12.47	1.709	
Benefits – initial	Control	57	8.46	2.010	0.153
	Experimental	58	8.93	1.485	
Benefits – 12 months	Control	57	8.30	1.908	0.131
	Experimental	58	8.79	1.565	
Barriers – initial	Control	57	30.09	4.505	0.618
	Experimental	58	29.67	4.410	
Barriers – 12 months	Control	57	24.53	3.728	0.545
	Experimental	58	24.09	4.045	
Self-efficacy – initial	Control	57	8.07	1.568	0.679
	Experimental	58	8.19	1.515	
Self-efficacy – 12 months	Control	57	9.00	1.309	0.941
	Experimental	58	8.98	1.162	

Test: Independent samples t-test.

Table 2.
Comparing control and experimental groups at initial evaluation and 12 months across different variables.

self-efficacy. There was no significant difference between the groups at the initial assessment, 12 months. P-values are above 0.05, indicating any observed difference is likely due to random chance. Therefore, both groups are comparable at both time points.

The present study collected data from 115 participants: 58 from the group under intervention and 57 from the non-intervention group. From the diagnostic results, all subjects had periodontal disease, including stage I, stage II, and stage III periodontitis. During the 3-month follow-up, four participants from the control group and one from the experimental group dropped out during the study period. One participant from the experiment group withdrew due to transportation problems. In the control group, four participants decided to discontinue treatment. Two moved temporarily from the country; one female participant got pregnant, and the last changed his mobile number, which could not be reached. In 6 months of follow-up, two participants were lost. One female from the experimental group got pregnant, and the other participant from the control group had business commitments. In a 12-month follow-up, only one participant was lost due to a car accident.

The HBM is a theoretical framework emphasizing risk perception and behavior assessment, as shown in **Figure 3**. Threat perception depends on two principles: perceived vulnerability to an illness or medical condition and the severity of its adverse effects. HBM also considers factors such as the quality of the dentist-patient relationship, previous therapy experiences, and the influence of family and peers.

In the HBM survey, no considerable change was found in all HBM arms, including self-efficacy, between the experimental and control groups. The oral hygiene practices of the participants were assessed according to the HBM survey, as well as their beliefs and attitudes toward their health. Most individuals brushed their teeth two times daily (71.3%), and 25.2% flossed their teeth once a day. About 96.2% used a manual toothbrush to clean their teeth, while 3.8% preferred electrical brushes. Moreover, 21.2% of the participants used interdental brushes, and 22.6% reported using tongue brushes.

In the final HBM survey, measuring scales were also included to assess the HBM parameters: perceived susceptibility, perceived severity, perceived benefits, perceived barriers, and perceived self-efficacy, which are highlighted in **Table 3**. The responses were in Likert Scales with options ranging from 1, strongly disagree to 5, strongly.

Susceptibility was calculated through questions, assessing the perceived consequences of the disease and susceptibility. The scale showed no change between the two groups ($p = 0.744$). In the research, the severity was calculated using three questions, where the respondents were asked about the perceived consequences of the disease. On the severity scale, no significant difference was found (p-value = 0.712). Two items were used to measure the benefits: brushing and flossing. The results imply that the scale was insignificant, with a p-value of 0.131. The eight-item scale was used to assess the barriers to cleaning and flossing. However, the scale was significant, with a p-value

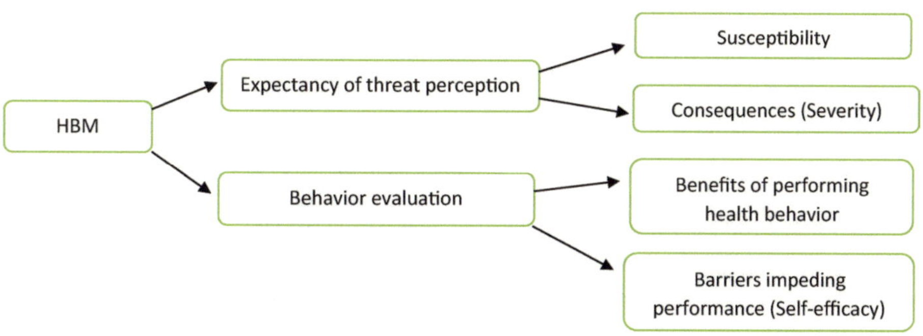

Figure 3.
HBM.

Variable	Experimental group		Control group		F	Partial Eta Squared	P-value
	EMM	SE	EMM	SE			
Susceptibility at 12 months	8.101	0.173	8.02	0.175	F (1, 112) = 0.107	0.001	0.744
Severity at 12 months	12.467	0.251	12.332	0.253	F (1, 112) = 0.143	0.001	0.706
Barriers at 12 months	24.211	0.368	24.399	0.371	F (1, 112) = 0.128	0.001	0.721
Benefits at 12 months	8.622	0.156	8.473	0.157	F (1, 112) = 0.447	0.004	0.505
Self-efficacy at 12 months	8.970	0.158	9.013	0.159	F (1, 112) = 0.036	0.001	0.851

Test: One-way ANCOVA, EMM – Estimated Marginal Means, SE – Standard Error, Covariates adjusted: Susceptibility_initial, Severity_initial, Barriers_initial, Benefits_initial, Self-efficacy_initial.

Table 3.
Comparing HBM factors between experimental and control groups.

of 0.545. Two self-efficacy questions for brushing and flossing were used to evaluate the self-efficacy. At a p-value of 0.941, the scale was found to be insignificant.

Table 3 shows the findings of a one-way ANCOVA analysis that compared the variables between the experimental and control groups 12 months after adjusting for the covariate effect of baseline (initial) measurement. The table compares the experimental and control groups regarding susceptibility, severity, obstacles, advantages, and self-efficacy. Estimated marginal means (EMM) and standard error (SE): These figures show the estimated mean scores and standard errors for each variable in the experimental and control groups. The F value is generated from ANCOVA, which compares the variables between the experimental and control groups after 12 months. The F values in the table correspond to various variables, including susceptibility, severity, barriers, advantages, and self-efficacy. The analysis shows no substantial change between the non-experimental and experimental groups in susceptibility (EMM = 8.02 vs. 8.101, p = 0.744), severity (EMM = 12.332 vs. 12.467, p = 0.706), barriers (EMM = 24.399 vs. 24.211, p = 0.721), benefits (EMM = 8.473 vs. 8.622, p = 0.505), and self-efficacy (9.013 vs. 8.970, p = 0.851) at 12 months.

Table 4 shows the independent samples t-test analysis findings that compared the variables between the experimental and control groups at each follow-up time point.

6.2 Change in bleeding on probing

Initially, at baseline, the participants in the control group had a mean of about 33.96% of bleeding on probing sites, while the experimental group participants had about 34.77%. After 3 months of review, the experimental group showed reduced bleeding on probing by approximately 50%, with only 19.76% on probing sites. In comparison, the control group percentage of BOP reduced to 24.63% with a reduction of 9.3% of total probing sites. Six months after the initial visit, the results of the BOP in the control group showed an increase in the mean value of 27.23%, while the experimental group showed a reduction of about 4%. At 12 months of follow-up,

Variable	Experimental group	Control group	P-value*
	Mean ± SD	Mean ± SD	
Bleeding – Initial (%)	34.77 ± 19.58	33.96 ± 17.73	0.818
Bleeding – 3 months (%)	19.76 ± 14.55	24.63 ± 16.00	0.091
Bleeding – 6 months (%)	15.96 ± 11.60	27.23 ± 17.56	<0.001*
Bleeding – 12 months (%)	17.72 ± 13.64	29.10 ± 14.96	<0.001*
Plaque – Initial (%)	69.29 ± 14.83	71.04 ± 15.41	0.535
Plaque – 3 months (%)	46.45 ± 20.40	54.42 ± 24.21	0.059
Plaque – 6 months (%)	38.04 ± 18.54	54.63 ± 25.53	<0.001*
Plaque – 12 months (%)	35.69 ± 22.77	52.87 ± 17.08	<0.001*
CAL – Initial	2.19 ± 0.30	2.31 ± 0.35	0.054
CAL – 3 months	1.87 ± 0.27	1.97 ± 0.28	0.066
CAL – 6 months	1.83 ± 0.27	2.00 ± 0.26	<0.001*
CAL – 12 months	1.85 ± 0.20	1.93 ± 0.29	0.095

**Statistically significant, CAL – Clinical Attachment Level, Test: Independent samples t-test.*

Table 4.
Comparison between the experimental group and control group at each follow-up time point.

BOP was substantially reduced in the experimental group in contrast to the non-experimental group (p < 0.001).

6.3 Change in plaque

At baseline visits, plaque scores for control and experimental groups were 71.04 and 69.29%, respectively. At 3 months follow-up, there was a 23% change in plaque score in the intervention group, dropping to 46.45%, while the control group's plaque score showed a 16.63% change, decreasing to 54.42%. During the 6-month review, the plaque percentage dropped by about 33% from the initial visit, with 38.04% in the experimental group and about a 16.42% change in the control group, demonstrating a considerable difference from the 3-month review. At 12 months of monitoring, a substantial change was found in the plaque percentage between the two groups (p < 0.001).

6.4 Change of CAL

The CAL measured at the initial assessment was 2.1 mm for the experimental and 2.3 mm for the control group. At 3 months of evaluation, the change in CAL in the experimental group was about 0.3 mm, and in the control group, there was about a 0.4 mm reduction in CAL. In 6 months of evaluation, the change in CAL in the experimental group and control was statistically significant (P < 0.001).

Both groups showed nearly no change in CAL at the 12-month evaluation, with the experimental group scoring CAL at 1.85 mm, while the CAL for the control group was 1.93 mm (p = 0.095).

Table 5 shows that at the end of 12 months of follow-up, the experimental group showed lower bleeding levels on probing, lower plaque accumulation, and clinical

Variable	Experimental group		Control group		F	Partial Eta Squared	P-value
	EMM	SE	EMM	SE			
Bleeding	21.798	1.715	30.291	1.781	F (1, 104) = 11.801	0.102	<0.001*
Plaque	47.857	1.915	60.840	1.989	F (1, 104) = 22.108	0.175	<0.001*
CAL	1.938	0.031	2.052	0.032	F (1, 104) = 6.666	0.060	0.011*

**Statistically significant, Test: Two-way mixed ANOVA, EMM – Estimated Marginal Means, SE – Standard Error, CAL – Clinical Attachment Level.*

Table 5.
A two-way mixed ANOVA analysis to examine the difference between the experimental group and the control group.

attachment loss compared to the control group ($p < 0.05$). This indicates that the experimental intervention had beneficial effects.

7. Discussion

According to the 2017 World Workshop Classification of Periodontitis, the diagnosis focuses on the several risk factors contributing to the disease's development along with the physical symptoms. Factors involved in the patient's past experiences with the disease and their response to the therapies [36]. Based on the location, the clinical health of the gingiva depends on the intact and reduced periodontium. Staging is based on four classes: clinical attachment loss, bone height, depth of the pocket, vertical bone defect, and loss of tooth. Three-level classification consists of grade A: low risk, grade B: moderate risk, and grade C: high progression risk [37].

Among all health behavior theories, HBM, suggested by Rosenstock in 1974, is the earliest and most broadly applied theory. The author discusses the connection between the opinions and behavior of an individual. The risk belief of the progression of the disease influences an individual's attitude [38]. In another study based on a descriptive-analytical study, 300 students underwent random selection. A conventional questionnaire for health beliefs was used to gather data, and the mean health attitude was moderate among students [22].

In a 2019 study by Lee C et al., action and coping planning greatly influence a person's behavior toward periodontal disease. Planning should be done in person or written form, and the individuals must specify how, when, and where they floss. Alternate attitudes should also be considered to prevent them from flossing [39]. Another study illustrated that experiments based on the social and cognitive structure help promote dental hygiene practices, leading to a healthy periodontal status. The structure comprises aims, planning, self-evaluation, and feedback [40].

Individuals who show no compliance with dental treatments are often observed to have depression incidents in life. The first response of a patient to a periodontal treatment depends on their public and empathetic skills. A greater degree of nervousness and reduced attention are linked to non-compliant attitudes. Therefore, dental practitioners must be able to recognize nervousness and agreeableness, leading to a non-compliant attitude [41, 42].

The HBM is an analytical structure that maintains the perception and attitude of an individual toward health. The study highlights that removing perceived barriers is necessary to encourage oral health behavior. Self-efficacy was an essential point of reference for brushing and flossing. Self-efficacy refers to an individual's self-confidence to carry out a task properly. This study suggests that higher self-efficacy is associated with improved compliance with plaque control attitudes. The study showed varying self-efficacies and perceived benefits of practicing plaque control measures. Adapting to behavior results in the person's concept of self-efficacy due to a sense of success that the behavior can be accomplished. These cognitive frameworks help to modify an individual's personality to follow the suggested dental hygiene instructions, therefore enhancing an individual's confidence.

The study assesses the principles of HBM in positively influencing individuals with periodontal disease to perform oral health practices. The results showed that the HBM structure has the potential to impact health-related behavior. The findings also focus on oral health practices and how it is hard to brush and floss. This indicates the significant effect on a person's behavior in complying with an oral hygiene routine. Individuals with increased self-efficacy were shown to be compliant with plaque control habits and willingly followed oral health routines. The outcomes of the results also highlight the altering relationship between cognitive framework and attitudes in altering an individual's behavior toward oral care habits. By revamping the treatment strategy per the individual's beliefs regarding susceptibility, severity, benefits, barriers, and self-efficacy, the practitioner can establish a stimulating atmosphere for longer-term alteration in the attitude.

The effects of an experiment on periodontal health have also been discussed through BOP, plaque accumulation, and CAL for 12 months. The baseline characteristics illustrated that about 34% of the areas showed BOP. After 3 months, bleeding reduced to 50% in the group undergoing intervention and 24.62% in the non-experimental group. Six months after the treatment, the BOP in the non-experimental group increased to 27.22%, whereas in the experimental group, it remained 4% lower. A constant regression in BOP in contrast to the control group ($p < 0.001$), was seen at 12 months in the experimental group. Plaque measurements follow the same pattern as BOP. Initially, each group showed an increased plaque level (>69%). At the end of 3 months, a significant regression of 23% was observed in the experimental group. At 6 months, plaque measurement reduced to 38.04%. The measurement of plaque accumulation in both groups stayed significant, indicating the positive effect of therapy at 12-month follow-up. The results on CAL demonstrate the experiment's potential in treating periodontal disease. At first assessment, CAL was lesser in the non-experimental group, about 2.3 mm, in contrast to the experimental group 2.1 mm. A better change was observed after 3 months, with a 0.3 mm regression in the experimental group and a 0.4 mm regression in the non-experimental group. A significant reduction in the CAL ($P < 0.001$) was seen, indicating that the experiment proved effective with an increase in time.

Despite using the HBM to encourage adherence to healthy behaviors as a professional recommends, there is a lack of research on periodontal patients' compliance with plaque control measures. Previous research may have evaluated chronic diseases of oral health. Still, fewer studies are performed on the effect of the components of HBM, like perceived severity, susceptibility, benefits, and barriers, on the behaviors and self-efficacy of periodontal patients. Also, there is a lack of high-quality RCT data that investigates the effectiveness of HBM-based interventions.

Several limitations include a small sample size and the inability to track long-term compliance with oral healthcare recommendations. It is important to highlight the significance of objective parameters, including clinical records and tests, since data alone provided by the patients is not enough and causes errors.

8. Conclusion

The study concludes a statistical increase in enhancing the plaque management routine and periodontal health in the group undergoing intervention. Individuals in the experimental group significantly decrease PI and GI scores. The study provided valuable knowledge on the impact of HBM on patients with periodontal diseases and their adherence to oral hygiene practices [43]. Furthermore, this study found that self-efficacy plays an important role in improving compliance behavior, revealing that participants with higher levels of self-efficacy complied with the suggested oral care schedule.

Funding

This study was funded by the Ministry of Higher Education (MHE) in Oman.

Conflict of interest

None disclosed.

Statements and declarations

Authorship

Dr. Zahra Mustafa Juma Al Lawati contributed to the collection of the data and design of the study.

Dr. Latfiya Al-Harthi revised the data critically and approved the final version of the draft.

Author details

Zahra Mustafa Juma Al Lawati[1]* and Latfiya Al Harthi[2]

1 Department of Periodontology, Ministry of Health, Muscat, Oman

2 Department of Periodontology, Medical City Hospital of Military and Security Services, Muscat, Oman

*Address all correspondence to: zahralawati88@gmail.com

References

[1] Jönsson B, Öhrn K, Lindberg P, Oscarson N. Cost-effectiveness of an individually tailored oral health educational programme based on cognitive behavioural strategies in non-surgical periodontal treatment. Journal of Clinical Periodontology. Jul 2012;**39**(7):659-665

[2] Kinane DF, Stathopoulou PG, Papapanou PN. Periodontal diseases. Nature Reviews Disease Primers. 22 Jun 2017;**3**(1):17038

[3] Wilson TG. Compliance and its role in periodontal therapy. Periodontology 2000. Oct 1996;**12**(1):16-23

[4] Kassebaum NJ, Bernabé E, Dahiya M, Bhandari B, Murray CJL, Marcenes W. Global burden of severe periodontitis in 1990-2010: A systematic review and meta-regression. Journal of Dental Research. Nov 2014;**93**(11):1045-1053

[5] Paquette DW. The Periodontal Infection-Systemic Disease Link: A Review of the Truth or Myth. - Abstract - Europe PMC [Internet]. 2002. Available from: https://europepmc.org/article/med/12670089 [Accessed: January 13, 2020]

[6] Tonetti MS DF. Periodontitis: From Local Infection to Systemic Diseases. - Abstract - Europe PMC [Internet]. 2005. Available from: https://europepmc.org/article/med/16848982 [Accessed: January 13, 2020]

[7] Scannapieco FA, Bush RB, Paju S. Periodontal disease as a risk factor for adverse pregnancy outcomes. A systematic review. Annals of Periodontology. 2003;**8**(1):70-78

[8] Al-Harthi LS, Cullinan MP, Leichter JW, Thomson WM. Periodontal diseases in an omani adult population: A preliminary study. Journal of Periodontology. May 2014;**85**(5):e104-e110

[9] Vyas T, Bhatt G, Gaur A, Sharma C, Sharma A, Nagi R. Chemical plaque control-a brief review. Journal of Family Medicine and Primary Care. 2021;**10**(4):1562-1568

[10] Lindhe. Long-term maintenance of patients treated for advanced periodontal disease*. Journal of Clinical Periodontology - Wiley Online Library [Internet]. 1984. Available from: https://onlinelibrary.wiley.com/doi/abs/10.1111/j.1600-051X.1984.tb00902.x [Accessed: July 19, 2025]

[11] Lindhe J, Westfelt E, Nyman S, Socransky SS, Haffajee AD. Long-term effect of surgical/non-surgical treatment of periodontal disease. Journal of Clinical Periodontology. 1984;**11**(7):448-458

[12] Shaddox LM, Walker CB. Treating chronic periodontitis: Current status, challenges, and future directions:13

[13] Macgregor IDM, Balding JW. Self-esteem as a predictor of toothbrushing behaviour in young adolescents. Journal of Clinical Periodontology. 1991;**18**(5):312-316

[14] Macgregor IDM, Regis D, Balding J. Self-concept and dental health behaviours in adolescents. Journal of Clinical Periodontology. 1997;**24**(5):335-339

[15] Tedesco LA, Keffer MA, Fleck-Kandath C. Self-efficacy, reasoned action, and oral health behavior reports: A social cognitive approach to compliance. Journal of Behavioral Medicine. Aug 1991;**14**(4):341-355

[16] Syrjälä AMH, Knuuttila MLE, Syrjälä LK. Self-efficacy perceptions in oral health behavior. Acta Odontologica Scandinavica. 1 Jan 2001;**59**(1):1-6

[17] Rosenstock IM. Historical origins of the health belief model. Health Education Monographs. 1 Dec 1974;**2**(4):328-335

[18] Bandura A. The explanatory and predictive scope of self-efficacy theory. Journal of Social and Clinical Psychology. Sep 1986;**4**(3):359-373

[19] Nasir EF, Suliman NM. Application of the health belief model in oral hygiene practice (brushing/flossing): A narrative review. Journal of International Oral Health. 2022;**14**(4):342-348

[20] Sanaeinasab H, Saffari M, Taghavi H, Karimi Zarchi A, Rahmati F, Al Zaben F, et al. An educational intervention using the health belief model for improvement of oral health behavior in grade-schoolers: A randomized controlled trial. BMC Oral Health. 2022;**22**(1):94

[21] Fini MB, Ryu Y, Mahaffey CC, Rhoads KE, Han H. Preventive dental Behaviors among U.S. college students: Application of the health belief model. American Journal of Health Behavior. 2023;**47**(6):167-178

[22] Chan CC, Chan AK, Chu C, Tsang Y. Theory-based behavioral change interventions to improve periodontal health. Frontiers in Oral Health. 2023;**4**:1067092

[23] Xiang B, Wong HM, Perfecto AP, McGrath CP. Modelling health belief predictors of oral health and dental anxiety among adolescents based on the health belief model: A cross-sectional study. BMC Public Health. 2020;**20**:1-12

[24] The Health Belief Model. The Wiley Encyclopedia of Health Psychology. Wiley Online Library [Internet]. Available from: https://onlinelibrary.wiley.com/doi/abs/10.1002/9781119057840.ch68 [Accessed: July 19, 2025]

[25] Luquis RR, Kensinger WS. Applying the health belief model to assess prevention services among young adults. International Journal of Health Promotion and Education. 2019;**57**(1):37-47

[26] Kühner MK, Raetzke PB. The effect of health beliefs on the compliance of periodontal patients with oral hygiene instructions. Journal of Periodontology. Jan 1989;**60**(1):51-56

[27] Barker T. Role of health beliefs in patient compliance with preventive dental advice. Community Dentistry and Oral Epidemiology. 1994;**22**(5PT1):327-336

[28] Vilar Doceda M, Petit C, Huck O. Behavioral interventions on periodontitis patients to improve oral hygiene: A systematic review. Journal of Clinical Medicine. Jan 2023;**12**(6):2276

[29] Bui FQ, Almeida-da-Silva CLC, Huynh B, Trinh A, Liu J, Woodward J, et al. Association between periodontal pathogens and systemic disease. Biomedical Journal. 1 Feb 2019;**42**(1):27-35

[30] Bulgakova AI, Vasilyeva NA, Vasilyev EA. The clinical and immunological rationale for the use of prolonged action dental ointment in periodontology. Journal of Advanced Pharmacy Education & Research. 2019;**9**(4):65-69

[31] Falcao A, Bullón P. A review of the influence of periodontal treatment in systemic diseases. Periodontology 2000. Wiley Online Library [Internet].

2019;**79**(1):117-128. Available from: https://onlinelibrary.wiley.com/doi/abs/10.1111/prd.12249 [cited 2025 Jul 19]

[32] Genco RJ, Sanz M. Clinical and public health implications of periodontal and systemic diseases: An overview. Periodontology 2000. Wiley Online Library [Internet]. 2020;**83**(1):7-13. Available from: https://onlinelibrary.wiley.com/doi/abs/10.1111/prd.12344 [Accessed: July 19, 2025]

[33] Nazir MA. Prevalence of periodontal disease, its association with systemic diseases and prevention. International Journal of Health Sciences. 2017;**11**(2):72-80

[34] Loos BG. Systemic markers of inflammation in periodontitis. Journal of Periodontology. Wiley Online Library [Internet]. 2005;**76**:2106-2115. Available from: https://aap.onlinelibrary.wiley.com/doi/abs/10.1902/jop.2005.76.11-s.2106 [Accessed: July 19, 2025]

[35] O'Leary TJ. The plaque control record. Journal of Periodontology. 1972;**43**:38

[36] Ravidà A, Travan S, Saleh MH, Greenwell H, Papapanou PN, Sanz M, et al. Agreement among international periodontal experts using the 2017 world workshop classification of periodontitis. Journal of Periodontology. 2021;**92**(12):1675-1686

[37] Solomon SM, Sufaru IG, Pasarin L, Martu S. Aspects regarding the new classification of periodontal diseases. Romanian Journal of Medical and Dental Education. 2019;**8**(3):1-6

[38] Glanz K, Bishop DB. The role of behavioral science theory in development and implementation of public health interventions. Annual Review of Public Health. 2010;**31**(1):399-418

[39] Lee C, Huang H, Sun T, Karimbux N. Impact of patient compliance on tooth loss during supportive periodontal therapy: A systematic review and meta-analysis. Journal of Dental Research. 2015;**94**(6):777-786

[40] Lin J-H, Huang Y-K, Lin K-D, Hsu Y-J, Huang W-F, Huang H-L. Randomized controlled trial on effects of a brief clinical-based intervention involving planning strategy on self-care behaviors in periodontal patients in dental practice. International Journal of Environmental Research and Public Health. 2019;**16**(20):3838

[41] Aquilanti L, Santarelli A, Mascitti M, Procaccini M, Rappelli G. Dental care access and the elderly: What is the role of teledentistry? A systematic review. International Journal of Environmental Research and Public Health. 2020;**17**(23):9053

[42] Fernández C, Maturana C, Coloma S, Carrasco-Labra A, Giacaman R. Teledentistry and mHealth for promotion and prevention of oral health: A systematic review and meta-analysis. Journal of Dental Research. [Internet]. 2021;**100**(9):914-927. Available from: https://journals.sagepub.com/doi/abs/10.1177/00220345211003828 [Accessed: July 19, 2025]

[43] Ferreira MC, Dias-Pereira A, Branco-de-Almeida L, Martins C, Paiva S. Impact of periodontal disease on quality of life: A systematic review. Journal of Periodontal Research. Wiley Online Library [Internet]. 2017;**52**(4):651-665. Available from: https://onlinelibrary.wiley.com/doi/abs/10.1111/jre.12436 [Accessed: July 19, 2025]

Chapter 5

Treatment of Peri-Implant Disease: Current Knowledge

Alexandre Perez and Tommaso Lombardi

Abstract

Peri-implant diseases represent serious complications after dental implant treatment, affecting both the surrounding soft and hard tissue. Regular, specific check-ups with the assessment and elimination of risk factors are effective precautions, and various conservative and surgical approaches are available for the treatment of peri-implant diseases. Early detection of clinical signs diseases and timely treatment are important for the success of dental implant treatment. Dentists must be familiar with the radiological and clinical characteristics of both conditions to make an accurate diagnosis and determine the appropriate treatment. The purpose of this chapter is to provide advice on the diagnosis and prevention of peri-implant disease for practitioners and to offer an overview of current knowledge on the treatment of peri-implant diseases.

Keywords: peri-implantitis, peri-implant mucositis, treatment, dental implants, periodontal disease

1. Introduction

Clinically, peri-implant mucositis is characterized by bleeding on gentle probing (<0.25 N), erythema, swelling, and/or suppuration [1–3]. As plaque is the primary etiological factor, effective treatment relies on mechanical plaque removal and ongoing plaque control, which can lead to significant improvement or complete resolution of the condition [4, 5]. The primary clinical endpoint in such interventions is the resolution of inflammation, typically assessed by the reduction or elimination of bleeding on probing, evaluated 2–3 months posttreatment [6, 7]. However, it is important to recognize that the development of peri-implant mucositis and its progression to peri-implantitis represent a pathological continuum. This dynamic may influence treatment outcomes and lesion responsiveness, particularly when distinguishing between short- and long-standing lesions [3].

Causative peri-implant mucositis treatment ideally comprises a combination of professionally administered mechanical or physical plaque removal and patient-administered plaque control [8, 9]. Professional nonsurgical treatment of peri-implant mucositis can be provided by dental hygienists, general dentists, and specialists [10]. While various treatment approaches are routinely employed in clinical practice, a universally accepted standard of care, apart from submarginal instrumentation, to treat peri-implant mucositis remains pending [2].

Professionally administered plaque removal (PAPR) aims to reduce soft tissue inflammation by removing inflammatory hard and soft deposits from the implant surface and/or superstructure [9]. Modalities and instruments that prevent damaging the smooth transmucosal components, potentially aggravating future plaque accumulation (e.g., implant collar, abutment), should be chosen [11]. Commonly used instruments and modalities include ultrasonic scalers with plastic or carbon fiber tips, air-polishing, plastic, carbon, or titanium curettes, rotating brushes, and lasers [12]. There is limited evidence to support or refute the effectiveness of repeated PAPR procedures in improving clinical parameters related to peri-implant mucositis [13]. Clinicians may also consider modifying the restorative contours, verifying the absence of excess cement, or motivating patients to cease smoking as part of the overall treatment strategy [10, 14, 15]. Furthermore, systematic reviews evidence low effectiveness of professional adjunctive photodynamic therapy, NaOCl, or chlorhexidine use as part of PAPR, while the administration of systemic antibiotics, whilst proving efficient, remains unjustifiable [10, 16, 17]. Although peri-implant mucositis is generally considered a reversible condition, complete resolution is rarely achieved across treatment modalities. Despite significant reductions in bleeding on probing and clinical signs of inflammation, residual signs of the disease frequently persist, highlighting a recurring limitation of current therapeutic approaches [4, 9, 18].

In addition to professional plaque removal, it is essential to implement and reinforce patient-administered plaque control (PAPC) routines [8]. The importance of PAPC has been illustrated within studies, demonstrating that peri-implant mucositis can be induced by oral hygiene routine suspension. In contrast, re-institution of oral hygiene has been shown to reverse disease after a period of >3 weeks [4, 19]. Individual routines comprise mechanical plaque removal using manual or powered toothbrushes, potentially in combination with oral irrigators or interdental brushes; chemical plaque control with adjunctive delivery of antimicrobials or probiotics, and triclosan-containing toothpaste. The application and combination of individual routines show great variability, without pronounced evidence to support a consensus for a single, specific standard of care, except for brushing [2, 8]. Some of the more recent reviews support the general additional benefit of adjuncts, comprising, for example, probiotics or oral irrigators as part of PAPC [18].

A recurring finding in peri-implant mucositis treatments is that complete disease resolution is unlikely to be achieved [2, 18]. This finding reinforces the importance of strict and periodic recall programs to ensure early detection and treatment to prevent disease progression [9, 18]. Patients may further benefit from individual oral hygiene instructions tailored to the individual patient profile and type of restoration to prevent plaque accumulation.

2. Treatment of peri-implantitis

The treatment of peri-implant pathologies remains a significant clinical challenge. While numerous studies have reported favorable outcomes, there is currently insufficient evidence to determine the most effective therapeutic modality or to define a universally accepted "gold standard" protocol [10, 20, 21]. Treatment approaches, techniques, and outcomes remain highly variable, reflecting the multifactorial and heterogeneous nature of peri-implantitis. This chapter aims to provide clinicians with a structured overview of current treatment strategies, modalities, and diagnostic criteria to support evidence-based decision-making.

2.1 General approach to peri-implantitis treatment

Despite distinct differences in treatment response, the treatment of peri-implantitis typically follows a stepwise approach, mirroring established protocols from periodontal therapy [22–24]. Initial causative, nonsurgical therapy aims at reducing the infection and peri-implant inflammation. This phase is—if indicated—followed by a corrective surgical therapy to reduce probing depths, restore tissue homeostasis, and improve access for maintenance. The third treatment phase consists of supportive Peri-Implant Therapy (SPIT). This phase represents the cornerstone of secondary prevention to ensure regular examination, professional hygiene, and reinforcement of oral hygiene routines to reduce the risk of disease recurrence (**Figure 1**) [10].

2.2 Phase I causative nonsurgical therapy

Initial-phase therapy mainly focuses on preserving the implant-supported restoration when clinically feasible. Its primary aim is to control infection and inflammation, manage potential risks, and ensure patient compliance before potentially escalating into more invasive interventions [22, 25, 26]. Initial nonsurgical therapy should also serve as an opportunity to identify, reassess, and manage existing and newly recognized risk factors. This includes correcting local contributing factors—such as removal of excess cement or modification of plaque-retentive prosthetic features—and reinforcing patient-related behavioral changes, including improved oral hygiene practices and support for smoking cessation. Additionally, systemic risk factors should be addressed, for example, by optimizing glycemic control in diabetic patients or initiating concurrent periodontal treatment in individuals with poorly controlled periodontitis [20, 22, 25–30].

The therapeutic principles of causative nonsurgical therapy are very similar to those applied during peri-implant mucositis treatment. Among available interventions, submucosal debridement using mechanical instrumentation—with or without adjunctive therapies—remains the most evidence-based approach.

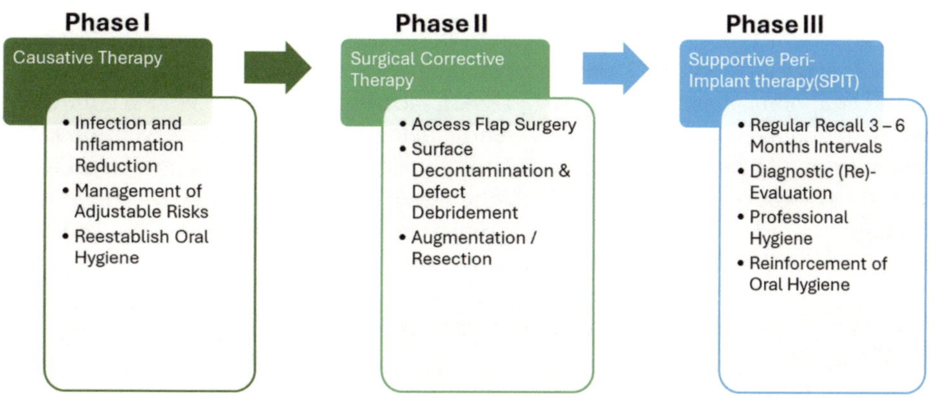

Figure 1.
Schematic overview of the stepwise treatment approach for peri-implantitis, comprising Phase I (causative therapy), Phase II (surgical corrective therapy), and Phase III (supportive peri-implant therapy, SPIT).

Adjuncts may include antiseptics, antibiotics, or laser applications, though current evidence suggests limited additional benefits compared to submarginal instrumentation alone [31]. Current treatment guidelines discourage the use of lasers [10]. While effective in biofilm disruption, air-polishing systems have been associated with a higher incidence of adverse effects, such as pain and subcutaneous emphysema, and should be used with caution [32–35]. Furthermore, the effect of adjunct systemic antibiotics has proven statistically significant and clinically meaningful, and may be carefully considered to improve treatment outcomes of nonsurgical therapy in severe cases [36, 37].

Clinical endpoints for nonsurgical peri-implantitis therapy should be assessed 6–12-weeks posttreatment and comprise the resolution of inflammation (absence of bleeding on probing and suppuration), the reduction in probing depths (ideally to ≤5 mm), improved plaque control and oral hygiene, and satisfactory cleanability of the prosthesis [20, 22, 25, 26]. While the complete resolution of the disease may not be achieved at this stage, stabilization of the condition, risk factor adjustment, and preparation for potential surgical intervention are key objectives of this treatment phase. In general, nonsurgical therapy may be effective in treating peri-implant mucositis and early-stage peri-implantitis while lacking efficiency in treating severe peri-implantitis [10, 24, 38–40].

2.3 Corrective surgical therapy

Refractory sites presenting with an increased probing depth of ≥5 mm, as well as persistent signs of inflammation, that is, BoP and suppuration, are indicated for corrective surgical therapy [10, 30]. This second phase of therapy comprises access flap surgery, potentially followed by reconstructive or resective procedures. Specifically, surgical therapy primarily aims to provide access to the implant surface to facilitate defect debridement, that is, removal of inflamed granulation tissue, as well as cleaning and decontaminating the implant surface from any bacterial deposits and calculus to achieve complete resolution of the inflammatory lesion [30]. Procedures may include tissue resection and/or augmentation of peri-implant osseous defects. They may vary based on the use of techniques and adjuncts for surface decontamination, the use of biomaterials, biologics, and their combination, and local or systemic adjunctive antibiotics and antimicrobials [10, 39] .

A reduction in probing depth to ≤5 mm and the absence of bleeding on probing (BoP) at 6 months post-surgery, along with the absence of progressive bone loss as assessed by radiographs at 12 months postoperatively, represent generally accepted clinical endpoints of surgical therapy [41, 42]. Notably, ensuring adequate compliance with oral hygiene procedures is essential before commencing intervention [24]. Clinicians should also be aware that, despite considerable improvement of clinical and radiographic parameters that may be achieved after surgical therapy, a considerably high rate (32–44%) of disease recurrence and a considerable rate (14–21%) of implant loss within 5 years posttreatment were reported [30, 41, 43, 44].

2.3.1 Anatomic factors affecting treatment outcomes: Peri-implantitis defect classifications

Attempts have been made to classify peri-implant osseous defects to describe disease severity and to estimate peri-implant-treatment effectiveness [44–46]. The most widely accepted peri-implant defect classifications differentiate between purely infraosseous (Class I), purely supracrestal, that is, horizontal (Class II), or combined defects, that is, presenting a horizontal and an infraosseous component (Class III). Furthermore, the infraosseous components are differentiated into buccal dehiscence (a-type), 2–3 defects (b-type), and circumferential saucer-shaped defects [47]. Finally, the defect depth extension below the implant neck, or the ratio of bone loss relative to the total length of the implant, may be used to differentiate between small (S) defects (3–4 mm), medium (M) (4–5 mm) to advanced (A) defect (≥ 6 mm) types (**Figure 2**).

Defect classification may help clinicians in guiding treatment decisions and estimating treatment prognosis. Small supracrestal Class II defects, for example, have shown to respond well to nonsurgical approaches or to access flap, resective surgery. Conversely, infraosseous Type Ic defects have responded better to guided bone regenerative approaches than buccal dehiscence defects (Class Ib) [46]. Advanced, i.e., > 7 mm deep defects, have been described as less responsive to surgical therapy (**Figure 3**) [48].

2.3.2 Peri-implant surface detoxification

Given the overwhelming evidence classifying peri-implantitis as a biofilm-associated disease, effective implant surface disinfection and complete decontamination appear crucial to achieving disease resolution [1, 20, 38, 49, 50]. Seminal studies have demonstrated that re-osseointegration and defect fill following regenerative approaches, even after implant surface decontamination, remain incomplete—highlighting the inherent challenge of achieving complete biofilm removal from contaminated implant surfaces [50–52]. Microroughened surface topographies, while established as the gold standard to promote osseointegration, may hinder effective decontamination further [53–55].

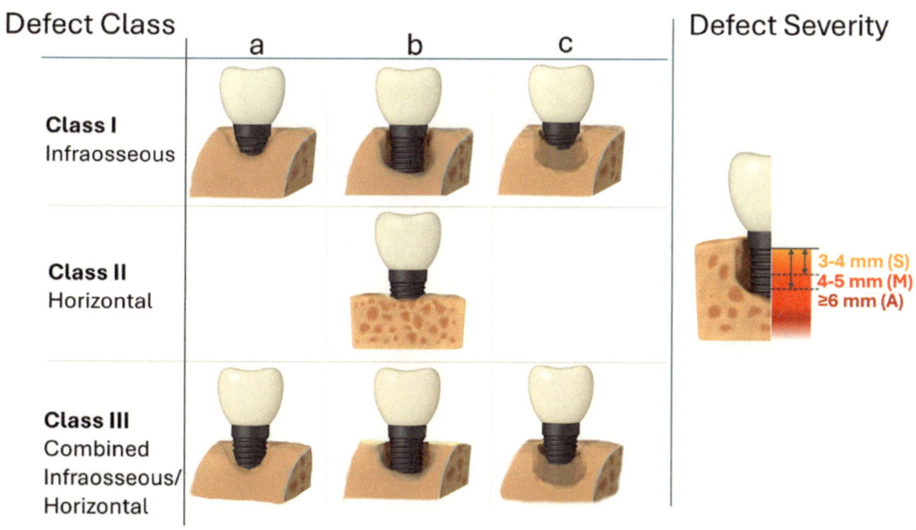

Figure 2.
Peri-implantitis defect type (left) and severity classification (right). Defect types are categorized by defect morphology: buccal dehiscence (a), 2–3-wall (b), and circumferential (contained) (c) defects and by the presence of infraosseous and/or supracrestal components (Class I–III). Defect severity is based on the vertical extension between the implant shoulder and the lesion's apex.

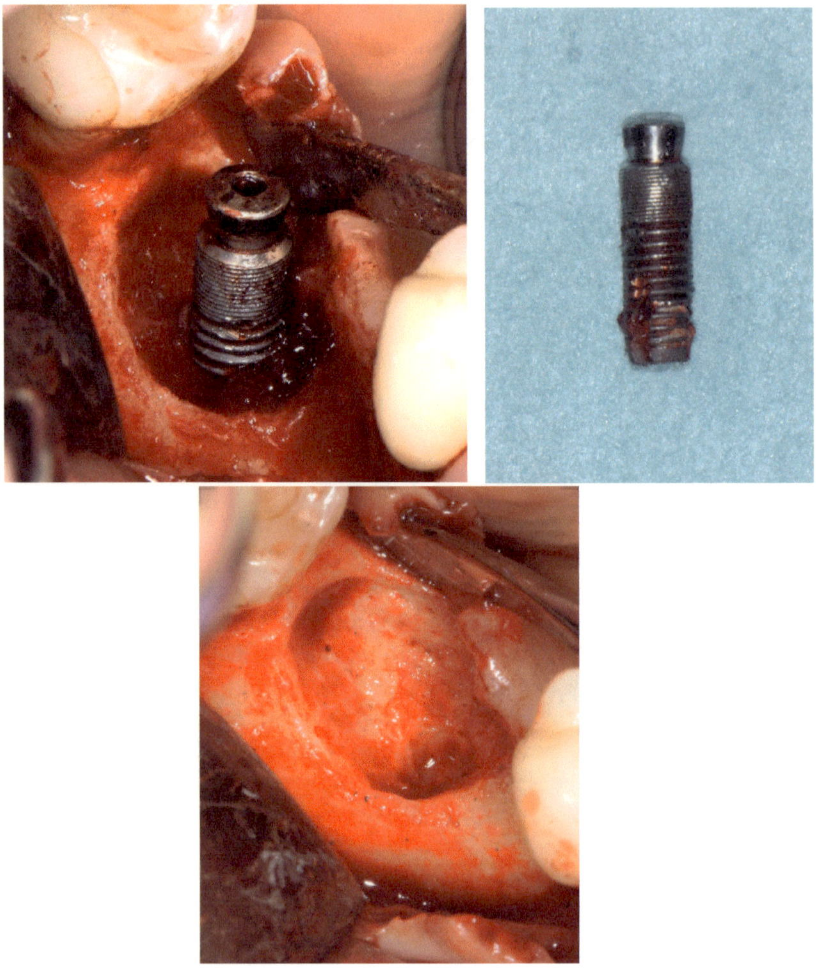

Figure 3.
Peri-implantitis defect type III (> 7 mm deep defects) and treatment (explantation).

A multitude of mechanical, chemical, and physical methods, with or without adjunctive local application of antiseptics or antibiotics, have been proposed [10, 39, 56, 57]. In contrast to nonsurgical approaches with limited access and visibility, open-flap mechanical instrumentation has been demonstrated as effective in removing plaque and calculus deposits [58]. Individual methods include scaling with metallic and nonmetallic scalers and rotating brushes or air powder abrasion. Implantoplasty using rotary instruments may be applied to remove the coronal implant threads and smooth the implant surfaces to prevent future plaque accumulation as part of apically repositioned flaps (APF) or guided bone regenerative (GBR) procedures [38, 59–61].

Residual biofilm following instrumentation has been described as common after mechanical debridement. The release of titanium particles remains a general concern [58, 62, 63]. Clinicians often complement mechanical methods with a second chemical or physical technique to improve surface decontamination [57, 58]. Physical methods include, for example, photodynamic therapy, laser-assisted techniques, or electrolytic methods. In contrast, chemical strategies may include rinsing with saline, application of hydrogen peroxide, ethylenediamine tetra acetate (EDTA) or local antibiotics or antiseptics, for example, tetracycline or chlorhexidine [57, 58, 64]. Despite considerable efforts to enhance implant surface decontamination as a prerequisite for re-osseointegration, evidence supporting the efficacy of individual techniques—or their combinations—in improving key clinical outcomes of surgical regenerative or resective approaches remains limited, except for modest support for the use of titanium brushes [39, 50, 57, 65, 66]. Notably, this finding may partly reflect the complex and heterogeneous nature of peri-implantitis, involving a broad spectrum of contributing factors, notably treatment site characteristics, implant design, defect morphology, and patient-specific risk profiles, including genetic predisposition (**Figure 4**) [3, 27, 67].

2.3.3 Regenerative peri-implantitis treatment

While some evidence supports using apically positioned flaps (APF) in combination with implantoplasty to restore peri-implant health, this approach may be unsuitable in esthetically sensitive areas [60, 61]. In such cases, regenerative surgical techniques are preferred to augment peri-implant lesions to support soft tissue contours [31, 68–70].

A wide range of biomaterials has been utilized to regenerate peri-implantitis defects across different healing modalities, including autologous bone, allografts, xenografts, and alloplasts, either alone or in combination with membranes and/or biologic or chemical agents [50, 68, 71]. High variability in outcome and high risk of bias have been reported throughout systematic reviews analyzing and comparing the effectiveness of regenerative procedures for peri-implantitis defects. This finding may be attributable to the complex and multifactorial nature of peri-implantitis, contributing to methodological heterogeneity, rendering it difficult to design low-bias, standardized comparative clinical trials [10, 31, 50, 68, 70]. There is currently no evidence suggesting that a specific material or

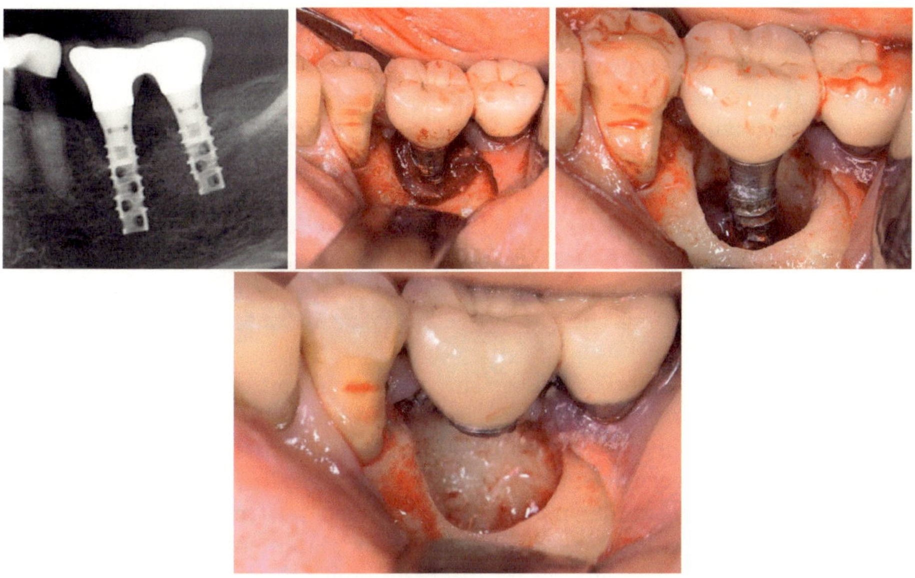

Figure 4.
Peri-implantitis at site 36, complex treatment: mechanical debridement, complex due to the hollow implant design, sectioning, and explantation of the implant.

material combination might be superior to others [50]. For example, there is no conclusion on the effectiveness of membranes in conjunction with bone grafts in augmenting peri-implantitis treatment. Experiments failed to show an increase in radiographic bone fill when using bone grafts with membranes compared to bone grafts alone [70, 72]. Also, there is currently no conclusion on the superiority of submerged vs. non-submerged healing as part of regenerative peri-implant therapy [68].

Compared to nonsurgical treatment, guided bone regeneration of peri-implantitis defects has been reported to result in 3.52 mm greater periodontal probing depth (PPD) reduction compared to nonsurgical therapy [31]. When comparing relative pocket depth (PD) reduction of individual approaches, values of 37.9% were reported for access flap and debridement, 33.4% for resective approach, 37.1% for augmenting with bone grafting materials, and 48.2% for GBR, suggesting marginal advantages of regenerative compared to non-regenerative approaches [70].

A mean PD reduction ranging from 2.0 to 4.5 mm and a mean reduction in BoP from 44.8 to 86% at 12 months post-therapy was recently reported for the regenerative peri-implant therapy using bone grafts [68, 69]. The mean radiographic bone fill was reported to be 2 mm [70]. Despite encouraging results superiority of regenerative therapy over access flap surgery without regenerative therapy in terms of clinical and esthetic outcomes needs to be established [10, 68, 69]. Finally, defect classification may affect treatment outcomes, with circumferential contained defects showing a better prognosis [46]. Regenerative techniques may be preferably adopted at intraosseous defects with a depth of ≥3 mm [68].

In conclusion, the mixed and often inconclusive outcomes of regenerative therapy compared to open-flap debridement alone underscore the current limitations of regenerative approaches and emphasize the need for individualized, clinically driven, and patient-centered treatment planning.

2.4 Implant removal and reimplantation

In cases where surgical peri-implant therapy is deemed ineffective or the prognosis is unfavorable, clinicians may consider implant removal and reimplantation as viable alternatives. The decision to remove an implant should be based on defect severity and overall treatment prognosis, considering both functional, esthetic, and patient-centered aspects.

Advanced peri-implantitis lesions affecting ≥50% of the implant length are relatively common, occurring in over 40% of cases, and have been associated with poor outcomes following surgical therapy [45, 73, 74]. After explantation, two primary strategies exist [1]: Immediate placement of a wider or longer implant when anatomical and prosthetic conditions allow, or [2] delayed placement following alveolar ridge augmentation and healing.

Immediate reimplantation has shown success rates of approximately 94%, with acceptable marginal bone loss (~0.9 mm) in selected cases [75]. However, in moderate to advanced defects involving ≥25% of the implant length, this approach carries a higher risk due to advanced alveolar bone loss and is generally not recommended. In such cases, bone grafting at the time of implant removal may be considered to preserve and restore ridge volume, with delayed implant placement typically planned for 3–6 months following augmentation [76]. Implant removal may also offer an opportunity to address additional site deficiencies, such as insufficient keratinized mucosa or compromised esthetic soft tissue contours [77–80]. In esthetically demanding regions, staged augmentation procedures and delayed implant placement, allowing for soft tissue conditioning, may be favored to achieve optimal esthetic outcomes. Systematic reviews report an implant survival rate of approximately 88% following delayed reimplantation over a mean follow-up of 40 months, with a ~ 15% reduction in survival rates observed in cases involving multiple reimplantation attempts [81].

From a procedural standpoint, the least invasive removal technique involves applying counter-clockwise torque with a removal tool compatible with the implant's internal or external connection [82, 83]. In selected cases, resectioning 1–2 mm of crestal cortical bone may facilitate explantation. Trephine burs and elevators remain effective but are more invasive alternatives, typically reserved for cases in which conservative approaches fail. Corticotomies may enhance healing potential, as bone at previously infected implant sites often exhibits reduced vascularity.

In summary, implant removal followed by reimplantation offers a viable alternative to regenerative or resective peri-implant therapy. Treatment strategies should be tailored to the individual case, considering defect morphology and severity, anatomical limitations, soft and hard tissue conditions, and esthetic demands following explantation (**Figure 5**).

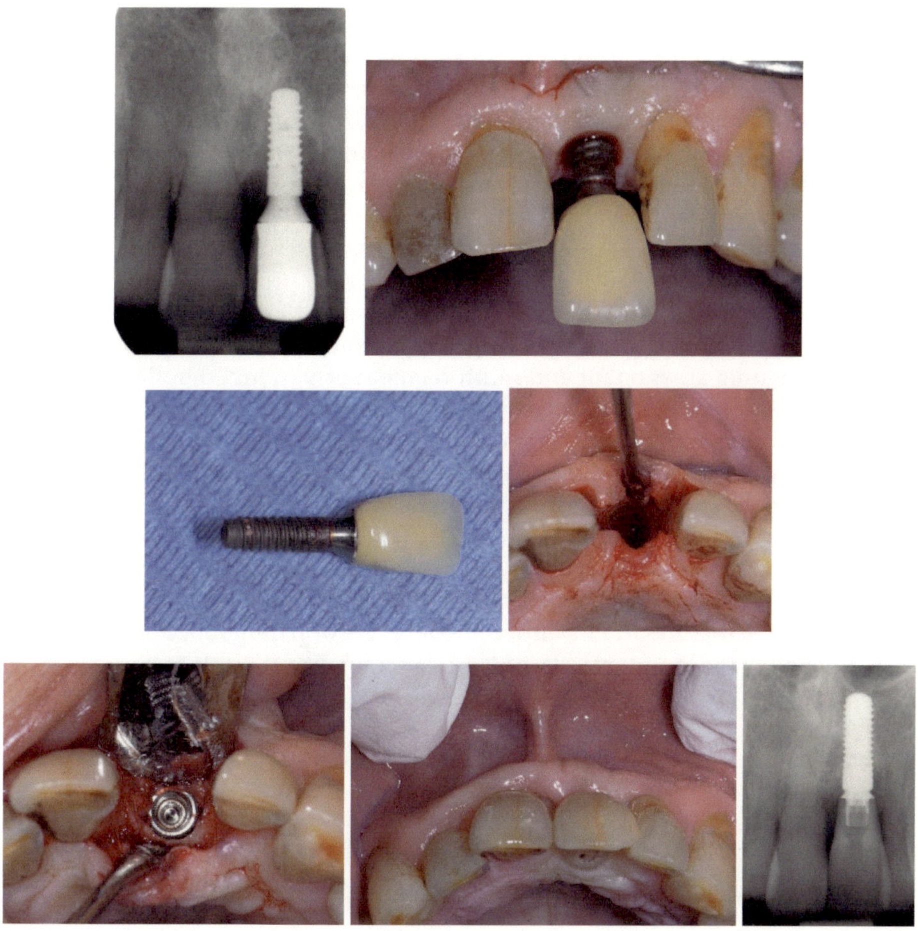

Figure 5.
Implant removal of unstable implant 21, mechanical debridement, reimplantation with simultaneous guide bone regeneration.

3. Prevention of peri-implantitis: Supportive peri-implant therapy

Due to the severity, rapid progression, and lack of consolidated treatment strategies, effective prevention of peri-implant diseases remains a cornerstone of implant therapy. Clinicians should recognize that prevention begins well before implant placement and extends throughout the lifetime of a prosthetic restoration [10, 38]. Prevention strategies target risk reduction at multiple levels—patient selection, treatment planning, surgical and prosthetic execution, and postoperative care. Once osseointegrated, supportive peri-implant care and therapy (SPIC, SPIT) play a critical role in maintaining peri-implant health. At the same time, secondary prevention aims at reducing the risk of disease recurrence after peri-implant treatment [10].

Primordial and primary prevention strategies aim to identify and manage modifiable risk factors and prevent risk factor development before and after implant placement, respectively [84]. Preventive measures include early patient risk profiling but also patient education on the importance of supportive peri-implant care (SPIC) recalls and oral health routines [85]. Furthermore, modifiable risk factors, comprising glycaemic control status, smoking but also the identification of parafunctional habits and bruxisms, are important at this stage [84]. From a treatment perspective, clinicians are advised to carefully plan and control ideal placement and deliver prosthetic designs that enable optimal hygiene routines and reduce the risk for plaque accumulation [86]. Finally, primordial prevention should also include the detection and treatment of any periodontal condition prior to implant placement [87].

SPIC and SPIT are regarded as crucial to prevent the onset or recurrence of peri-implant disease following successful implant integration and active or completed therapy, respectively [88–91]. Corresponding protocols should be individualized and regularly re-evaluated, with risk assessment tools available to guide patient-specific preventive strategies [92]. These protocols should include professional mechanical plaque removal at 3- to 6-month intervals, monitoring peri-implant health using gentle probing (0.2 N) and any signs of plaque accumulation, and ongoing assessment and reinforcement of patient compliance with oral hygiene instructions [10, 27, 28]. Early detection of peri-implant disease to enable timely intervention and prevent progression to peri-implantitis is a key objective of SPIC [2, 90]. Baseline periapical radiographs obtained after initial physiological bone remodeling serve as essential references for confirming disease presence and monitoring its progression over time [1].

Finally, secondary and tertiary prevention aim to reduce the risk of peri-implant disease recurrence and prevent complications in patients who have completed or are undergoing active treatment. Preventive measures are of paramount importance and remain integral to the long-term success and sustainability of implant therapy.

Author details

Alexandre Perez[1*] and Tommaso Lombardi[2]

1 Unit of Oral Surgery and Implantology, Division of Oral and Maxillofacial Surgery, Department of Surgery, Faculty of Medicine, University of Geneva and University Hospitals of Geneva, Geneva, Switzerland

2 Unit of Oral Medicine and Oral Maxillofacial Pathology, Division of Oral and Maxillofacial Surgery, Department of Surgery, Faculty of Medicine, University of Geneva & Geneva University Hospitals, Geneva, Switzerland

*Address all correspondence to: alexandre.perez@hug.ch

References

[1] Lang NP, Berglundh T. On behalf of working group 4 of the seventh European workshop on periodontology. Periimplant diseases: Where are we now? – Consensus of the seventh European workshop on periodontology. Journal of Clinical Periodontology. 2011;**38**:178-181

[2] Jepsen S, Berglundh T, Genco R, Aass AM, Demirel K, Derks J, et al. Primary prevention of peri-implantitis: Managing peri-implant mucositis. Journal of Clinical Periodontology. 2015;**42**(Suppl 16):S152-S157

[3] Heitz-Mayfield LJA, Salvi GE. Peri-implant mucositis. Journal of Clinical Periodontology. 2018;**45**:S237-S245

[4] Salvi GE, Aglietta M, Eick S, Sculean A, Lang NP, Ramseier CA. Reversibility of experimental peri-implant mucositis compared with experimental gingivitis in humans. Clinical Oral Implants Research. 2012;**23**:182-190

[5] Pontoriero R, Tonelli MP, Carnevale G, Mombelli A, Nyman SR, Lang NP. Experimentally induced peri-implant mucositis. A clinical study in humans. Clinical Oral Implants Research. 1994;**5**:254-259

[6] Monje A, Amerio E, Farina R, Nart J, Ramanauskaite A, Renvert S, et al. Significance of probing for monitoring peri-implant diseases. International Journal of Oral Implantology. 2021;**14**:385-399

[7] Sanz M, Chapple IL. On behalf of working group 4 of the VIII European workshop on periodontology. Clinical research on peri-implant diseases: Consensus report of working group 4. Journal of Clinical Periodontology. 2012;**39**:202-206

[8] Salvi GE, Ramseier CA. Efficacy of patient-administered mechanical and/or chemical plaque control protocols in the management of peri-implant mucositis. A systematic review. Journal of Clinical Periodontology. 2015;**42**(Suppl 16):S187-S201

[9] Schwarz F, Becker K, Sager M. Efficacy of professionally administered plaque removal with or without adjunctive measuresfor the treatment of peri-implant mucositis. A systematic review and meta-analysis. Journal of Clinical Periodontology. Apr 2015;**42**(Suppl. 16):S202-S213. DOI: 10.1111/ jcpe.12349

[10] Herrera D, Berglundh T, Schwarz F, Chapple I, Jepsen S, Sculean A, et al. The EFP workshop participants and methodological consultant. Prevention and treatment of peri-implant diseases—The EFP S3 level clinical practice guideline. Journal of Clinical Periodontology. 2023;**50**:4-76

[11] Yen Nee W, Raja Awang RA, Hassan A. Effects on the titanium implant surface by different hygiene instrumentations: A narrative review. Cureus. 30 Oct 2022;**14**(10):e30884. DOI: 10.7759/cureus.30884

[12] Verket A, Koldsland OC, Bunæs D, Lie SA, Romandini M. Non-surgical therapy of peri-implant mucositis—Mechanical/physical approaches: A systematic review. Journal of Clinical Periodontology. 2023;**50**:135-145

[13] Riben-Grundstrom C, Norderyd O, André U, Renvert S. Treatment of peri-implant mucositis using a glycine powder air-polishing or ultrasonic device: A randomized clinical trial. Journal of Clinical Periodontology. 2015;**42**:462-469

[14] de Tapia B, Bonnin M, Valles C, Mozas C, Herrera D, Sanz M, et al. Clinical outcomes and associated factors in the treatment of peri-implant mucositis, combining mechanical debridement and prosthesis modification: A 30-month follow-up prospective case series. Journal of Clinical Periodontology. 2022;**49**:1357-1365

[15] Heitz-Mayfield LJA, Salvi GE, Botticelli D, Mombelli A, Faddy M, Lang NP. On behalf of the implant complication research group (ICRG). Anti-infective treatment of peri-implant mucositis: A randomised controlled clinical trial: Treatment of peri-implant mucositis. Clinical Oral Implants Research. 2011;**22**:237-241

[16] Dommisch H, Hoedke D, Valles C, Vilarrasa J, Jepsen S, Pascual La Rocca A. Efficacy of professionally administered chemical agents as an adjunctive treatment to sub-marginal instrumentation during the therapy of peri-implant mucositis. Journal of Clinical Periodontology. 2023;**50**:146-160

[17] Hallström H, Persson GR, Lindgren S, Olofsson M, Renvert S. Systemic antibiotics and debridement of peri-implant mucositis. A randomized clinical trial. Journal of Clinical Periodontology. 2012;**39**:574-581

[18] Gennai S, Bollain J, Ambrosio N, Marruganti C, Graziani F, Figuero E. Efficacy of adjunctive measures in peri-implant mucositis. A systematic review and meta-analysis. Journal of Clinical Periodontology. 2023;**50**(Suppl 26):161-187

[19] Schierano G, Pejrone G, Brusco P, Trombetta A, Martinasso G, Preti G, et al. TNF- α TGF- β 2 and IL-1 β levels in gingival and peri-implant crevicular fluid before and after de novo plaque accumulation. Journal of Clinical Periodontology. 2008;**35**:532-538

[20] Schwarz F, Derks J, Monje A, Wang H-L. Peri-implantitis. Journal of Periodontology. 2018;**89**(Suppl 1): S267-S290

[21] Papathanasiou E, Finkelman M, Hanley J, Parashis AO. Prevalence, etiology and treatment of Peri-implant Mucositis and Peri-Implantitis: A survey of periodontists in the United States. Journal of Periodontology. 2016;**87**:493-501

[22] Cosgarea R, Gasparik C, Dudea D, Culic B, Dannewitz B, Sculean A. Peri-implant soft tissue colour around titanium and zirconia abutments: A prospective randomized controlled clinical study. Clinical Oral Implants Research. 2015;**26**:537-544

[23] Newman M, Takei H. Newman and Carranza's Clinical Periodontology. 13th ed. Philadelphia: Elsevier; 2019

[24] Sanz M, Herrera D, Kebschull M, Chapple I, Jepsen S, Beglundh T, et al. EFP workshop participants and methodological consultants. Treatment of stage I-III periodontitis-the EFP S3 level clinical practice guideline. Journal of Clinical Periodontology. 2020;**47**(Suppl 22):4-60

[25] de Waal YCM, Winning L, Stavropoulos A, Polyzois I. Efficacy of chemical approaches for implant surface decontamination in conjunction with sub-marginal instrumentation, in the non-surgical treatment of peri-implantitis: A systematic review. Journal of Clinical Periodontology. 2023;**50**:212-223

[26] Liñares A, Sanz-Sánchez I, Dopico J, Molina A, Blanco J, Montero E. Efficacy of adjunctive measures in the non-surgical treatment of peri-implantitis:

A systematic review. Journal of Clinical Periodontology. 2023;**50**:224-243

[27] Berglundh T, Armitage G, Araujo MG, Avila-Ortiz G, Blanco J, Camargo PM, et al. Peri-implant diseases and conditions: Consensus report of workgroup 4 of the 2017 world workshop on the classification of periodontal and Peri-implant diseases and conditions. Journal of Periodontology. 2018;**89**:S313-S318

[28] Serino G, Ström C. Peri-implantitis in partially edentulous patients: Association with inadequate plaque control. Clinical Oral Implants Research. 2009;**20**:169-174

[29] Tormena M, Matarazzo F, De Oliveira BM, Pereira O, Previdelli I, Araújo MG. The effect of inadequate access to peri-implant hygiene on marginal bone level. A 4-year cohort prospective study. Clinical Oral Implants Research. 2020;**31**:836-845

[30] Karlsson K, Trullenque-Eriksson A, Tomasi C, Derks J. Efficacy of access flap and pocket elimination procedures in the management of peri-implantitis: A systematic review and meta-analysis. Journal of Clinical Periodontology. 2023;**50**:244-284

[31] Faggion CM, Listl S, Frühauf N, Chang H-J, Tu Y-K. A systematic review and Bayesian network meta-analysis of randomized clinical trials on non-surgical treatments for peri-implantitis. Journal of Clinical Periodontology. 2014;**41**:1015-1025

[32] Alonso V, García-Caballero L, Couto I, Diniz M, Diz P, Limeres J. Subcutaneous emphysema related to air-powder tooth polishing: A report of three cases. Australian Dental Journal. 2017;**62**:510-515

[33] Bassetti M, Bassetti R, Sculean A, Salvi GE. Subkutanes Emphysem nach nicht chirurgischer Periimplantitistherapie nach der Anwendung einer Air-Flow-Einheit: Ein Fallbericht. The Swiss Dental Journal SSO. 2014;**124**:807-817

[34] Bruckmann C, Bruckmann L, Gahleitner A, Stavropoulos A, Bertl K. Pneumocephalus as result of nonsurgical peri-implantitis treatment with an air-polishing device for submucosal debridement—A case report. Clinical and Experimental Dental Research. 2022;**8**:632-639

[35] Merli M, Bernardelli F, Giulianelli E, Carinci F, Mariotti G, Merli M, et al. Short-term comparison of two non-surgical treatment modalities of peri-implantitis: Clinical and microbiological outcomes in a two-factorial randomized controlled trial. Journal of Clinical Periodontology. 2020;**47**:1268-1280

[36] Shibli JA, Ferrari DS, Siroma RS, Figueiredo LCD, Faveri MD, Feres M. Microbiological and clinical effects of adjunctive systemic metronidazole and amoxicillin in the non-surgical treatment of peri-implantitis: 1 year follow-up. Brazilian Oral Research. 30 Sep 2019;**33**(Suppl. 1):e080. DOI: 10.1590/1807-3107bor-2019.vol33.0080

[37] Blanco C, Pico A, Dopico J, Gándara P, Blanco J, Liñares A. Adjunctive benefits of systemic metronidazole on non-surgical treatment of peri-implantitis. A randomized placebo-controlled clinical trial. Journal of Clinical Periodontology. 2022;**49**:15-27

[38] Scarano A, Khater AGA, Gehrke SA, Serra P, Francesco I, Di Carmine M, et al. Current status of Peri-implant diseases: A clinical review for evidence-based decision making. JFB. 2023;**14**:210

[39] Cosgarea R, Roccuzzo A, Jepsen K, Sculean A, Jepsen S, Salvi GE. Efficacy

of mechanical/physical approaches for implant surface decontamination in non-surgical submarginal instrumentation of peri-implantitis. A systematic review. Journal of Clinical Periodontology. 2023;**50**:188-211

[40] Romandini M, Laforí A, Pedrinaci I, Baima G, Ferrarotti F, Lima C, et al. Effect of sub-marginal instrumentation before surgical treatment of peri-implantitis: A multi-Centre randomized clinical trial. Journal of Clinical Periodontology. 2022;**49**:1334-1345

[41] Carcuac O, Abrahamsson I, Derks J, Petzold M, Berglundh T. Spontaneous progression of experimental peri-implantitis in augmented and pristine bone: A pre-clinical in vivo study. Clinical Oral Implants Research. 2020;**31**:192-200

[42] Karlsson K, Derks J, Håkansson J, Wennström JL, Petzold M, Berglundh T. Interventions for peri-implantitis and their effects on further bone loss: A retrospective analysis of a registry-based cohort. Journal of Clinical Periodontology. 2019;**46**:872-879

[43] Heitz-Mayfield LJA, Salvi GE, Mombelli A, Loup P-J, Heitz F, Kruger E, et al. Supportive peri-implant therapy following anti-infective surgical peri-implantitis treatment: 5-year survival and success. Clinical Oral Implants Research. 2018;**29**:1-6

[44] Schwarz F, Herten M, Sager M, Bieling K, Sculean A, Becker J. Comparison of naturally occurring and ligature-induced peri-implantitis bone defects in humans and dogs. Clinical Oral Implants Research. 2007;**18**:161-170

[45] Monje A, Pons R, Insua A, Nart J, Wang H, Schwarz F. Morphology and severity of peri-implantitis bone defects. Clinical Implant Dentistry and Related Research. Aug 2019;**21**(4):635-643. cid.12791

[46] Schwarz F, Sahm N, Schwarz K, Becker J. Impact of defect configuration on the clinical outcome following surgical regenerative therapy of peri-implantitis. Journal of Clinical Periodontology. 2010;**37**:449-455

[47] Mordini L, Sun N, Chang N, De Guzman J-P, Generali L, Consolo U. Peri-Implantitis regenerative therapy: A review. Biology. 2021;**10**:773

[48] Serino G, Turri A. Outcome of surgical treatment of peri-implantitis: Results from a 2-year prospective clinical study in humans: Outcome of surgical treatment of peri-implantitis. Clinical Oral Implants Research. 2011;**22**:1214-1220

[49] Berglundh T, Wennström JL, Lindhe J. Long-term outcome of surgical treatment of peri-implantitis. A 2-11-year retrospective study. Clinical Oral Implants Research. 2018;**29**:404-410

[50] Renvert S, Polyzois I, Maguire R. Re-osseointegration on previously contaminated surfaces: A systematic review. Clinical Oral Implants Research. 2009;**20**:216-227

[51] Persson LG, Araújo MG, Berglundh T, Gröndahl K, Lindhe J. Resolution of peri-implantitis following treatment. An experimental study in the dog. Clinical Oral Implants Research. 1999;**10**:195-203

[52] Persson LG, Ericsson I, Berglundh T, Lindhe J. Osseintegration following treatment of peri-implantitis and replacement of implant components: An experimental study in the dog. Journal of Clinical Periodontology. 2001;**28**:258-263

[53] Ichioka Y, Virto L, Nuevo P, Gamonal JD, Derks J, Larsson L, et al. Decontamination of biofilm-contaminated implant surfaces: An in

vitro evaluation. Clinical Oral Implants Research. 2023;**34**:1058-1072

[54] Teughels W, Van Assche N, Sliepen I, Quirynen M. Effect of material characteristics and/or surface topography on biofilm development. Clinical Oral Implants Research. 2006;**17**:68-81

[55] Bosshardt DD, Chappuis V, Buser D. Osseointegration of titanium, titanium alloy and zirconia dental implants: Current knowledge and open questions. Periodontology 2000. 2000;**2017**(73):22-40

[56] Roccuzzo A, De Ry SP, Sculean A, Roccuzzo M, Salvi GE. Current approaches for the non-surgical Management of Peri-implant Diseases. Current Oral Health Reports. 2020;**7**:274-282

[57] Valderrama P, Wilson TG Jr. Detoxification of implant surfaces affected by Peri-implant disease: An overview of surgical methods. International Journal of Dentistry. 2013;**2013**:1-9

[58] Monje A, Amerio E, Cha JK, Kotsakis G, Pons R, Renvert S, et al. Strategies for implant surface decontamination in peri-implantitis therapy. International Journal of Oral Implantology. 2022;**15**:257-265

[59] Baima G, Citterio F, Romandini M, Romano F, Mariani GM, Buduneli N, et al. Surface decontamination protocols for surgical treatment of peri-implantitis: A systematic review with meta-analysis. Clinical Oral Implants Research. 2022;**33**:1069-1086

[60] Esteves Lima RP, Abreu LG, Belém FV, Pereira GHDM, Brant RA, Costa FO. Is Implantoplasty efficacious at treating Peri-Implantitis? A systematic review and meta-analysis. Journal of Oral and Maxillofacial Surgery. 2021;**79**:2270-2279

[61] Romeo E, Lops D, Chiapasco M, Ghisolfi M, Vogel G. Therapy of peri-implantitis with resective surgery. A 3-year clinical trial on rough screw-shaped oral implants. Part II: Radiographic outcome. Clinical Oral Implants Research. 2007;**18**:179-187

[62] Sahrmann P, Ronay V, Hofer D, Attin T, Jung RE, Schmidlin PR. In vitro cleaning potential of three different implant debridement methods. Clinical Oral Implants Research. 2015;**26**:314-319

[63] Asa'ad F, Thomsen P, Kunrath MF. The role of titanium particles and ions in the pathogenesis of Peri-Implantitis. Journal of Bone Metabolism. 2022;**29**:145-154

[64] Schlee M, Naili L, Rathe F, Brodbeck U, Zipprich H. Is complete Re-Osseointegration of an infected dental implant possible? Histologic results of a dog study: A short communication. JCM. 2020;**9**:235

[65] Ramanauskaite A, Fretwurst T, Schwarz F. Efficacy of alternative or adjunctive measures to conventional non-surgical and surgical treatment of peri-implant mucositis and peri-implantitis: A systematic review and meta-analysis. International Journal of Implant Dentistry. 2021;**7**:112

[66] Ramanauskaite A, Schwarz F, Cafferata EA, Sahrmann P. Photo/mechanical and physical implant surface decontamination approaches in conjunction with surgical peri-implantitis treatment: A systematic review. Journal of Clinical Periodontology. 2023;**50**:317-335

[67] Derks J, Tomasi C. Peri-implant health and disease. A systematic

review of current epidemiology. Journal of Clinical Periodontology. 2015;**42**:S158-S171

[68] Donos N, Calciolari E, Ghuman M, Baccini M, Sousa V, Nibali L. The efficacy of bone reconstructive therapies in the management of peri-implantitis. A systematic review and meta-analysis. Journal of Clinical Periodontology. 2023;**50**:285-316

[69] Tomasi C, Regidor E, Ortiz-Vigón A, Derks J. Efficacy of reconstructive surgical therapy at peri-implantitis-related bone defects. A systematic review and meta-analysis. Journal of Clinical Periodontology. 2019;**46**:340-356

[70] Chan H, Lin G, Suarez F, MacEachern M, Wang H. Surgical Management of Peri-Implantitis: A systematic review and meta-analysis of treatment outcomes. Journal of Periodontology. 2014;**85**:1027-1041

[71] Mercado F, Hamlet S, Ivanovski S. Regenerative surgical therapy for peri-implantitis using deproteinized bovine bone mineral with 10% collagen, enamel matrix derivative and doxycycline-a prospective 3-year cohort study. Clinical Oral Implants Research. 2018;**29**:583-591

[72] Roos-Jansåker A-M, Persson GR, Lindahl C, Renvert S. Surgical treatment of peri-implantitis using a bone substitute with or without a resorbable membrane: A 5-year follow-up. Journal of Clinical Periodontology. 2014;**41**:1108-1114

[73] Monje A, Alcoforado G, Padial-Molina M, Suarez F, Lin G, Wang H. Generalized aggressive periodontitis as a risk factor for dental implant failure: A systematic review and meta-analysis. Journal of Periodontology. 2014;**85**:1398-1407

[74] Ravidà A, Siqueira R, Saleh I, Saleh MHA, Giannobile A, Wang HL. Lack of clinical benefit of Implantoplasty to improve implant survival rate. Journal of Dental Research. 2020;**99**:1348-1355

[75] Anitua E, Piñas L, Begoña L, Alkhraisat MH. Prognosis of dental implants immediately placed in sockets affected by Peri-implantitis: A retrospective pilot study. The International Journal of Periodontics & Restorative Dentistry. 2017;**37**:713-719

[76] Pons R, Carreño M, Amerio E, Gargallo-Albiol J, Nart J, Monje A. Hard tissue dimensional changes following implant removal due to peri-implantitis: A retrospective study. Clinical Implant Dentistry and Related Research. 2021;**23**:432-443

[77] Monje A, Blasi G. Significance of keratinized mucosa/gingiva on peri-implant and adjacent periodontal conditions in erratic maintenance compliers. Journal of Periodontology. 2019;**90**:445-453

[78] Ueno D, Nagano T, Watanabe T, Shirakawa S, Yashima A, Gomi K. Effect of the keratinized mucosa width on the health status of Periimplant and contralateral periodontal tissues: A cross-sectional study. Implant Dentistry. 2016;**25**:796-801

[79] Perussolo J, Souza AB, Matarazzo F, Oliveira RP, Araújo MG. Influence of the keratinized mucosa on the stability of peri-implant tissues and brushing discomfort: A 4-year follow-up study. Clinical Oral Implants Research. 2018;**29**:1177-1185

[80] Mahardawi B, Jiaranuchart S, Damrongsirirat N, Arunjaroensuk S, Mattheos N, Somboonsavatdee A, et al. The lack of keratinized mucosa as a risk

factor for peri-implantitis: A systematic review and meta-analysis. Scientific Reports. 2023;**13**:3778

[81] Oh S-L, Shiau HJ, Reynolds MA. Survival of dental implants at sites after implant failure: A systematic review. The Journal of Prosthetic Dentistry. 2020;**123**:54-60

[82] Monje A, Nart J. Management and sequelae of dental implant removal. Periodontology. 2000;**2022**(88):182-200

[83] Masaki C, Kondo Y, Tomoeda K, Nodai T, Munemasa T, Mukaibo T, et al. Treatment strategies for dental implant removal: A literature review. Japanese Dental Science Review. 2024;**60**:120-127

[84] Carra MC, Blanc-Sylvestre N, Courtet A, Bouchard P. Primordial and primary prevention of peri-implant diseases: A systematic review and meta-analysis. Journal of Clinical Periodontology. 2023;**50**:77-112

[85] Cortellini S, Favril C, De Nutte M, Teughels W, Quirynen M. Patient compliance as a risk factor for the outcome of implant treatment. Periodontology. 2000;**2019**(81):209-225

[86] Katafuchi M, Weinstein BF, Leroux BG, Chen Y, Daubert DM. Restoration contour is a risk indicator for peri-implantitis: A cross-sectional radiographic analysis. Journal of Clinical Periodontology. 2018;**45**:225-232

[87] Aguirre-Zorzano LA, Estefanía-Fresco R, Telletxea O, Bravo M. Prevalence of peri-implant inflammatory disease in patients with a history of periodontal disease who receive supportive periodontal therapy. Clinical Oral Implants Research. 2015;**26**:1338-1344

[88] Roccuzzo M, Layton DM, Roccuzzo A, Heitz-Mayfield LJ. Clinical outcomes of peri-implantitis treatment and supportive care: A systematic review. Clinical Oral Implants Research. 2018;**29**:331-350

[89] Rokn A, Aslroosta H, Akbari S, Najafi H, Zayeri F, Hashemi K. Prevalence of peri-implantitis in patients not participating in well-designed supportive periodontal treatments: A cross-sectional study. Clinical Oral Implants Research. 2017;**28**:314-319

[90] Costa FO, Takenaka-Martinez S, Cota LOM, Ferreira SD, Silva GLM, Costa JE. Peri-implant disease in subjects with and without preventive maintenance: A 5-year follow-up. Journal of Clinical Periodontology. 2012;**39**:173-181

[91] Monje A, Wang H-L, Nart J. Association of Preventive Maintenance Therapy Compliance and Peri-Implant Diseases: A cross-sectional study. Journal of Periodontology. 2017;**88**:1030-1041

[92] Heitz-Mayfield LJA, Heitz F, Lang NP. Implant disease risk assessment IDRA–a tool for preventing peri-implant disease. Clinical Oral Implants Research. 2020;**31**:397-403

Section 2

State of the Art

Chapter 6

The Immunobiological and Dense Collagen Fibrous Connective Tissue Barriers: The Gate to Periodontal and Peri-Implant Health and Longevity

Itzhak Binderman, Michal Halperin-Sternfeld and Alberto Miselli

Abstract

Periodontal disease is the primary cause of alveolar bone loss and tooth loss, with pathogenesis rooted in microbial invasion and immune dysregulation. Despite advances in periodontal therapy and implantology, peri-implantitis has emerged as a significant clinical challenge due to the absence of natural protective barriers around implants. This chapter explores the structural and immunobiological roles of two key periodontal defense systems: the supracrestal gingival tissue (SGT) and the periodontal organ (PO). The PO's fibrous barrier, comprising collagen fibers and mechanically strained fibroblasts, is critical for maintaining periodontal health. Its degradation, mediated mainly by matrix metalloproteinases (MMPs), leads to compromised mechanical integrity, dysfunction of fibroblasts, adenosine triphosphate (ATP) release, and inflammatory bone resorption. In contrast, peri-implant tissues lack this organized fibrous attachment, relying instead on a vulnerable epithelial interface, making them highly susceptible to peri-implantitis. We describe novel strategies to mimic the fibrous attachment of natural dentition by bioengineering periosteal integration onto implant abutments. Additionally, we highlight emerging therapeutic approaches, including MMP inhibition and purinergic receptor blockade, to preserve soft tissue barriers and prevent bone loss. Overall, maintaining the structural and mechanobiological integrity of SGT and PO is essential for both periodontal and peri-implant health. Future therapies must target both the microbial and molecular pathways that compromise these barriers.

Keywords: immunobiological supracrestal barrier, collagen supraalveolar barrier, periosteum, periodontal organ, matrix metalloproteinases

1. Introduction

Periodontal disease remains the leading cause of alveolar bone loss and the subsequent loss of natural dentition. Although it is well established that the disease is initiated by pathogenic bacteria colonizing the gingival crevices, current therapeutic and preventive strategies, while capable of slowing disease progression, are largely unable to halt or reverse the condition entirely. Replacement of extracted teeth by placing dental implants that enable esthetic and functional prosthetic restoration has become the state of the art in dentistry. Recently, it became apparent that peri-implant bone loss dramatically endangers prosthetic restorations, albeit it has become a major prognostic problem. This condition, known as peri-implantitis, is characterized by a chronic inflammatory response triggered either by bacterial invasion or a foreign body reaction that incites an immunoinflammatory cell population, ultimately leading to progressive bone loss around the implant.

In this chapter, we focus on two critical defense structures in the periodontium: the immunobiological barrier of the supracrestal gingival tissue (SGT) and the fibrous barrier of the periodontal organ (PO). While the PO dense fibrous barrier is created in tooth development, the SGT, composed of supracrestal soft connective tissue and epithelial attachment, is established as the tooth erupts. Both form the initial line of defense against microbial biofilms. Dental implants, however, lack the PO; therefore, their defense depends solely on the SGT.

We emphasize the pivotal role of matrix metalloproteinases (MMPs), whose elevated enzymatic activity degrades the fibrous PO barrier and acts as a key driver of alveolar bone loss. Disruption of this barrier leads to a loss of physiological tensile strain, which in turn diminishes mechanical stimulation of fibroblasts aligned along collagen fibers. These fibroblasts respond by releasing ATP, a signal implicated in the pathogenesis of both alveolar and peri-implant bone resorption. Given the absence of a natural fibrous barrier in peri-implant soft tissues, we have developed a novel abutment design that supports the biological attachment of the periosteum to its surface. This innovation facilitates the formation of a fibrous barrier, where collagen fibers and mechanically strained fibroblasts replicate the protective architecture found in natural dentition.

2. Establishment of the periodontal organ (PO)

Tooth development in humans begins around the fifth week of gestation as epithelial thickenings in the oral cavity, known as the dental lamina. These thickenings result from the ingrowth of oral ectoderm into the underlying neural crest-derived ectomesenchyme. Development proceeds through a sequence of epithelial-mesenchymal interactions that culminate in the formation of the tooth germ and supporting periodontium structures. Tooth buds develop from the dental lamina and are embedded within the jawbone, surrounded by mesenchymal progenitor cells that give rise to cementum, periodontal ligament (PDL), and alveolar bone. During root development, and even before tooth eruption, bundles of collagen and elastin fibers extend from the alveolar bone crest's periosteum to insert into the cervical cementum, forming a dense fibrous barrier that determines and regulates the PO function and stability (**Figure 1**). This fibrous network is overlaid by a syncytium of fibroblasts and immune cells, connected *via* adherens junctions, and subjected to continuous physiological tensile strain, termed "isometric tensile prestress" by Ingber [1].

The periosteum has a dual function: an inner osteogenic layer adjacent to the alveolar bone and an outer fibrous layer that interfaces with the SGT (**Figure 1**). Also, transseptal fibers connect the cementum of neighboring teeth, maintaining the integrity of the dental arch. These components form a physical and immunological barrier

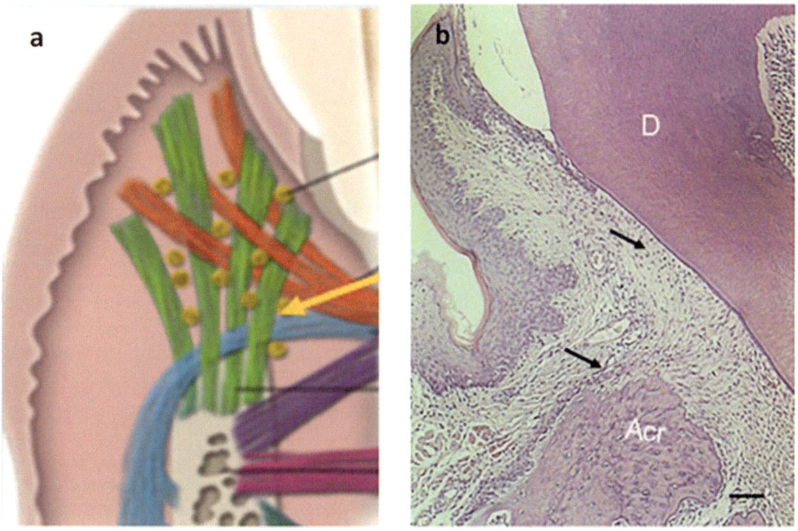

Figure 1.
A schematic illustration of collagen bundles inserted into the cementum (a) and a corresponding histological section showing the fibers and the strained cells along their course (b). In (a), the blue band represents the periosteum extending over the alveolar bone crest and papilla, forming the PO barrier as it inserts into the root cementum, features also visible in the histological section (b).

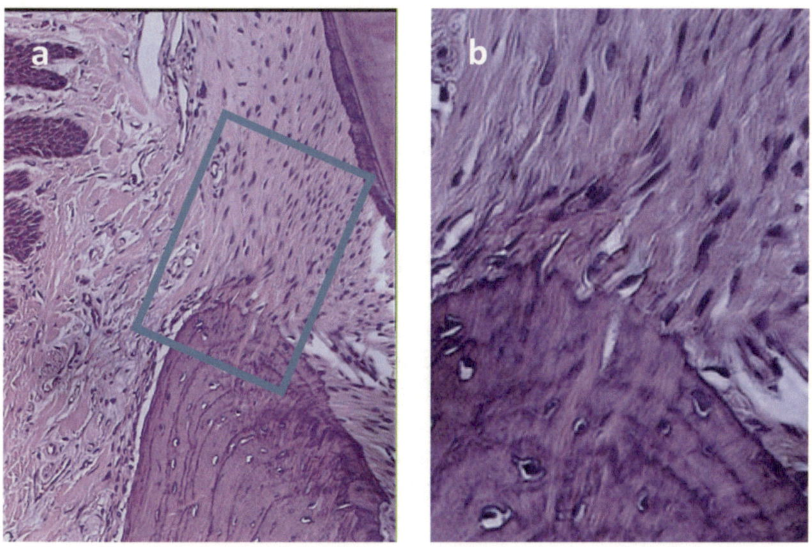

Figure 2.
Histological section of the rat molar periodontium showing Sharpey's collagen fibers emerging from the crest of the alveolar bone and extending toward the cervical root cementum (a). The boxed area in (a) is enlarged in (b), illustrating the Sharpey fibers and associated elongated fibroblasts aligned in the direction of fiber insertion into the cementum.

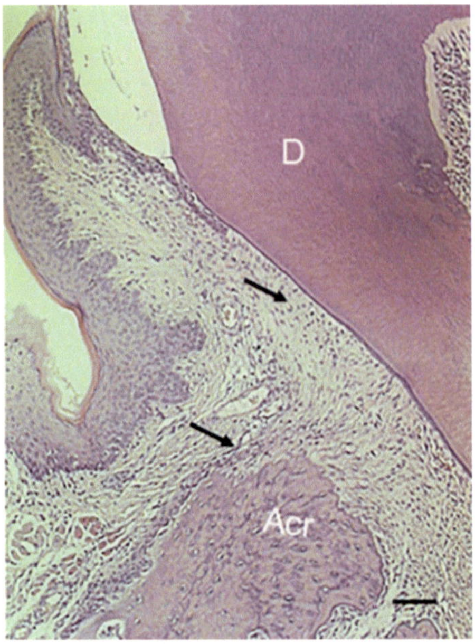

Figure 3.
In the present histological section, the papilla and its connective tissue represent the SGT barrier. The alveolar bone crest (Acr), covered by periosteum (black arrows), shows periosteal fibers and cells inserted into the root cementum and root dentin, forming the PO barrier (D).

essential for periodontal function. In addition, Sharpey's collagen fibers, extending from the alveolar bone crest and inserted into the cementum, facilitate vertical alveolar bone growth during tooth eruption (**Figure 2**). Altogether, the barrier that protects the PO consists of dense layers of collagen fibers interlaced with fibroblasts and an innate immune cell system.

The collective unit of alveolar bone, PDL, cementum, and fibrous connective tissue forms the PO, a structural and immunological shield critical for oral health. As the tooth erupts, the SGT, composed of supracrestal soft connective tissue and epithelial attachment, interfaces with the oral cavity, forming the initial line of defense against microbial biofilms (**Figure 3**).

3. Establishment of the supracrestal gingival tissue (SGT)

Tooth eruption is a highly regulated process by which teeth traverse the oral mucosa to attain their final occlusal position. During this process, the reduced enamel epithelium transforms into the junctional epithelium, a nonkeratinized structure that adheres to the enamel surface and connects with the oral epithelium. The gingival sulcus is established between the enamel and the free gingiva. Upon complete eruption, the SGT, which comprises the free marginal gingiva and the epithelial attachment, forms a vital interface between the fibrous connective tissue of the SGT and the oral environment. Collagen fibers from the cementum extend into the free marginal gingiva, surrounded by vasculature, nerves, fibroblasts, and immune cells, all covered by basal lamina and stratified squamous epithelium. Due to its direct exposure to the biofilm, the SGT serves as a frontline immunobiological barrier. Its efficacy relies on sufficient tissue volume, robust blood supply, and the functionality of resident immune cells. In healthy conditions, a coordinated population of T cells, neutrophils, and macrophages maintains mucosal immunity [2]. However, when the microbial challenge exceeds the immune capacity, dysregulation may occur, leading to chronic inflammation.

4. Breakdown of physical and immune barriers

The SGT and its junctional epithelium are under constant microbial challenge in the narrow space between the oral epithelium and the tooth enamel surface. Their integrity depends on coordinated immune surveillance by T cells, neutrophils, and macrophages. When immune responses are overwhelmed, a persistent inflammatory cascade ensues. Both resident and recruited inflammatory cells upregulate the production of MMPs, particularly collagenases, leading to the degradation of collagen fibers and extracellular matrix (ECM) components [3]. Degradation of ECM by MMPs can be derived from both bacteria in dental plaque and host cellular sources.

MMP activity is markedly higher in periodontitis compared to gingivitis. While gingivitis presents limited tissue degradation, periodontitis is characterized by extensive breakdown of the collagen fibrous PO barrier and increased cytokine production [4]. Under physiological conditions, MMP activity is regulated by tissue inhibitors of metalloproteinases (TIMPs). An imbalance between MMPs and TIMPs promotes excessive degradation of collagen fibers, disrupting the SGT and PO barriers and leading to progression to periodontal disease [5, 6].

Our previous studies have demonstrated that surgical disruption of the periodontal organ (PO) fibrous matrix, such as through elevation of a mucoperiosteal flap, can initiate molecular pathways leading to alveolar bone remodeling and resorption along the PDL aspect, similar to the enzymatic activity of matrix metalloproteinases (MMPs) observed in periodontitis [3, 7].

Under physiological conditions, fibroblasts and immune cells within the supracrestal gingival tissue (SGT) and PO exert traction forces through their interactions with fibronectin-collagen fibers via transmembrane integrins. These integrins are linked to the intracellular cytoskeleton through adhesion complexes, forming a dynamic molecular connectivity network essential for maintaining tensile strain. This ECM-cellular framework, along with intercellular molecular communication, is critical for supporting the structural and functional integrity of the dentition and periodontium [1]. Such mechanical connectivity enables the transduction of ECM-derived signals into cellular responses, including differentiation, migration, and immune activation [8, 9].

Disruption of this molecular architecture, whether due to inflammation, surgical intervention, or MMP activity, results in the abrupt loss of cellular tensile strain. This deformation induces the release of adenosine triphosphate (ATP) from affected cells, which then activates purinergic P2X and P2Y receptors on immune cells. This ATP-mediated signaling cascade promotes inflammatory responses and osteoclastic activity, ultimately leading to alveolar bone loss [10, 11].

This mechanobiological model aligns with systemic diseases characterized by impaired cytoskeletal function and reduced tensile strain. For example, osteoarthritis has been linked to ECM and cytoskeletal disorganization stemming from abnormal mechanical loading [12, 13]. Similarly, we propose that adult periodontitis is a cytoskeletal disorder marked by a breakdown in cellular tension and loss of cytoskeletal integrity [11]. In this context, preserving the molecular tensile connectivity between cells and the ECM within the SGT and PO is critical for maintaining periodontal health.

5. Peri-implant SGT and residual bone crest tissue

The tissues surrounding implants differ completely from the structure of the PO of natural dentition. Implants are inserted into a residual bone ridge to attain maximum mechanical stability. The surface of their cervical part is in intimate contact with a dense matrix of cortical bone, while the rough surface of the implant body is integrated within the regenerating trabecular bone, providing optimal integration. The implant abutment's smooth surface usually faces the oral epithelium, which covers soft connective tissue, similar to SGT. The epithelium grows along the basal membrane until it reaches the cervical abutment surface, forming a kind of hemidesmosome attachment. It is, therefore, inevitable that the junctional epithelium, which separates the soft connective tissue from the abutment surface, becomes a nesting space for bacteria.

In contrast to the dense fibrous and strained cellular attachment of periosteum to root cementum, the PO barrier of natural dentition, no such barrier is generated above the bone crest and the abutment. Then, the SGT immune system becomes the primary guard that can withstand challenging bacterial ingression. The immune response capacity and integrity of SGT cellular immune populations are the only efficient antibacterial and anti-inflammatory system. It seems reasonable for clinicians to advocate to form a bed of soft connective tissue, at least 4 mm of SGT width facing the abutment surface, in order to increase the capacity and volume of antibacterial immune cell populations.

Risk factors such as poor oral hygiene, smoking, and inadequate maintenance must be systematically addressed to ensure long-term implant success [14]. Additionally, the design of implants and the type of implant-abutment connection have been shown to influence marginal bone preservation. Features such as platform switching, internal conical connections, and moderately rough implant surfaces help reduce crestal bone remodeling by minimizing micro-gaps and micromovements at the bone-implant interface. It is well-accepted that platform switching, internal conical connections, and moderately rough implant surfaces help minimize crestal bone remodeling by reducing micro-gaps and micromovements at the bone interface [15]. Precise three-dimensional implant positioning buccolingually, mesiodistally, and apicocoronally is critical for maintaining surrounding bone integrity. Improper placement can compromise the thin buccal plate, limit prosthetic flexibility, and contribute to early bone loss or soft tissue recession [16]. Maintaining the integrity of the supracrestal tissue complex, including the junctional epithelium and connective tissue zone attachment, is essential for establishing a stable biological seal. Repeated disconnection and reconnection of the abutment can disrupt this seal, leading to marginal bone remodeling [17]. Furthermore, an adequate band of keratinized mucosa and sufficient tissue thickness around implants provide a protective barrier against bacterial challenges and mechanical trauma. In cases of deficiency, soft tissue grafting may be indicated to increase volume and improve long-term stability [18].

6. Management and therapies

The SGT and the PO form a dynamic, interconnected structure that is central to periodontal health. These structures not only provide mechanical support but also serve as immunological sentinels. Preservation of their integrity, particularly their fibrous, collagen-rich barriers and cellular strain networks, is critical in preventing disease initiation and progression. Disruption of these systems by MMP activity or surgery leads to altered signaling, inflammatory responses, and eventual alveolar bone loss. Local application of MMP inhibitors or blocking MMP activity can prevent or stop the degradation of collagen fiber barriers and prevent bone loss. Chlorhexidine has limited anti-collagenase activity. Additionally, N-acetylcysteine (NAC), an antioxidant, is also an anti-collagenase. Many more drugs should be used for this purpose. Another key factor is that extracellular ATP can be inhibited by blocking the P2X receptor for ATP. We have shown that blocking the purinoreceptors in a rat model where surgical disruption of the mucoperiosteum was performed significantly reduced alveolar bone resorption [19].

Since the peri-implant tissues lack a fibrous barrier, it becomes challenging to prevent peri-implantitis. Control of bacterial plaque and professional maintenance are critical in preventing mucositis and peri-implantitis, both of which are directly linked to progressive bone loss. Inflammatory cytokines such as IL-1β, TNF-α, and IL-6 have been associated with tissue destruction around implants when the host response is deregulated [20]. Additionally, implant surface characteristics and surgical trauma influence early immune cell behavior and healing potential [21], while the innate immune system's activation through NLRP3 inflammasome pathways has also been implicated in chronic inflammation [22]. We have recently experimented the possibility of creating a periosteum extension that could be biologically bound to the abutment surface. We have shown that coating the abutment with biological glue and fibronectin generated a fibrous and cellular attachment directly to the abutment surface, thus mimicking the PO fibrous barrier (**Figure 4**).

In conclusion, we described here the basic epithelial and immune-biological barrier present in the supracrestal gingiva tissue (SGT) and the very specific dense collagen fibrous barrier of the periodontium organ: alveolar bone, PDL, and cementum (PO) present in the healthy periodontium, while in the peri-implant tissues, a poor epithelial barrier is present and no fibrous barrier. Therefore, peri-implant breakdown depends mainly on the immune-biological barrier capacity and volume in the SGT. Therapies should be developed to inhibit the enzymatic degradation of ECM and the signaling pathways of chronic inflammatory cytokines. It is a challenge to generate a biological attachment of fibrous tissue to the implant abutment.

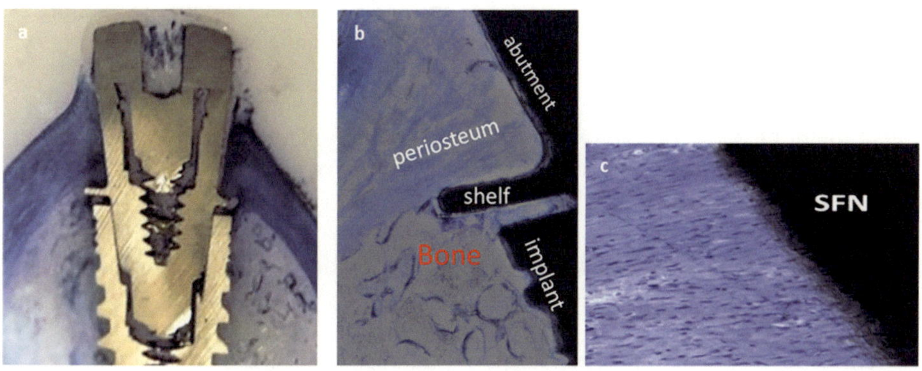

Figure 4.
Histological sections from a mini pig's lower jaw demonstrate the placement of a dental implant with a conical abutment featuring a lateral extension ("shelf") positioned slightly below the alveolar crest and covered by mucoperiosteum (a). (b) shows the osseointegration up to the shelf level and periosteum with dense fibers attaching biologically to the abutment surface, as also demonstrated in (c). For the first time, a true biological attachment of connective tissue to the titanium surface of the abutment and its shelf, which was coated with glue and fibronectin. Strained fibroblasts are aligned along collagen fibers running into the titanium surface (SFN). This study was performed and funded by MIS Implants Technologies LTD, Israel.

Author details

Itzhak Binderman[1*], Michal Halperin-Sternfeld[1,2] and Alberto Miselli[3]

1 Department of Oral Biology, The Maurice and Gabriela Goldschleger School of Dental Medicine, Gray Faculty of Medical and Health Sciences, Tel Aviv University, Tel Aviv, Israel

2 Department of Periodontology and Implant Dentistry, The Maurice and Gabriela Goldschleger School of Dental Medicine, Gray Faculty of Medical and Health Sciences, Tel Aviv University, Tel Aviv, Israel

3 Department of Prosthodontics, Universidad Central de Venezuela, Caracas, Venezuela

*Address all correspondence to: binderman.itzhak@gmail.com

References

[1] Ingber D. Mechanobiology and diseases of mechanotransduction. Annals of Medicine. 2003;**35**(8):564-577

[2] Dutzan N et al. On-going mechanical damage from mastication drives homeostatic Th17 cell responses at the oral barrier. Immunity. 2017;**46**(1):133-147

[3] Binderman I, Bahar H, Yaffe A. Strain relaxation of fibroblasts in the marginal periodontium is the common trigger for alveolar bone resorption: A novel hypothesis. Journal of Periodontology. 2002;**73**(10):1210-1215

[4] Séguier S et al. Is collagen breakdown during periodontitis linked to inflammatory cells and expression of matrix metalloproteinases and tissue inhibitors of metalloproteinases in human gingival tissue? Journal of Periodontology. 2001;**72**(10):1398-1406

[5] Kubota T et al. Altered gene expression levels of matrix metalloproteinases and their inhibitors in periodontitis-affected gingival tissue. Journal of Periodontology. 2008;**79**(1):166-173

[6] Luchian I et al. The role of matrix metalloproteinases (MMP-8, MMP-9, MMP-13) in periodontal and Peri-implant pathological processes. International Journal of Molecular Sciences. 2022;**23**(3):1806-1824

[7] Yaffe A, Fine N, Binderman I. Regional accelerated phenomenon in the mandible following mucoperiosteal flap surgery. Journal of Periodontology. 1994;**65**(1):79-83

[8] Discher DE, Janmey P, Wang Y-L. Tissue cells feel and respond to the stiffness of their substrate. Science. 2005;**310**(5751):1139-1143

[9] Engler AJ et al. Matrix elasticity directs stem cell lineage specification. Cell. 2006;**126**(4):677-689

[10] Yu H, Ferrier J. Mechanisms of ATP-induced Ca2+ signaling in osteoclasts. Cellular Signalling. 1994;**6**(8):905-914

[11] Binderman I, Gadban N, Yaffe A. Extracellular ATP is a key modulator of alveolar bone. Advances in Dental Research. 2017;**26**(1):23-29

[12] Blain EJ. Involvement of the cytoskeletal elements in articular cartilage homeostasis and pathology. International Journal of Experimental Pathology. 2009;**90**(1):1-15

[13] Loeser RF. Osteoarthritis year in review 2013: Biology. Osteoarthritis and Cartilage. 2013;**21**(10):1436-1442

[14] Heitz-Mayfield LJA, Salvi GE. Peri-implant mucositis. Journal of Clinical Periodontology. 2018;**45**(S20):S237-S245

[15] Berglundh T et al. Peri-implant diseases and conditions: Consensus report of workgroup 4 of the 2017 world workshop on the classification of periodontal and Peri-implant diseases and conditions. Journal of Clinical Periodontology. 2018;**45**:S286-S291

[16] Buser D, Martin W, Belser UC. Optimizing esthetics for implant restorations in the anterior maxilla: Anatomic and surgical considerations. The International Journal of Oral & Maxillofacial Implants. 2004;**19**(Suppl.):43-61

[17] Abrahamsson I et al. Tissue reactions to abutment shift: An experimental study

in dogs. Clinical Implant Dentistry and Related Research. 2003;**5**(2):82-88

[18] Linkevicius T et al. Influence of vertical soft tissue thickness on crestal bone changes around implants with platform switching: A comparative clinical study. Clinical Implant Dentistry and Related Research. 2015;**17**(6):1228-1236

[19] Yaffe A, Bahar H, Binderman I. Topical application of drugs influencing cytoskeleton and cell contractility affects alveolar bone loss in rats. Journal of Periodontology. 2006;**77**(5):826-831

[20] Belibasakis GN et al. Applications of the oral microbiome in personalized dentistry. Archives of Oral Biology. 2019;**104**:7-12

[21] Schwarz F et al. Peri-implantitis. Journal of Clinical Periodontology. 2018;**45**:S246-S266

[22] Salvi GE, Cosgarea R, Sculean A. Prevalence and mechanisms of peri-implant diseases. Journal of Dental Research. 2017;**96**(1):31-37

Chapter 7

Periodontal Pathogens and their Involvement in the Oral Carcinogenesis Process

Alexandra Roi, Ciprian Ioan Roi, Mircea Rivis, Ruxandra Luca, Simina Boia and Laura-Cristina Rusu

Abstract

Periodontal disease is a current pathology with a rising incidence among the population, being characterized by persistent, chronic inflammation that determines a progressive destruction of the soft tissue and, eventually, the alveolar bone. An important mechanism particular to the periodontal pathogens is their involvement and modulation of the immune response of the host. The development of periodontal disease depends on keystone microbial infections, and in recent years, it has been described that important genetic and immunological pathways, along with other risk factors, contribute to the pathogenesis of this pathology. The chronic inflammation is considered one of the main mechanisms that contributes to the initiation of the carcinogenesis process. Based on this fact, oral carcinogenesis is seen as a complex interaction between multiple factors and the host immune system. The biofilms encountered in oral cancer are represented by anaerobic bacteria, highlighting their importance in the development of this malignancy. The characteristic microbial involvement and the triggered interactions determined by the periodontal disease reveal its potential involvement in the pathogenesis of oral cancer. The periodontal pathogens could be seen as important key factors, exhibiting a potential role of biomarkers for the development of oral cancer.

Keywords: periodontal disease, periodontal pathogens, oral cancer, chronic inflammation, oral dysbiosis, oral carcinogenesis process

1. Introduction

Oral cancer is considered worldwide a major challenge for the healthcare system, with the main histopathological form of oral squamous cell carcinoma. It was reported that this type of cancer is responsible for 2% of all diagnosed cancer cases, and the deaths related to this pathology represent 1.9% of all cancer deaths [1]. While discussing the major risk factors, research outlined the implications of alcohol and tobacco in most of the cases; the occurrence of oral cancer was observed in situations when these factors are not associated.

The role of infectious agents has gained attention during the past years and has been linked to the occurrence, promotion, and progression of oral cancer. The microbial instability encountered in the oral environment and the changed dynamics between the bacterial species have direct repercussions on the cellular interactions and features [2]. One of the first study directions regarding bacterial infections and their possible implications in the carcinogenesis process was related to *Helicobacter pylori* [3], causing gastritis and a persistent inflammatory response as well, being known to be implicated in the occurrence of gastric cancer [3].

The existing studies describe the implications of the inflammatory response toward bacterial infections as being a main cause in the development of cancers. This aspect is explained by the fact that bacteria can directly target the host cell and influence its integrity, determining the tumor formation during the interactions that occur in different stages of the cellular development [4]. These pathological alterations occur through the actions upon the surface molecules by the bacterial toxins and proteins that induce a deoxyribonucleic acid (DNA) change, which modifies the signaling pathways and favors the malignant cell development [5].

It was reported that approximately 15% of all cancers are determined by existing infections, and the implicated microorganisms determine the cancer initiation and progression through the inflammation they cause [6]. Taking into consideration the fact that periodontal disease is responsible for inducing a chronic inflammation [7], the specific oral periodontal pathogens may have a direct role in the development of oral cancer, progression, and prognosis [8]. Research has highlighted the link between chronic periodontitis and an increased risk of oral cancer, a meta-analysis describing a 2-fold increased risk of oral cancer in patients diagnosed with periodontal disease [9]. Also, diagnosed cancer patients who are unable to maintain proper oral hygiene due to the chemotherapy or radiotherapy treatment side effects, a fact that can increase the gingival inflammation and determine further periodontal complications [10].

It appears that the oral biofilm of oral squamous cell carcinoma patients contains a high quantity of anaerobic bacteria that is encountered in periodontal disease [11]. The results of several studies have linked the poor oral hygiene status with the incidence of oral cancer, as well as the link between periodontal pathogens and the incidence of different cancer types, among which is oral cancer [12]. There has been identified an implication of the periodontal pathogen *Fusobacterium nucleatum* in the chemoresistance of colorectal cancer cells, by having an action upon the autophagy process [13]. Also, it was reported that *Porphyromonas gingivalis* contributes to and induces the invasiveness of oral cancer cells by promoting the secretion of IL-8 and controlling the regulation of the matrix metalloproteinases (MMPs) [14].

An important aspect that is related to the development of oral cancer is the impact of several risk factors upon the oral cavity and the existing predisposing agents like chemicals, pesticides, or heavy metals that have an impact upon the epigenetic alterations and pro-oncogenic interactions, inducing oral cancer development [15, 16]. Nevertheless, among these factors the oral infections and dysbiosis are considered a key factor in the etiopathogenesis of oral malignant lesions [17].

There are over 600 bacterial species that form the oral microbiome, and until recently, with the help of sequencing technology, the identification of the bacterial communities that are encountered in the oral environment and have an implication in oral and general health was a difficult task [18]. Their identification and characterization allowed the analysis of the interactions between different bacterial species and their involvement in multiple physiological processes [19]. There are results that describe that the gut microbiota is involved in the incidence of different general pathologies, mainly represented by chronic degenerative disorders, neurovascular diseases, and malignancies [20–22]. From all malignancies, the relationship between oral cancer and the oral and gut microbiome has been intensively studied, and the results outline a direct involvement of these microbiomes in the incidence of this type of cancer. Studies reveal that among the most common oral pathogens associated with oral squamous cell carcinoma are *Porphyromonas gingivalis*, *Prevotella intermedia,* and *Fusobacterium nucleatum,* bacterial species that are linked to periodontal disease as well [22–24].

Oral bacteria determine changes that influence their impact upon the general health, causing multiple pathologies [18]. Studies have discussed the possibility that the oral pathogens could contribute to the initiation of oral squamous cell carcinoma (OSCC) by targeting the metabolism of the cells, promoting carcinogenesis. These metabolic changes are represented by alterations in the concentration of vitamins and nutrients, a fact that will induce the release of several cytokines that can be linked to the incidence of different pathologies [22].

There has been identified a link that reveals the role of the interaction between multiple oral bacteria and the incidence of the oral carcinogenesis process. Nevertheless, a direct causative relation cannot be established between only a certain oral pathogen and the occurrence of oral malignancy [22]. Moreover, there is a need to identify potential microbial biomarkers that could be linked to different stages of oral malignancy development [4].

Nevertheless, important interactions occur between the microbial communities and the oral homeostasis, influencing the general and local response of the host, a fact that will facilitate the repercussions upon the oral epithelium. Existing studies suggest that the periodontal pathogens can facilitate oral cancer progression, influencing the cell survival, the proliferation rate, the apoptosis and the invasion potential of the tumor. This action mechanism includes both direct bacterial effects and secondary inflammatory responses.

An important aspect that was highlighted was that the early undiagnosed cancer or precancerous lesions have the potential to enable the colonization and proliferation of the oral bacteria, with a direct action upon the tumor progression, suggesting the importance of constantly reviewing patients diagnosed with periodontal disease as having a high risk for oral malignancy development.

2. Periodontal diseases and its pathogens

Periodontal disease is known for its chronic evolution, currently having an incidence among different age groups. It was reported that in Europe, the prevalence is 5–20% among the age group 35–44 years and 40% in the case of elderly patients belonging to the age group 65–74 years old [25]. Mainly, the etiology of the periodontal disease is represented by an inflammatory response toward the pathogens of the dental plaque, as a prolonged accumulation of a bacterial community. Firstly, the inflammatory response is represented by the occurrence of gingivitis, which, as a pathological progression, can develop into periodontitis, with permanent destruction of the periodontal ligaments and bone structure [26]. The evolution toward periodontitis represents an individual susceptibility that has an important link to the immune response toward the microbial community, the existent dysbiosis, the oral hygiene status and other preexisting chronic diseases that could trigger the

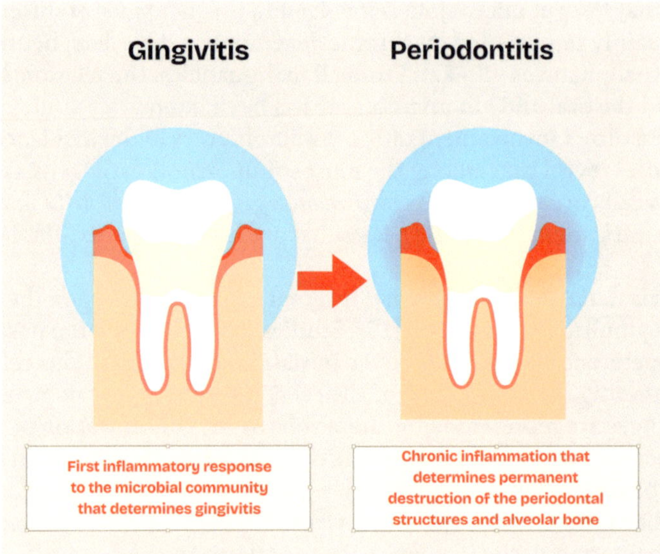

Figure 1.
The characteristics of the evolution from gingivitis to periodontal disease.

immune-inflammatory response (**Figure 1**) [27, 28]. During the characterization of the periodontal disease, the predominant species are the gram-negative species, which determining a dysbiosis of the oral environment, promoting the evolution of this pathology [29].

Chronic periodontitis can be classified based on the involvement of the teeth, being localized or generalized, and the environmental and genetic factors play an important role in its incidence [30]. Severe periodontal disease is currently the 11th most prevalent condition, affecting 10% of the adult population. Based on the incidence related to this age group, it could explain the higher cancer risk associated with this population [31]. Also, the inflammation caused by periodontal diseases seems to influence and increase the incidence of other systemic diseases or their associated complications [30]. The identified systemic diseases that are linked to the periodontal diseases are cardiovascular disease, Alzheimer's disease, diabetes mellitus, rheumatoid disease, inflammatory pathologies, or several types of cancers [32].

The role of dental plaque as a main etiological factor of periodontal disease has been discussed, approved, and taken into consideration while assessing each clinical case. In the study performed by Loe et al. [33], where on a human cohort they induced an "experimental gingivitis" by having an abstinence from oral hygiene, determining an accumulation of dental plaque that induced an inflammation of the gingiva that led to the diagnosis of gingivitis. Reinforced the oral hygiene habits showing that the dental plaque is reduced, and the signs of gingival inflammation decrease [33].

The analysis of the composition of the dental plaque in these cases showed the evolution of the microbial community, from gram-positive cocci to gram-negative ones, containing a high amount of fusobacteria, spirochetes, and filaments. It appears that these changes in the microbial community occur during the mild gingivitis phase [34]. Describing the microbial community composition during the phase of gingivitis and evolving to periodontal disease is an important step in acknowledging the implication of specific pathogens.

Periodontal disease is dependent on the composition of the subgingival biofilm that determines, in certain cases, severe destruction of the periodontal tissue. While analyzing the specific role of different periodontal pathogens, studies have outlined the essential bacterial triggers of this disease, specifically *Aggregatibacter actinomycetemcomitans, P. gingivalis, P. intermedia, T. forsythia* and *F. nucleatum* were among the most identified species [35, 36]. Currently, their identification is possible by using specific DNA-based technologies that can target and validate specific microorganisms [37, 38]. The microbiological evaluation helps the clinician to implement the proper treatment and evaluate the treatment accordingly to the existing microbiological situation [39].

When an imbalance occurs in the oral microbial communities, it is referred to as an oral dysbiosis. Within this environment, researchers have established that there are several bacteria that, when combined, can determine specific changes of the entire microbiota, changes that are linked to a disease-inducing microbiota, by inducing a chronic inflammatory response [40]. In the areas where inflammation occurs, nutrients appear as a response to the tissue alterations, being constantly a further source for the pathogens that are linked to the inflammatory process, sustaining the continuous dysbiosis of the oral environment [41].

Studies have discussed the existence of a specific "keystone pathogen" that is represented by *Porphyromonas gingivalis*, which is apparently responsible for the inflammatory process in the periodontium, a condition that will continue to convert the symbiotic relationships between the existing microorganisms into dysbiotic ones. Taking into consideration this action, it is considered that *Porphyromonas gingivalis* is one of the main pathogens responsible for periodontal disease [42]. From several existing hypotheses regarding the initiation of the inflammatory process within the periodontal tissue and the implications of the bacterial community and plaque changes, several discussions highlight the presence of *Porphyromonas gingivalis*, suggesting that even a small amount could significantly alter the subgingival profile, sustaining the dysbiosis [42].

Nevertheless, there is evidence that the dysbiosis state associated with periodontal disease is determined by gram-negative bacteria, which become dominant over species that are associated with a healthy environment [5]. Studies revealed the fact that the red-complex triad formed by *Porphyromonas gingivalis*, *Tannerella forsythia*, and *Treponema denticola* is frequently encountered in periodontal disease (**Figure 2**) [5, 6]. The most common subgingival pathogens that were identified in patients diagnosed with chronic periodontal disease and are responsible for producing periodontal abscesses were reported to be *Fusobacterium nucleatum*, *Prevotella intermedia/nigrescens*, *Porphyromonas gingivalis*, and *Aggregatibacter actino-mycetemcomitans* [7, 8].

Additionally, the progress and persistence of periodontal disease leads to the development of a more diverse microbiota population, based on the fact that there is an increase in the variety of nutrients that are accessible to the bacterial community, as a consequence of the persistence of inflammation and an inefficient immunity response, fact that lead to an uncontrolled bacterial growth [5]. As a further response to the prolonged immune response [9], the tumor necrosis factor (TNF), cytokines IL-1, and prostaglandin E2 (PGE-2) will activate and stimulate the osteoclasts, encourage the initiation of bone loss [10] through the receptor activator of nuclear factor kappa-B ligand (RANKL) pathway (**Figure 3**).

The altered salivary levels of IL-1beta and PGE-2 appear to have a strong correlation with the severity of the periodontal disease, making them potential biomarkers of the therapy efficiency [11]. Several diseases due to their immunocompromising actions, such as diabetes mellitus, exacerbate the progression of the periodontal

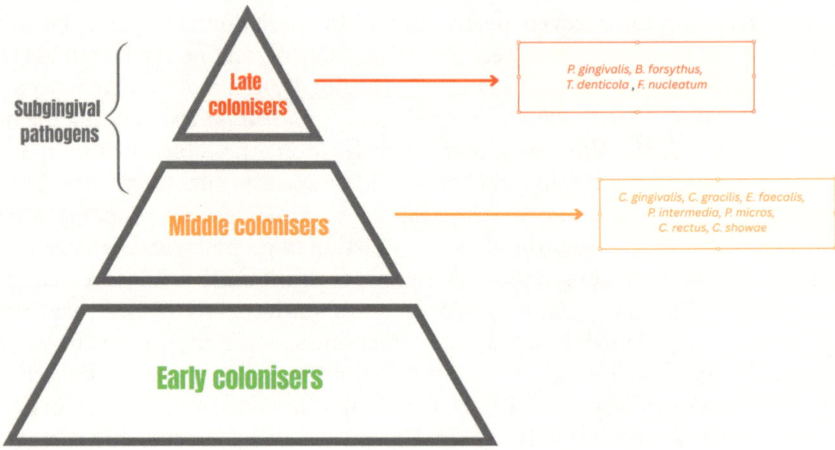

Figure 2.
The microbial community associated with the subgingival plaque.

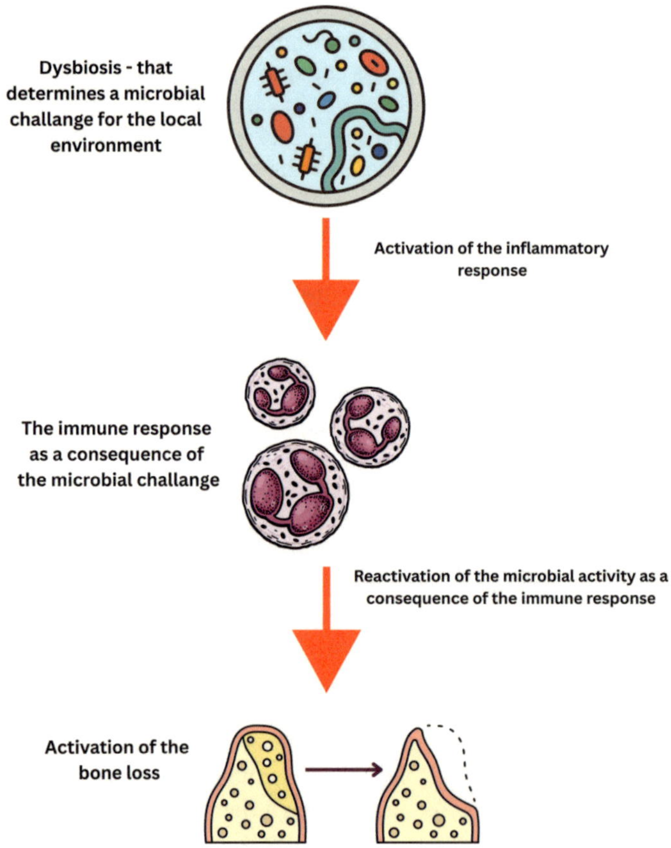

Figure 3.
The interdependent events associated with periodontal disease.

disease [9] having a negative impact on the aggressive evolution [8]. Also, patients who undergo chemotherapy or radiation therapy have the risk that their periodontal disease may exacerbate, needing to reinforce their oral hygiene practices and refer to a specialist for a check-up. Taking into consideration that radiotherapy affects the oral tissue and chemotherapy determines immunosuppression and xerostomia, these treatments can increase the incidence of periodontal disease and its severity in patients diagnosed with cancer [12].

Understanding the complete pathophysiology of the periodontal disease and the degree of inflammation that it produces allows the evaluation of its impact upon the incidence of the induced systemic inflammation [43].

In the etiology of periodontal disease multiple factors co-exist, factors that contribute to the initiation and progress of this pathology. Among these factors the host environmental factors, the keystone periodontal bacteria and the host immunity are reported to play a crucial role. An essential contribution to this process is linked to specific genetic profiles that will determine an individual's susceptibility to the development of inflammatory responses [44]. The oral microbiome and the dysbiosis encountered in periodontal disease can determine an increase in the level of proinflammatory mediators, such as many cytokines and C-reactive protein [45]. Nevertheless, in certain studies, these oral bacteria were identified in the atheromatous plaques, outlining the dissemination potential that can trigger and influence the severity of systemic pathologies [46, 47]. It is discussed that in the periodontal microcirculation, signaling molecules like interleukin-1, tumor necrosis factor, and interleukin-6 can be found in the bloodstream and migrate to other organs [48]. The chronic inflammation, similar to that encountered in periodontal disease, can induce the malignant transformation of various cells, which is known as a risk factor for cancer [49].

The periodontal pathogens induce an abnormal immune response, which will promote the pathogenic invasion and produce specific metabolites, such as lactic acid and valine [50]. All of the changes specific to the dysbiosis observed in periodontal disease can influence the processes that control cell replication and repair, and those that are responsible for the membrane transport and metabolism of amino acids and fatty acids [51, 52]. The pathogenic bacteria specific for the periodontal disease, which determines an inflammatory state that can be responsible for inducing DNA damage within the epithelial cell layer, being linked to cancer progression [53].

3. Oral carcinogenesis process

The process that represents the shift from healthy oral tissue develops into malignant tissue is known as oral carcinogenesis. The normal cellular functions, including cell division, differentiation, and cell death, are disrupted by this intricate and multistep process that involves multiple genetic and epigenetic changes. Carcinogenesis is very complex, being influenced by individual susceptibility and associated environmental factors [54].

3.1 Genetic alterations

It appears that approximately 6–10 genetic events are implicated in the oral carcinogenesis process. Cell division, differentiation, and senescence are basic biological processes that are governed by several regulators. An accumulation of alterations within different cellular pathways, which can occur at any level of a specific route, determines oral cancer. Tumor cells are able to divide more quickly, use the blood vessels to fuel their growth, and delete or amplify signals to produce abnormal structural and functional changes. After these events, the cancerous cells have the potential to invade the surrounding normal tissue or to disseminate to distant sites [55].

The genetic alterations can be represented by:

- In case of well-differentiated tumors, the chromosomes 3p, 5q, and 9p were deleted with a 3q gain; in poorly differentiated tumors, chromosomes 4q, 8p, 11q, 13q, 18q, and 21q were deleted with a gain in 1p, 11q, 13, 19, and 22q, indicating a possible correlation with tumor development [56].

- An allelic imbalance at chromosome 3p and 9p.

- The loss of heterozygosity and the presence of microsatellite instability at 9p21–p22 [57].

- Chromosome breakpoints in centromeric regions of chromosomes 1, 3, 8, 14, 15, 1p22, 11q13, and 19p13 [58].

- p53 gene mutations and inactivation.

Methylation is the primary epigenetic alteration encountered in the malignant tumors of the oral cavity. In the development of cancer, both promoter hypermethylation and genome-wide hypomethylation are important. Epigenetic changes are crucial for the existing genomic processes that occur during carcinogenesis and are often linked to the loss of genetic expression. These types of changes can inactivate the DNA-repairing genes, allowing for the malignant process to develop.

A methylation-specific polymerase chain reaction (PCR) revealed in case of head and neck carcinomas samples aberrant hypermethylation patterns in the p16, methylguanine-DNA methyltransferase (MGMT), and death-associated protein kinase (DAP-K) gene methylation patterns [59, 60].

3.2 Stages of oral carcinogenesis

The process begins in a normal epithelium or already altered ones, such as oral potentially malignant disorder-leukoplakia, erythroplakia, leukoerythroplakia, erosive lichen planus, oral submucous fibrosis, or actinic keratosis [61].

Histologically, the lesion goes through many stages (preneoplastic damage) before eventually developing into a malignancy. Reactive epithelial alterations (like hyperkeratosis, hyperplasia, and acanthosis) or preneoplastic changes (like mild, moderate, and severe dysplasia) can be used in order to categorize lesions that occur in the epithelium throughout the carcinogenesis process before the invasive carcinoma [61].

The development of oral cancer begins as an epithelial dysplasia, which is characterized by the abnormal growth of dysplastic squamous cells. This event leads to the degradation of the subepithelial basement membrane (BM). The local destruction of tissues and the metastasis are basically the consequence of BM degradation [62].

3.2.1 Oral epithelial dysplasia

It is defined by cytological and architectural changes that represent the absence of the typical surface epithelium maturation and stratification pattern [63]. Removing the triggering stimuli may cause the dysplastic changes to return to normal. Also, the development of oral malignant tumors, followed by invasion and metastasis, is the result of multiple cumulative events, influenced by the genetic alterations known as carcinogenesis of the epithelium [64].

Although longitudinal studies indicate that this has minimal relevance in predicting risk, clinicians could believe that the degree of dysplasia is proportionate to the chance of malignant transformation. It is not possible to correctly identify which instances of oral epithelial dysplasia may progress to cancer using the standard grading system of mild, moderate, and severe dysplasia [64].

3.2.2 Carcinoma in situ

In the early stage of oral cancer, also known as oral intraepithelial carcinoma, or oral squamous cell carcinoma *in situ*, occurs when the malignant cells are localized within the epithelium and have not yet affected the deeper tissues. It is frequently referred to as stage 0 oral cancer and is considered a precancerous stage [65]. Carcinoma *in situ* is not yet an invasive cancer, but if left untreated, it has a significant chance of developing into invasive oral squamous cell carcinoma (OSCC).

3.2.3 Invasive carcinoma

Malignant epithelial cells infiltrate the deeper tissues of the oral cavity, destroying the basement membrane that divides the surface epithelium from the connective tissue localized under it, a characteristic of invasive oral carcinomas. Based on their level of cellular differentiation, invasive carcinomas are histologically categorized from well-differentiated (looking like normal squamous epithelium) to poorly differentiated (exhibiting profound cellular and nuclear atypia, with minimal similarity to normal tissue). There are two types of invasive patterns: Erosive (a wide, pushing front) and infiltrative (cell nests and cords) [66].

3.3 Risk factors

The chronic use of alcohol and tobacco is the main risk factor for the initiation and progression of oral cancer in case of Western nations. Although smoking and drinking are separate risk factors, if they are combined it will significantly raise the risk. A high incidence of oral cancer in Asian nations is caused by the use of smokeless tobacco products like gutkha and betel quid [54].

3.3.1 Tobacco

Tobacco consumption has a lot of forms, depending on the culture and social status of the patients. Since 1985, the International Agency for Research on Cancer (IARC) has classified tobacco in all of its forms—including smoke, snuff, and chew—as carcinogenic to humans (Group 1) [67]. The risk increases with daily cigarette use and duration of tobacco use, and it falls proportionately with the amount of time after quitting.

The thickened, hyperkeratotic modification of the palatal mucosa is known as nicotine stomatitis, and it is most commonly linked to pipe smoking, while milder cases can also arise as a result of cigar smoking. Sometimes, the palatal mucosa develops a thick, fissured surface and becomes hyperkeratotic. Frequently, on this surface the inflammation of the minor salivary glands can occur determining the appearance of a red-centered area [68]. These lesions are areas of oral mucosa where the carcinogenic factors can determine changes. Tobacco is considered one of the main risk factors for recurrence and second primary occurrence, being also linked to a lower chance of survival.

3.3.2 Alcohol

Alcohol is also categorized as a category 1 carcinogen classified by the International Agency for Research on Cancer (IARC). By oxidizing ethanol into acetaldehyde, an intermediate metabolite that interacts with DNA, the alcohol dehydrogenase (ADH) enzyme may be responsible for alcohol-associated carcinogenesis. In order to cause cancer, it either alters DNA or prevents its production. Additionally, many carcinogens use ethanol as a solvent, a fact that increases the amount of different chemicals that enter the oral cells [69, 70]. Certain carcinogenic contaminants, such as nitrosamines and polycyclic aromatic hydrocarbons, are also present in alcohol.

3.3.3 Synergistic effect of tobacco and alcohol

Studies revealed that heavy smokers have the habit of drinking more compared to light smokers, and heavy drinkers smoke more than light drinkers. When alcohol and tobacco are consumed together, their effects will be synergic and multiply rather than add up. The combination of alcohol and smoke increases the formation of acetaldehyde, which could be the explanation for the synergy that has been identified. Additionally, ethanol may make mucosa's permeable to other carcinogens higher [71].

3.3.4 HPV infection

Particularly in those who do not have alcohol and tobacco as risk factors, human papillomavirus (HPV), specifically HPV type 16, may be the etiological factor.

Numerous processes determine HPV's carcinogenicity, including cell immortalization, genomic instability, a lack of DNA damage repair, and anti-apoptotic activity. One important process that takes part in the development of the viral oncogenes E6 and E7 is the integration of HPV DNA into the host genome. E6 protein inhibits the anti-oncogenic function of p53 protein by attaching to it and preventing it from binding to the DNA [72].

4. Mechanisms linking periodontal pathogens to carcinogenesis

By releasing substances with a carcinogenic potential, also interfering with the different cell signaling pathways, altering the eukaryotic cell cycle, and causing persistent local inflammation, periodontal infections can have an implication in the development of cancer. All of these processes have the potential to accelerate the growth and spread of local malignant tumors, outlining the importance and need for good oral hygiene in preventing cancer.

4.1 Chronic inflammation

Chronic or dysregulated inflammation, identified as a crucial process in tumor formation, development, invasion, and metastasis, is determined by the implication of cytokines, chemokines, prostaglandins, and the accumulation of reactive oxygen and nitrogen radicals within the oral tissue microenvironment [73, 74].

Persistent inflammatory substances can stimulate cell proliferation and determine an increased cell survival by activating oncogenes and inactivating the tumor suppressor genes. Periodontal pathogenic bacteria, especially *Fusobacterium, Veillonella, Actinomyces, Clostridium, Haemophilus, and Enterobacteriaceae,* sustain a persistent chronic inflammatory response, leading to the degradation of periodontal tissue and determining the development of oral cancer [75]. They also elevate the levels of numerous proinflammatory cytokines, including TNF-α, multiple interleukins, and matrix metalloproteinases (MMPs).

Inflammatory cells have a significant influence on tumor progression. In the first stages of neoplasia, these cells serve as potent tumor promoters, creating a specific environment for tumor proliferation, increasing genomic instability, and influencing angiogenesis. Within the tumorigenic process, neoplastic cells use inflammatory pathways to promote their dissemination and metastasis potential.

Despite the expectation that inflammatory responses should be anti-tumor, cancer patients often have deficiencies in these responses. In periodontitis, the immune response is initiated when an antigen reaches the epithelial surfaces. Antigens will ultimately interact with macrophages or certain other types of antigen-presenting cells, including B cells, monocytes, dendritic cells, and Langerhans cells [76].

Macrophages are cells that originate from the mononuclear phagocyte system, essential for antimicrobial immunity, tissue homeostasis, and organ development. The study of tumor stroma, as a vital mediator of cancer-related inflammation, identified tumor-associated macrophages (TAM) as a significant element of leukocyte infiltration in the majority of malignancies, influencing the disease prognosis [77, 78]. These cells are known to promote tumor growth, angiogenesis, and metastasis.

The tumor-associated neutrophils (TAN) are the first responders to inflammation and can also release factors that promote tumor growth and metastasis. Often found in tumors, they have been overlooked in the context of cancer-related inflammation, primarily due to their short lifespan and fully differentiated status. The role of neutrophils in tumor progression remains unknown, with evidence supporting both pro-tumoral and anti-tumoral functions [79, 80].

Mast cells play a complex and multifaceted role in oral cancer development and its progression. Increased microvessel density and mast cell density have been observed in OSCC, potentially contributing to a poor prognosis. The role of mast cells in tumor promotion is primarily attributed to their angiogenic properties. Studies utilizing various mouse models have demonstrated evidence of degranulation and angiogenesis associated with mast cells in premalignant conditions.

The interaction between cancer cells and their microenvironment is crucial for tumor progression and growth inhibition. Mast cells exhibit direct mitogenic activities on tumor cells and indirectly influence the microenvironment by enhancing its invasive potential. This phenomenon is primarily induced by heparin and TNF-α [81, 82]. The density of mast cells and the presence of specific subtype are correlated with prognosis in oral cancer [83].

Eosinophils frequently represent the predominant inflammatory leukocytes infiltrating the sites of oral squamous carcinoma. Oral carcinomas secrete prostaglandins, which may play a role in the eosinophil infiltration. Tumor-associated tissue eosinophilia (TATE) is a well-established pathological characteristic linked to oral squamous cell carcinoma (OSCC) [84]. Evidence suggests a favorable prognosis linked to eosinophil infiltration in grade II and III tumors. Nevertheless, in well-differentiated oral cancer of grades III and IV, the presence of TATE signifies a poor prognosis [85].

Activated T lymphocytes are essential in the immune response to oral cancer, especially oral squamous cell carcinoma (OSCC). Certain T cell subtypes, such as CD8+, T helper 1 cells, and NK cells, are linked to anti-tumor responses, while others, such as CD4+ T cells, including T helper 2 and regulatory T cells, may facilitate tumor progression. The balance and activation status of T cell populations in the tumor microenvironment (TME) significantly affect the progression and prognosis of OSCC [86, 87].

4.2 Interference with cell signaling pathways

Periodontal pathogens may disrupt various mechanisms that regulate the proliferative response in normal cells across OSCC. The activation of certain immunological and inflammatory responses in the host by *P. gingivalis* is regarded as the fundamental mechanism. Moreover, *Porphyromonas gingivalis* has been shown to infiltrate and enter several epithelial cells, allowing it to modify some genes in response to persistent infection [88]. It is responsible for the initiation of a sequence of signaling cascades and other molecular interactions, resulting in immune evasion, proliferation, invasion, metastasis, inflammation, and heightened aggressiveness of oral cancer cells. *Porphymonas gingivalis* stimulates the expression of B7-H1 and B7-DC receptors on host cells, resulting in immune evasion. It further facilitates OSCC proliferation by stimulating the expression of epidermal growth factor receptor (EGFR) and cyclin D1 *via* the miR-21/PDCD4/AP-1 signaling pathway. *P. gingivalis* stimulates the production of MMP-9 by activating the protease-activated receptor (PAR)-2/nuclear factor kappa-light-chain-enhancer of activated B cells (NF-κB), p38/heat shock protein 27 (HSP27), and ERK1/2-Ets1 pathways, facilitating the invasion [89].

P. gingivalis has been demonstrated to activate both the JAK/Stat and PI3K/Akt pathways, thereby inhibiting the intrinsic apoptotic pathway by averting mitochondrial membrane depolarization and obstructing cytochrome c release. This is accompanied by the downregulation of pro-apoptotic genes (caspase 3, caspase 9, Bad, and Bax) and the upregulation of anti-apoptotic genes (survivin, Bcl-2, bcl-XL, and Bfl-1) in gingival epithelial cells (GEC) [90],

P. gingivalis, F. nucleatum, and T. denticola were shown to enhance migration, invasion, and stemness, hence fostering an aggressive phenotype of OSCC *via* the overexpression of integrin αV by TL4/MyD88-mediated stimulation [91].

F. nucleatum significantly influences cancer formation and progression by altering cellular signaling pathways that regulate cell proliferation and immunological responses, hence facilitating tumor growth, metastasis, and immune evasion. *F. nucleatum* may activate oncogenes such as STAT3, JAK1, and myelocytomatosis (MYC), which enhance cell survival, proliferation, and suppress apoptosis [92]. Another mechanism used by *F. nucleatum* is the promotion of epithelial-mesenchymal transition (EMT), a process where the cancer cells relinquish their epithelial properties and acquire mesenchymal ones, hence increasing their capacity for invasion and metastasis [93]. *F. nucleatum* may enhance the expression of matrix metalloproteinases (MMPs), enzymes responsible for the degradation of the extracellular matrix, hence promoting cancer cell invasion and metastasis. Also, it may enhance cancer cell proliferation by elevating lactate synthesis *via* the GLUT1 transporter, hence facilitating tumor development [94].

4.3 Production of carcinogenic substances

Periodontal diseases may generate carcinogenic agents, such as reactive oxygen species (ROS), reactive nitrogen species (RNS), and volatile sulfur compounds (VSCs). These compounds may induce DNA damage, inflammation, and eventually, the onset of oral cancer. These highly reactive chemicals may inflict damage on DNA, proteins, and lipids, possibly resulting in cellular mutations and facilitating oral cancer progression.

Periodontitis elicits increased reactive oxygen species generation in periodontal tissue. Upon the onset of periodontitis, reactive oxygen species generated in the periodontal lesion infiltrate the bloodstream, leading to the oxidation of blood molecules and the manifestation of circulating oxidative stress [95, 96].

Certain periodontal infections generate volatile sulfur compounds, such as hydrogen sulfide, methyl mercaptan, and dimethyl sulfide. Although mostly recognized for inducing halitosis, volatile sulfur compounds (VSCs) may also be detrimental to oral tissues and may foster an inflammatory milieu conducive to cancer progression [97].

5. Clinical implications of periodontal pathogens in oral cancer

Multiple research studies that were conducted in the last 10 years have offered new insights regarding the link between different oral bacteria to the incidence of oral squamous cell carcinoma (OSCC). The correlations between OSCC and the oral pathogens were identified through the comparison of the oral bacterial DNA obtained from OSCC patients and the one obtained from normal participants, using 16S rRNA sequencing [98].

It is considered that a higher risk for the development of OSCC is linked to the existing periodontal pathogenic bacteria that studies encountered in high levels in the samples provided by these patients, identifying *Campylobacter*, *Filifactor*, *Pseudomonas*, *Capnocytophaga*, and *Fusobacterium*. As a consequence, the samples of the diagnosed cancer patients revealed higher levels of certain proinflammatory mediators, such as lipopolysaccharide, that are released by the periodontal pathogens [99]. Among all the periodontal pathogens, *Fusobacterium nucleatum* exhibited the most encountered changes linked to malignancy from all the microorganisms [100, 101]. Nevertheless, it appeared that Fusobacterium was identified in high levels in those OSCC patients in stage four [102].

The role of *Fusobacterium nucleatum* has been intensively studied, and some researchers consider that it plays an important role in the bacterial interaction in the case of OSCC patients, based on its ability to adhere to other bacterial species and form a complex network that will promote inflammation and further changes in OSCC patients [103]. As other anaerobic bacteria such as *Campylobacter*, *Parvimonas*, and *Peptostreptococcus* have been associated with the development of colorectal cancer [104], the *Capnocytophaga* and *Filifactor* appear to be involved in the pathogenesis of lung cancer [105].

Furthermore, it is not completely known how these anaerobic bacteria contribute to the development of OSCC, and more research is required in order to establish the exact interactions. *Pseudomonas* has important virulence characteristics that can determine the carcinogenesis process by damaging the epithelium, while *Pseudomonas aeruginosa* can induce DNA changes that target the epithelial cells [106, 107].

The implications of the periodontal pathogens are directly related to the compositional shift existing in the tumor sites, being explained through their capacity, especially in the case of *Fusobacterium nucleatum*, to adhere and generate inflammation, causing DNA damage to the epithelial cells. Although different bacteria encountered in the oral environment can determine various alterations, the periodontal pathogens appear to be directly linked to OSCC. The studies reveal that a lower quantity of bacteria, such as *Firmicutes, Streptococcus,* and *Actinobacteria*, was found in the case of OSCC samples, compared to the healthy group [100, 103].

In case of OSCC, within the carcinogenesis process, it was observed that the early colonization of *Streptococcus*, while *Fusbacterium nucleatum* is a transitional bacterium that co-aggregates in the early and late stages of colonization [108, 109]. Additionally, as a controversy, it appears that *Streptococcus* has the possibility to reduce the proinflammatory process that is induced by *Fusobacterium nucleatum* in the epithelial layer [110]. Also, the presence of Firmicutes and Actinobacteria was negatively associated with the precancerous stage, suggesting that their levels may change in the early stage of cancer development [111, 112]. Taking this into consideration, it could be stated that Firmicutes and Actinobacteria, in the case of the early stages of oral cancer, exhibit a lower percentage that is combined with a higher amount of *Fusobacterium nucleatum*, fact that can suggest the presence of a precancerous or a malignant state [113].

Several studies have encountered changes between the normal, precancerous, and cancerous lesions, as well as changes in the case of the periodontal pathogens identified, revealing that bacteria can play an important role as biomarkers of specific stages. Certain microbial combinations have been evaluated as possible biomarkers for OSCC, some of them showing a high specificity [111]. In their study, Zhao et al. [100] showed that *Fusobacterium nucleatum* has a high potential for predicting OSCC. Another study conducted by Yang et al. [102] reported that a certain combination of *Porphyromonas pasteri, Fusobacterium periodonticum*, and *Streptococcus mitis* could discriminate the OSCC patients in stage four from healthy controls.

The bacterial community suffers changes during the various stages of carcinogenesis, from the normal epithelial to the precancerous and eventually to the cancerous state. They will suffer changes and adapt in order to offer and sustain a proper tumor microenvironment that can provide the support for the further development. There is a sequence within the bacterial community, and the first step in generating the necessary dysbiosis and environment for the carcinogenesis process is obtained through the production of specific products that damage the DNA and may cause oral cancer. This step is achieved by the so-called "drivers-passengers" theory, the " drivers" being the first that appear in the early stages of oral cancer [114, 115]. *Porphyromonas gingivalis* could be considered a "driver" since it is present in the early stages of carcinogenesis, and the damage it produces can directly harm the DNA by producing lipopolysaccharides that represent an important inflammatory chemical that promotes oral carcinogenesis [116]. The conducted studies that focused on the bacterial community and its changes observed an important shift in *Porphyromonas gingivalis* levels in the OSCC development, highlighting its most frequent implication in the early stages of OSCC [117].

The passengers are represented by the bacteria that are present in healthy conditions, but in case of the occurrence of the dysbiosis, this community will benefit from the newly developed tumor microenvironment [115]. This category of bacteria is responsible for the development and further spread of the malignant process. As studies have reported, it appears that *Fusobacterium nucleatum* could be an important bacterium in the " passenger" category. Although it is present also in small amounts in healthy oral environments, it appears to be mostly encountered in OSCC patients [118]. The bacterial composition suffers changes in the different stages of the oral carcinogenesis, allowing the different processes to take place, such as the multiplication of the cancer cells, the invasion rate, and the metastasis occurrence [119–121]. Therefore, *Fusobacterium nucleatum* could be considered a marker for the malignant transformation of oral epithelial cells.

As an important step in the carcinogenesis, the aberrant cell proliferation is one of the most important processes that is disturbed and that can be controlled by the microbial agents. As a consequence, the periodontal pathogens can influence the different pathways that control the proliferation rate of the normal cells in most cancers. *Porphyromonas gingivalis* produces FimA, a protein that can accelerate the progress of the cell cycle, reducing at the same time the activity of the p53 tumor suppressor, and increasing the levels of phosphoinositide 3-kinase (PI3K) and of phosphoinositide-dependent protein-serine kinase 1 (PDK1) [122]. In a study conducted by Behzadi et al. [123], the exposure of the epithelial cells to *Porphyromonas gingivalis* and *Fusobacterium nucleatum* triggers a specific receptor that activates the IL-6 production, which will further activate the STAT3, which will induce the OSCC cell multiplication. Also, *Porphyromonas gingivalis* decreases the level of p53, which will sustain the cell growth. Another implication of the pathogens is through the regulation of the β-catenin signaling that controls the tumorgenesis and proliferation, *Porphyromonas gingivalis* inducing its activation, determining important changes in the cell cycle [124].

Another impact of *Porphyromonas gingivalis* is upon the gene expression of α-defensins, those being responsible for the division process of the oral cancer cells through a direct control of the epidermal growth factor receptor (EGFR), activating the dermal keratinocytes [125]. Nevertheless, *A. actinomycetemcomitans* has been identified to control cell apoptosis, having an opposite effect upon the oral cancer cell and their proliferative characteristics [125]. Most of the existing studies outline the implication of *Porphyromonas gingivalis* in the cell proliferation process, contributing to the oral carcinogenesis initiation. There are studies that discuss the fact that this bacterium would suppress the cell proliferation in the G1 phase, inducing autophagy by the formation of reactive oxygen species [126].

The inhibition of cell apoptosis in oral cancer is an important mechanism that allows the tumoral growth and invasion. There is evidence that this process can be determined also by oral pathogens that will inhibit the apoptosis and promote the tumorigenesis. *Porphyromonas gingivalis* was identified as having an implication in activating the apoptosis through intrinsic mitochondrial pathways, enhancing the activity of the anti-apoptotic factors, and inhibiting the proapoptotic ones [127].

The periodontal pathogens can increase the survival of the tumor cells through several extracellular and intracellular approaches that will avoid the apoptosis process. The autophagy activity appears to be increased in patients diagnosed with periodontitis compared to healthy individuals [128]. It has been discussed that the autophagy process in a proper way sustains angiogenesis, protects the periodontal cells from apoptosis, and in the case of *Porphyromonas gingivalis*, it facilitates its escape from the host's immune interaction [128]. There is evidence that shows that oral cancer cells can promote autophagy as a response to the bacterial invasion, limiting in this manner the toxic environment and helping the malignant cells to survive [129]. The autophagy process is analyzed by Chen et al. [130], and they concluded that it could be a determining factor for the increased IL-1 production in the case of cancer cells that were infected with *P. gingivalis*.

The pathogenic bacteria specific for periodontal disease have an important immune-regulatory action, controlling the cytokines, the growth factors, and chemokines, disrupting the normal immune response of the host [131]. This action allows the promotion of carcinogenesis, the dissemination of the cancerous cells, while sustaining the multiplication of the periodontal pathogens [132]. *Porphyromonas gingivalis* has proven an intense immunosuppressive action through the activation of STAT3, a fact that will promote the production of immunosuppressive myeloid-derived tumor cells that will allow the proliferation of OSCC [133]. The immune control performed by the periodontal pathogenic agents, by reprogramming the immune cells, including the polymononuclear neutrophils, determines the continuous evolution of the gingival inflammation, a fact that can influence the development of OSCC [134].

Data from existing *in vitro* studies support the affirmation that the periodontal pathogens can promote the oral cancer progression. Extending the research by performing *in vivo* studies using an oral carcinoma mouse model, it revealed that *Fusobacterium nucleatum* exhibited the highest upregulation effect upon the oncogenes and IL-8 secretion, while *Porphyromonas gingivalis* showed a direct effect upon the MMP1, MMP9, and MYC. Nevertheless, in the case of the combined infection with both periodontal pathogens, the results were potentiated, showing that the mice that were in contact with both pathogens had more oral lesions compared to the group of mice that interacted with only one pathogen separately [135, 136].

Over time, multiple studies aimed to identify and characterize the microbial community associated with OSCC, using the next-generation sequencing (NGS) method [50, 137, 138]. Among the first links that have been found was in the study conducted by Nagy et al. [139], where high levels of *Porphyromonas* and *Fusobacterium* were observed in the OSCC samples compared to the controls. Nevertheless, currently, with the help of NGS, a complete profile of the tumor-specific microbial community can be performed in order to identify the specific bacteria within the samples.

In case of periodontal disease, all the results point out the importance of the bacterial community as a pathogen and trigger of oral cancer. The promotion of oral cancer and its progression is influenced by *Porphyromonas gingivalis* and *Fusobacterium nucleatum* [140]. However, in certain conditions, the interaction of *Porphyromonas gingivalis* can be antagonized by *Streptococcus gordonii* [141]. Nevertheless, there are more antagonistic actions present within the oral microbiome, and an important one is the interaction between *Lactobacillus plantarum,* which is part of the healthy flora, and *Porphyromonas gingivalis*, inhibiting its growth and oral cancer development by inducing cell apoptosis [142].

All these interactions between the oral microbial community will, at a certain point, determine a dysbiosis, a fact that will facilitate the periodontal disease development and a prolonged chronic inflammation that will promote the carcinogenic changes specific to oral cancer. It appears that the metabolic activities of the oral bacteria exhibit a bigger role in the pathogenesis of a disease than the bacterial community composition.

6. Conclusions

The presence of dysbiosis in the supra- and subgingival biofilm is an important trigger for chronic inflammation, contributing to the pathogenesis of periodontal disease. The presence of these periodontal pathogens is an important factor that has been linked to multiple oral and systemic diseases, through the persistence of inflammation, the modulation of the immune response, and the angiogenesis process.

The role of the periodontal pathogens has been acknowledged as a keystone, and numerous epidemiological studies discuss the link between periodontal disease and oral cancer. According to the results of multiple studies, periodontal pathogens could influence the development of cancer by controlling all the important mechanisms, such as proliferation, invasion, cell survival, and apoptosis, having a direct bacterial effect.

There are described certain combinations of different oral pathogens that have been proposed as indicators for the diagnosis of oral cancer. The development of OSCC is characterized by multiple processes, including abnormal cell proliferation, perturbed immune surveillance, a high invasion and metastasis capability, and a modified intrinsic cell apoptosis and angiogenesis process. It has been highlighted that certain oral bacteria, like *Fusobacterium nucleatum* and *Porphyromonas gingivalis*, are involved in the majority of the carcinogenesis pathways, sustaining the development of OSCC. Therefore, the dysbiosis of the oral environment, the diagnosis of periodontal diseases should be seen as a complex interaction between the oral pathogens and the host immune system, an interaction that, under certain conditions, could represent a risk factor for the development of oral cancer.

Author details

Alexandra Roi[1], Ciprian Ioan Roi[2]*, Mircea Rivis[2], Ruxandra Luca[3], Simina Boia[4] and Laura-Cristina Rusu[1]

1 University Clinic of Oral Pathology, Multidisciplinary Center for Research, Evaluation, Diagnosis and Therapies in Oral Medicine, “Victor Babeș” University of Medicine and Pharmacy, Timisoara, Romania

2 University Clinic of Anesthesiology and Oral Surgery, Research Center of Dento-Alveolar Surgery, Anesthesia and Sedation in Dental Medicine, “Victor Babes” University of Medicine and Pharmacy, Timișoara, Romania

3 University Clinic of Oral Rehabilitation and Dental Emergencies, Interdisciplinary Research Center for Dental Medical Research, Lasers and Innovative Technologies, “Victor Babes” University of Medicine and Pharmacy, Timișoara, Romania

4 University Clinic of Periodontology, Anton Sculean Research Center for Periodontal and Peri-Implant Diseases, “Victor Babes” University of Medicine and Pharmacy, Timișoara, Romania

*Address all correspondence to: ciprian.roi@umft.ro

References

[1] Bray F, Ferlay J, Soerjomataram I, Siegel RL, Torre LA, Jemal A. Global cancer statistics 2018: GLOBOCAN estimates of incidence and mortality worldwide for 36 cancers in 185 countries. CA: A Cancer Journal for Clinicians. 2018;**68**:394-424. DOI: 10.3322/caac.21492

[2] Perera M, Al-Hebshi N, Perera I, Ipe D, Ulett G, Speicher D. Inflammatory bacteriome and oral squamous cell carcinoma. Journal of Dental Research. 2018;**97**:725-732. DOI: 10.1177/0022034518767118

[3] Ranjbar R, Behzadi P, Farshad S. Advances in diagnosis and treatment of helicobacter pylori infection. Acta Microbiologica et Immunologica Hungarica. 2017;**64**:273-292. DOI: 10.1556/030.64.2017.008

[4] Li TJ, Hao YH, Tang YL, Liang XH. Periodontal pathogens: A crucial link between periodontal diseases and oral cancer. Frontiers in Microbiology. 2022;**13**:919633

[5] Mager DL. Bacteria and cancer: Cause, coincidence or cure? A review. Journal of Translational Medicine. 2006;**28**(4):14

[6] Perera M, Al-Hebshi NN, Speicher DJ, et al. Emerging role of bacteria in oral carcinogenesis: A review with special reference to perio-pathogenic bacteria. Journal of Oral Microbiology. 2016;**8**:32762

[7] D'Aiuto F, Parkar M, Andreou G, et al. Periodontitis and systemic inflammation: Control of the local infection is associated with a reduction in serum inflammatory markers. Journal of Dental Research. 2004;**83**:156-160

[8] Meyer MS, Joshipura K, Giovannucci E, et al. A review of the relationship between tooth loss, periodontal disease, and cancer. Cancer Causes & Control. 2008;**19**:895-907

[9] Ye L, Jiang Y, Liu W, et al. Correlation between periodontal disease and oral cancer risk: A meta-analysis. Journal of Cancer Research and Therapeutics. 2016;**12**:C237-CC40

[10] Holmes S. The oral complications of specific anticancer therapy. International Journal of Nursing Studies. 1991;**28**:343-360

[11] Yost S, Stashenko P, Choi Y, et al. Increased virulence of the oral microbiome in oral squamous cell carcinoma revealed by metatranscriptome analyses. International Journal of Oral Science. 2018;**12**(10):32

[12] Oji C, Chukwuneke F. Poor oral hygiene may be the sole cause of oral cancer. Journal of Oral and Maxillofacial Surgery. 2012;**11**:379-383

[13] Yu T, Guo F, Yu Y, et al. *Fusobacterium nucleatum* promotes chemoresistance to colorectal cancer by modulating autophagy. Cell. 2017;**27**(170):548-63e16

[14] Ha NH, Park DG, Woo BH, et al. *Porphyromonas gingivalis* increases the invasiveness of oral cancer cells by upregulating IL-8 and MMPs. Cytokine. 2016;**10**(86):64-72

[15] Falzone L, Marconi A, Loreto C, Franco S. Spandidos dA and Libra M: Occupational exposure to carcinogens: Benzene, pesticides and fibers (review). Molecular Medicine Reports. 2016;**14**:4467-4474

[16] Rapisarda V, Ledda C, Matera S, Fago L, Arrabito G, Falzone L, et al. Absence of t(14,18) chro- mosome translocation in agricultural workers after short-term exposure to pesticides. Molecular Medicine Reports. 2017;**15**:3379-3382

[17] Banna GL, Torino F, Marletta F, Santagati M, Salemi R, Cannarozzo E, et al. Lactobacillus rhamnosus GG: An overview to explore the rationale of its use in cancer. Frontiers in Pharmacology. 2017;**8**:603

[18] Dewhirst FE, Chen T, Izard J, Paster BJ, Tanner AC, Yu WH, et al. The human oral microbiome. Journal of Bacteriology. 2010;**192**:5002-5017

[19] Human Microbiome Project Consortium. A framework for human microbiome research. Nature. 2012;**486**:215-221

[20] Vesty A, Gear K, Biswas K, Radcliff FJ. Taylor MW and Douglas RG: Microbial and inflammatory-based salivary biomarkers of head and neck squamous cell carcinoma. Cllinical and Experimental Dental Research. 2018;**4**:255-262

[21] Yang T, Zubcevic J. Gut-brain axis in regulation of blood pressure. Frontiers in Physiology. 2017;**8**:845

[22] Atanasova KR, Yilmaz O. Looking in the *Porphyromonas gingivalis* cabinet of curiosities: The microbium, the host and cancer association. Molecular Oral Microbiology. 2014;**29**:55-66

[23] Katz J, Onate MD, Pauley KM, Bhattacharyya I, Cha S. Presence of *Porphyromonas gingivalis* in gingival squamous cell carcinoma. International Journal of Oral Science. 2011;**3**:209-215

[24] Mager DL, Haffajee AD, Devlin PM, Norris CM, Posner MR, Goodson JM. The salivary microbiota as a diagnostic indicator of oral cancer: A descriptive, non-randomized study of cancer- free and oral squamous cell carcinoma subjects. Journal of Translational Medicine. 2005;**3**:27

[25] WHO Regional Office for Europe. Available from: https://www.euro.who.int/en/health-topics/disease-prevention/oral-health/data-and-statistics

[26] Gopinath D, Menon RK, Veettil SK, Botelho MG, Johnson NW. Periodontal diseases as putative risk factors for head and neck cancer: Systematic review and meta-analysis. Cancers. 1893;**2020**:12

[27] Cardoso EM, Reis C, Manzanares-Céspedes MC. Chronic periodontitis, inflammatory cytokines, and interrelationship with other chronic diseases. Postgraduate Medicine. 2018;**130**:98-104

[28] Mehrotra N, Singh S. Periodontitis. Treasure Island, FL, USA: StatPearls Publishing; 2021

[29] Curtis MA, Diaz PI, van Dyke TE. The role of the microbiota in periodontal disease. Periodontology. 2000;**2020**(83):14-25

[30] Kinane DF, Stathopoulou PG, Papapanou PN. Periodontal dis- eases. Nature Reviews. Disease Primers. 2017;**3**:17038

[31] Janakiram C, Dye BA. A public health approach for prevention of periodontal disease. Periodontology 2000. 2000;**2020**(84):202-214

[32] Hajishengallis G, Chavakis T. Local and systemic mechanisms linking periodontal disease and inflammatory comorbidities. Nature Reviews Immunology. 2021;**21**:426-440

[33] Loe H, Theilade E, Jensen SB. Experimental gingivitis in man. Journal of Periodontology. 1930;**1965**(36):177-187

[34] Belstrom D, Damgaard C, Kononen E, Gursoy M, Holmstrup P, Gursoy UK. Salivary cytokine levels in early gingival inflammation. Journal of Oral Microbiology. 2017;**9**(1):1364101

[35] Bao K, Li X, Poveda L, et al. Proteome and microbiome mapping of human gingival tissue in health and disease. Frontiers in Cellular and Infection Microbiology. 2020;**10**:588155

[36] Shi M, Wei Y, Nie Y, et al. Alterations and correlations in microbial community and metabolome characteristics in generalized aggres- sive periodontitis. Frontiers in Microbiology. 2020;**11**:573196

[37] Van der Weijden F, Rijnen M, Valkenburg C. Comparison of three qPCR-based commercial tests for detection of periodontal patho- gens. Scientific Reports. 2021;**11**(1):6141

[38] Belstrom D, Paster BJ, Fiehn NE, Bardow A, Holmstrup P. Salivary bacterial fingerprints of established Oral disease re- vealed by the human Oral microbe identification using next generation sequencing (HOMINGS) technique. Journal of Oral Microbiology. 2016;**8**:30170

[39] Claesson R, Johansson A, Belibasakis GN. Clinical laboratory diag- nostics in dentistry: Application of microbiological methods. Frontiers in Oral Health. 2022;**3**:983991

[40] Hajishengallis G, Lamont RJ. Beyond the red complex and into more complexity: The polymicrobial synergy and dysbiosis (PSD) model of periodontal disease etiology. Molecular Oral Microbiology. 2012;**27**(6):409-419

[41] Hajishengallis G. The inflammophilic character of the periodontitis-associated microbiota. Molecular Oral Microbiology. 2014;**29**(6):248-257

[42] Hajishengallis G, Darveau RP, Curtis MA. The keystone-pathogen hypothesis. Nature Reviews. Microbiology. 2012;**10**(10):717-725

[43] Sedghi LM, Bacino M, Kapila YL. Periodontal disease: The good, the bad, and the unknown. Frontiers in Cellular and Infection Microbiology. 2021;**11**:766944

[44] Soder B, Yakob M, Meurman JH, Andersson LC, Klinge B, Soder PO. Periodontal disease may associate with breast cancer. Breast Cancer Research and Treatment. 2011;**127**(2):497-502

[45] Janket SJ, Javaheri H, Ackerson LK, Ayilavarapu S, Meurman JH. Oral infections, metabolic inflammation, genetics, and Cardiometabolic diseases. Journal of Dental Research. 2015;**94**(Suppl. 9):119S-127S

[46] Virtanen E. Degree ThesisChronic Dental Diseases and Systemic Health: Cardiovascular Diseases and Cancer. Helsinki: University of Helsinki and Helsinki University Hospital; 2018

[47] Pejcic A, Kesic L, Milasin J. Association between periodontopathogens and CRP levels in patients with periodontitis in Serbia. Journal of Dental Research Dental Clinics Dental Prospects. 2011;**5**:10-16

[48] Lamster IB, Lalla E, Borgnakke WS, Taylor GW. The relationship between oral health and diabetes mellitus. Journal of the American Dental Association (1939). 2008;**139**(Suppl.):19S-24S

[49] Nwizu N, Wactawski Wende J, Genco RJ. Periodontal disease and

cancer: Epidemiologic studies and possible mechanisms. Periodontology 2000. 2000;**83**(1):213-233

[50] Perera M, Al-Hebshi NN, Speicher DJ, Perera I, Johnson NW. Emerging role of bacteria in oral carcinogenesis: A review with special reference to perio-pathogenic bacteria. Journal of Oral Microbiology. 2016;**9**:8. DOI: 10.3402/jom.v8.32762

[51] Wei J, Xie G, Zhou Z, Shi P, Qiu Y, Zheng X, et al. Salivary metabolite signatures of oral cancer and leukoplakia. International Journal of Cancer. 2011;**129**:2207-2217. DOI: 10.1002/ijc.25881

[52] Huang M, ZhenZhao H, Chu G, Yang X, Ran S, Hu B, et al. Variations in oral microbiota associated with oral cancer. Scientific Reports. 2017;**7**:11773. DOI: 10.1038/s41598-017-11779-9

[53] Lee WH, Chen HM, Yang SF, Liang C, Peng CY, et al. Bacterial alterations in salivary microbiota and their association in oral cancer. Scientific Reports. 2017;**7**:16540

[54] Tanaka T, Ishigamori R. Understanding carcinogenesis for fighting oral cancer. Journal of Oncology. 2011;**2011**:603740. DOI: 10.1155/2011/603740

[55] Todd R, Donoff RB, Wong DT. The molecular biology of oral carcinogenesis: Toward a tumor progression model. Journal of Oral and Maxillofacial Surgery. 1997;**55**(6):613-623

[56] Bockmühl U, Wolf G, Schmidt S, Schwendel A, Jahnke V, Dietel M, et al. Genomic alterations associated with malignancy in head and neck cancer. Head & Neck. 1998;**20**(2):145-151. DOI: 10.1002/(sici)1097-0347(199803)20:2<145::aid-hed8>3.0.co;2-2

[57] Partridge M, Emilion G, Pateromichelakis S, A'Hern R, Lee G, Phillips E, et al. The prognostic significance of allelic imbalance at key chromosomal loci in oral cancer. British Journal of Cancer. 1999;**79**(11-12):1821-1827. DOI: 10.1038/sj.bjc.6690290

[58] Williams HK. Molecular pathogenesis of oral squamous carcinoma. Molecular Pathology. 2000;**53**(4):165-172. DOI: 10.1136/mp.53.4.165

[59] Ram H, Sarkar J, Kumar H, Konwar R, Bhatt ML, Mohammad S. Oral cancer: Risk factors and molecular pathogenesis. Journal of Oral and Maxillofacial Surgery. 2011;**10**(2):132-137. DOI: 10.1007/s12663-011-0195-z

[60] Gasche JA, Goel A. Epigenetic mechanisms in oral carcinogenesis. Future Oncology. 2012;**8**(11):1407-1425. DOI: 10.2217/fon.12.138

[61] Rivera C, Venegas B. Histological and molecular aspects of oral squamous cell carcinoma (review). Oncology Letters. 2014;**8**:7-11

[62] Jerjes W, Hamdoon Z, Rashed D, Hopper C. Advancing non-invasive diagnosis of Oral epithelial dysplasia: Comparative insights from In vivo optical coherence tomography and histopathology. Journal of Clinical Medicine. 2025;**14**(4):1118. DOI: 10.3390/jcm14041118

[63] Ho PS, Chen PL, Warnakulasuriya S, Shieh TY, Chen YK, Huang IY. Malignant transformation of oral potentially malignant disorders in males: A retrospective cohort study. BMC Cancer. 2009 Jul;**30**(9):260. DOI: 10.1186/1471-2407-9-260

[64] Gale N, Michaels L, Luzar B, Poljak M, Zidar N, Fischinger J, et al. Current review on squamous

intraepithelial lesions of the larynx. Histopathology. 2009;**54**(6):639-656. DOI: 10.1111/j.1365-2559.2008.03111.x

[65] Pitiyage G, Tilakaratne WM, Tavassoli M, Warnakulasuriya S. Molecular markers in oral epithelial dysplasia: Review. Journal of Oral Pathology & Medicine. 2009;**38**(10):737-752. DOI: 10.1111/j.1600-0714.2009.00804.x

[66] Baqai N, Amin R, Fatima T, Ahmed Z, Faiz N. Expression profiling of EMT transcriptional regulators ZEB1 and ZEB2 in different histopathological grades of Oral squamous cell carcinoma patients. Current Genomics. 2024;**25**(2):140-151. DOI: 10.2174/011389202928 4920240212091903

[67] Secretan B, Straif K, Baan R, Grosse Y, El Ghissassi F, Bouvard V, et al. WHO International Agency for Research on Cancer monograph working group. A review of human carcinogens-part E: Tobacco, areca nut, alcohol, coal smoke, and salted fish. The Lancet Oncology. 2009;**10**(11):1033-1034. DOI: 10.1016/s1470-2045(09)70326-2

[68] Chamoli A, Gosavi AS, Shirwadkar UP, Wangdale KV, Behera SK, Kurrey NK, et al. Overview of oral cavity squamous cell carcinoma: Risk factors, mechanisms, and diagnostics. Oral Oncology. 2021;**121**:105451. DOI: 10.1016/j.oraloncology.2021.105451

[69] Stornetta A, Guidolin V, Balbo S. Alcohol-derived acetaldehyde exposure in the Oral cavity. Cancers (Basel). 2018;**10**(1):20. DOI: 10.3390/cancers10010020

[70] Kawakita D, Matsuo K. Alcohol and head and neck cancer. Cancer Metastasis Reviews. 2017;**36**(3):425-434. DOI: 10.1007/s10555-017-9690-0

[71] Nokovitch L, Maquet C, Crampon F, Taihi I, Roussel L-M, Obongo R, et al. Oral cavity squamous cell carcinoma risk factors: State of the art. Journal of Clinical Medicine. 2023;**12**(9):3264. DOI: 10.3390/jcm12093264

[72] Melo BAC, Vilar LG, Oliveira NR, Lima PO, Pinheiro MB, Domingueti CP, et al. Human papillomavirus infection and oral squamous cell carcinoma - a systematic review. Brazilian Journal of Otorhinolaryngology. 2021;**87**(3):346-352. DOI: 10.1016/j.bjorl.2020.10.017

[73] Feller L, Altini M, Lemmer J. Inflammation in the context of oral cancer. Oral Oncology. 2013;**49**(9):887-892. DOI: 10.1016/j.oraloncology.2013.07.003

[74] Mantovani A, Pierotti MA. Cancer and inflammation: A complex relationship. Cancer Letters. 2008;**267**(2):180-181. DOI: 10.1016/j.canlet.2008.05.003

[75] Li TJ, Hao YH, Tang YL, Liang XH. Periodontal pathogens: A crucial link between periodontal diseases and Oral cancer. Frontiers in Microbiology. 2022;**30**(13):919633. DOI: 10.3389/fmicb.2022.919633. PMID: 35847109; PMCID: PMC9279119

[76] Pendyala G, Joshi S, Chaudhari S, Gandhage D. Links demystified: Periodontitis and cancer. Dental Research Journal. 2013;**10**(6):704-712

[77] Allavena P, Sica A, Solinas G, Porta C, Mantovani A. The inflammatory micro-environment in tumor progression: The role of tumor-associated macrophages. Critical Reviews in Oncology/Hematology. 2008;**66**(1):1-9. DOI: 10.1016/j.critrevonc.2007.07.004

[78] Bingle L, Brown NJ, Lewis CE. The role of tumour-associated macrophages

in tumour progression: Implications for new anticancer therapies. The Journal of Pathology. 2002;**196**(3):254-265. DOI: 10.1002/path.1027

[79] Geng S, Matsushima H, Okamoto T, Yao Y, Lu R, Page K, et al. Emergence, origin, and function of neutrophil-dendritic cell hybrids in experimentally induced inflammatory lesions in mice. Blood. 2013;**121**(10):1690-1700. DOI: 10.1182/blood-2012-07-445197

[80] Matsushima H, Geng S, Lu R, Okamoto T, Yao Y, Mayuzumi N, et al. Neutrophil differentiation into a unique hybrid population exhibiting dual phenotype and functionality of neutrophils and dendritic cells. Blood. 2013;**121**(10):1677-1689. DOI: 10.1182/blood-2012-07-445189

[81] Johansson A, Rudolfsson S, Hammarsten P, et al. Mast cells are novel independent prognostic markers in prostate cancer and represent a target for therapy. The American Journal of Pathology. 2010;**177**:1031-1041. DOI: 10.2353/ajpath.2010.100070

[82] Gudiseva S, Santosh ABR, Chitturi R, Anumula V, Poosarla C, Baddam VRR. The role of mast cells in oral squamous cell carcinoma. Contemporary Oncology. 2017;**21**(1):21-29. DOI: 10.5114/wo.2017.65157

[83] Cai XJ, Peng CR, Zhang JY, Li XF, Wang X, Han Y, et al. Mast cell infiltration and subtype promote malignant transformation of Oral Precancer and progression of Oral cancer. Cancer Research Communications. 2024;**4**(8):2203-2214. DOI: 10.1158/2767-9764.CRC-24-0169

[84] Davoine F, Sim A, Tang C, Fisher S, Ethier C, Puttagunta L, et al. Eosinophils in human oral squamous carcinoma; role of prostaglandin D2. Journal of Inflammation. 2013;**10**(1):4. DOI: 10.1186/1476-9255-10-4

[85] Dorta RG, Landman G, Kowalski LP, Lauris JR, Latorre MR, Oliveira DT. Tumour-associated tissue eosinophilia as a prognostic factor in oral squamous cell carcinomas. Histopathology. 2002;**41**:152-157

[86] Sutera S, Furchì OA, Pentenero M. Investigating tumor-infiltrating lymphocytes in the microenvironment of Oral squamous cell carcinoma (OSCC) and Oral potentially malignant disorders (OPMDs): Can they shift our perspective? A scoping review. Journal of Clinical Medicine. 2025;**14**(2):606. DOI: 10.3390/jcm14020606

[87] Quan H, Shan Z, Liu Z, Liu S, et al. The repertoire of tumor-infiltrating lymphocytes within the microenvironment of oral squamous cell carcinoma reveals immune dysfunction. Cancer Immunology, Immunotherapy. 2020;**69**(3):465-476

[88] Sayehmiri F, Sayehmiri K, Asadollahi K, et al. The prevalence rate of *Porphyromonas gingivalis* and its association with cancer: A systematic review and meta-analysis. International Journal of Immunopathology and Pharmacology. 2015;**28**:160-167

[89] Zhou Y, Meyle J, Groeger S. Periodontal pathogens and cancer development. Periodontology 2000. 2000;**96**(1):112-149. DOI: 10.1111/prd.12590

[90] Sobocki BK, Basset CA, Bruhn-Olszewska B, Olszewski P, Szot O, Kaźmierczak-Siedlecka K, et al. Molecular mechanisms leading from periodontal disease to cancer. International Journal of Molecular Sciences. 2022;**23**(2):970. DOI: 10.3390/ijms23020970

[91] Kamarajan P, Ateia I, Shin JM, Fenno JC, Le C, Zhan L, et al. Periodontal pathogens promote cancer aggressivity via TLR/MyD88 triggered activation of integrin/FAK signaling that is therapeutically reversible by a probiotic bacteriocin. PLoS Pathogens. 2020;**16**:e1008881. DOI: 10.1371/journal.ppat.1008881

[92] McIlvanna E, Linden GJ, Craig SG, Lundy FT, James JA. *Fusobacterium nucleatum* and oral cancer: A critical review. BMC Cancer. 2021;**21**(1):1212. DOI: 10.1186/s12885-021-08903-4

[93] Krisanaprakornkit S, Iamaroon A. Epithelial-mesenchymal transition in Oral squamous cell carcinoma. ISRN Oncology. 2012;**2012**:681469-681410. DOI: 10.5402/2012/681469

[94] Sun J, Tang Q, Yu S, Xie M, Zheng W, Chen G, et al. *F. nucleatum* facilitates oral squamous cell carcinoma progression via GLUT1-driven lactate production. eBioMedicine. 2023;**88**:104444. DOI: 10.1016/j.ebiom.2023.104444

[95] Tomofuji TI, Koichiro SA, Toshihiro A, Tetsuji E, Daisuke T, Naofumi Y, et al. Periodontitis and increase in circulating oxidative stres. Japanese Dental Science Review. 2009;**45**:46-51. DOI: 10.1016/j.jdsr.2008.12.002

[96] Nakamura H, Takada K. Reactive oxygen species in cancer: Current findings and future directions. Cancer Science. 2021;**112**(10):3945-3952. DOI: 10.1111/cas.15068

[97] Basic A, Dahlén G. Microbial metabolites in the pathogenesis of periodontal diseases: A narrative review. Frontiers in Oral Health. 2023;**14**(4):1210200. DOI: 10.3389/froh.2023.1210200

[98] Guerrero-Preston R, Godoy-Vitorino F, Jedlicka A, Rodríguez-Hilario A, et al. 16S rRNA amplicon sequencing identifies microbiota associated with oral cancer, human papilloma virus infection and surgical treatment. Oncotarget. 2016;7:51320-51334

[99] Perera M, Al-Hebshi NN, Perera I, Ipe D, et al. Inflammatory Bacteriome and Oral squamous cell carcinoma. Journal of Dental Research. 2018;**97**:725-732

[100] Zhao H, Chu M, Huang Z, Yang X, et al. Variations in oral microbiota associated with oral cancer. Scientific Reports. 2017;**7**:11773

[101] Al-Hebshi NN, Nasher AT, Maryoud MY, Homeida HE, et al. Inflammatory bacteriome featuring fusobacterium nucleatum and Pseudomonas aeruginosa identified in association with oral squamous cell carcinoma. Scientific Reports. 1834;**2017**:7

[102] Yang CY, Yeh YM, Yu HY, Chin CY, et al. Oral microbiota community dynamics associated with Oral squamous cell carcinoma staging. Frontiers in Microbiology. 2018;**9**:862

[103] Schmidt BL, Kuczynski J, Bhattacharya A, Huey B, Corby PM, et al. Changes in abundance of oral microbiota associated with oral cancer. PLoS One. 2014;**9**:e98741

[104] Long X, Wong CC, Tong L, Chu ESH, Ho Szeto C, et al. Peptostreptococcus anaerobius promotes colorectal carcinogenesis and modulates tumour immunity. Nature Microbiology. 2019;**4**:2319-2330

[105] Wang K, Huang Y, Zhang Z, Liao J, Ding Y, Fang X, et al. A preliminary

study of microbiota diversity in saliva and Bronchoalveolar lavage fluid from patients with primary bronchogenic carcinoma. Medical Science Monitor. 2019;**25**:2819-2834

[106] Gellatly SL, Hancock RE. Pseudomonas aeruginosa: New insights into pathogenesis and host defenses. Pathogens and Disease. 2013;**67**:159-173

[107] Elsen S, Collin-Faure V, Gidrol X, Lemercier C. The opportunistic pathogen Pseudomonas aeruginosa activates the DNA double-strand break signaling and repair pathway in infected cells. Cellular and Molecular Life Sciences. 2013;**70**:4385-4397

[108] Nobbs AH, Jenkinson HF, Jakubovics NS. Stick to your gums: Mechanisms of oral microbial adherence. Journal of Dental Research. 2011;**90**:1271-1278

[109] Zhang G, Chen R, Rudney JD. Streptococcus cristatus modulates the fusobacterium nucleatum-induced epithelial interleukin-8 response through the nuclear factor-kappa B pathway. Journal of Periodontal Research. 2011;**46**:558-567

[110] Theilade E, Wright WH, Jensen SB, Loe H. Experimental gingivitis in man. II. A longitudinal clinical and bacteriological investigation. Journal of Periodontal Research. 1966;**1**:1-13

[111] Yang SF, Huang HD, Fan WL, Jong YJ, Chen MK, Huang CN, et al. Compositional and functional variations of oral microbiota associated with the mutational changes in oral cancer. Oral Oncology. 2018;**77**:1-8

[112] Takahashi Y, Park J, Hosomi K, Yamada T, et al. Analysis of oral microbiota in Japanese oral cancer patients using 16S rRNA sequencing. The Journal of Oral Biosciences. 2019;**61**:120-128

[113] Mok SF, Karuthan C, Cheah YK, Ngeow WC, et al. The oral microbiome community variations associated with normal, potentially malignant disorders and malignant lesions of the oral cavity. The Malaysian Journal of Pathology. 2017;**39**:1-15

[114] Geng J, Song Q, Tang X, Liang X, Fan H, Peng H, et al. Co-occurrence of driver and passenger bacteria in human colorectal cancer. Gut Pathogens. 2014;**6**:26

[115] Li Q, Hu Y, Zhou X, Liu S, Han Q, Cheng L. Role of oral bacteria in the development of oral squamous cell carcinoma. Cancers. 2020;**12**(10):2797

[116] Ikebe M, Kitaura Y, Nakamura M, Tanaka H, et al. Lipopolysaccharide (LPS) increases the invasive ability of pancreatic cancer cells through the TLR4/MyD88 signaling pathway. Journal of Surgical Oncology. 2009;**100**:725-731

[117] Kuboniwa M, Hasegaw Y, Ma S, Shizukuishi S, Amano A, Lamont RJ, et al. Gingivalis accelerates gingival epithelial cell progression through the cell cycle. Microbes and Infection. 2008;**10**:122-128

[118] Bronzato JD, Bomfim RA, Edwards DH, Crouch D, Hector MP, Gomes B. Detection of fusobacterium in oral and head and neck cancer samples: A systematic review and meta-analysis. Archives of Oral Biology. 2020;**112**:104669

[119] Abdulkareem AA, Shelto RM, Landini G, Cooper PR, Milward MR. Periodontal pathogens promote epithelial-mesenchymal transition in oral squamous carcinoma cells in vitro. Cell Adhesion & Migration. 2018;**12**:127-137

[120] Binder Gallimidi A, Fischman S, Revach B, Bulvik R, Maliutina A, Rubinstein AM, et al. Periodontal pathogens *Porphyromonas gingivalis* and fusobacterium nucleatum promote tumor progression in an oral-specific chemical carcinogenesis model. Oncotarget. 2015;**6**:22613-22623

[121] Zhang L, Liu Y, Zheng HJ, Zhang CP. The Oral microbiota may have influence on Oral cancer. Frontiers in Cellular and Infection Microbiology. 2019;**9**:476

[122] Kuboniwa M, Hasegawa Y, Mao S, Shizukuishi S, Amano A, Lamont RJ. P. Gingivalis accelerates gingival epithelial cell progression through the cell cycle. Microbes and Infection. 2008;**10**:122-128. DOI: 10.1016/j.micinf.2007.10.011

[123] Behzadi P, Sameer AS, Nissar S, Banday MZ, Gajdács M, García-Perdomo HA, et al. Toll-like receptors: General molecular and structural biology. Journal of Immunology Research. 2021;**1**:1-21. DOI: 10.1155/2021/9914854

[124] Zhou Y, Sztukowska M, Wang Q, Inaba H, Potempa J, Scott DA. Noncanonical activation of β-catenin by *Porphyromonas gingivalis*. Infection and Immunity. 2015;**83**:3195-3203. DOI: 10.1128/IAI.00302-15

[125] Hoppe T, Kraus D, Novak N, Probstmeier R, Frentzen M, Wenghoefer M. Oral pathogens change proliferation properties of oral tumor cells by affecting gene expression of human defensins. Tumour Biology. 2016;**37**:13789-13798. DOI: 10.1007/s13277-016-5281-x

[126] Cho TJ, Wee SW, Woo VH, Choi JI, Kim SJ, Shi HI. *Porphyromonas gingivalis*-induced autophagy suppresses cell proliferation through G1 arrest in oral cancer cells. Archives of Oral Biology. 2014;**59**:370-378. DOI: 10.1016/j.archoralbio.2014.01.001

[127] Yao L, Jermanus C, Barbetta B, Choi C, Verbeke P, Ojcius DM. *Porphyromonas gingivalis* infection sequesters pro-apoptotic bad through Akt in primary gingival epithelial cells. Molecular Oral Microbiology. 2010;**25**:89-101. DOI: 10.1111/j.2041-1014.2010.00569.x

[128] Wei W, An Y, Fei D, Wang Q. Activation of autophagy in periodontal ligament mesenchymal stem cells promotes angiogenesis in periodontitis. Journal of Periodontology. 2018;**89**:718-727. DOI: 10.1002/JPER.17-0341

[129] Huang J, Brumell JH. Bacteria–autophagy interplay: A battle for survival. Nature Reviews. Microbiology. 2014;**12**:101-114. DOI: 10.1038/nrmicro3160

[130] Chen MF, Lu MS, Hsieh CC, Chen WC. *Porphyromonas gingivalis* promotes tumor progression in esophageal squamous cell carcinoma. Cellular Oncology. 2021;**2021**(44):373-384. DOI: 10.1007/s13402-020-00573-x

[131] Hajishengallis G, Lambris JD. Complement and Dysbiosis in periodontal disease. Immunobiology. 2012;**2012**(217):1111-1116. DOI: 10.1016/j.imbio.2012.07.007

[132] Elebyary O, Barbour A, Fine N, Tenenbaum HC, Glogauer M. The crossroads of periodontitis and Oral squamous cell carcinoma: Immune implications and tumor promoting capacities. Frontiers in Oral Health. 2021;**2021**:1. DOI: 10.3389/froh.2020.584705

[133] Arjunan P, Meghil MM, Pi W, Xu J, Lang L, et al. Oral Pathobiont

activates anti-apoptotic pathway, promoting both immune suppression and oncogenic cell proliferation. Scientific Reports. 2018;**8**:16607. DOI: 10.1038/s41598-018-35126-8

[134] Lewkowicz N, Mycko MP, Przygodzka P, Ćwiklińska H, et al. Induction of human IL-10-producing neutrophils by LPS-stimulated Treg cells and IL-10. Mucosal Immunology. 2016;**9**:364-378. DOI: 10.1038/mi.2015.66

[135] Binder Gallimidi A, Fischman S, Revach B, et al. Periodontal pathogens *Porphyromonas gingivalis* and *Fusobacterium nucleatum* promote tumor progression in an oral-specific chemical carcinogenesis model. Oncotarget. 2015;**8**(6):22613-22623

[136] Rossa C Jr, D'Silva NJ. Immune-relevant aspects of murine models of head and neck cancer. Oncogene. 2019;**29**(38):3973-3988

[137] Pushalkar S, Mane SP, Ji X, Li Y, Evans C, Crasta OR, et al. Microbial diversity in saliva of oral squamous cell carcinoma. FEMS Immunology and Medical Microbiology. 2011;**61**(3):269-277. DOI: 10.1111/j.1574-695X.2010.00773.x

[138] Pushalkar S, Ji X, Li Y, Estilo C, Yegnanarayana R, Singh B, et al. Comparison of oral microbiota in tumor and non-tumor tissues of patients with oral squamous cell carcinoma. BMC Microbiology. 2012;**12**(1):144. DOI: 10.1186/1471-2180-12-144

[139] Nagy K, Sonkodi I, Szöke I, Nagy E, Newman H. The microflora associated with human oral carcinomas. Oral Oncology. 1998;**34**:304-308

[140] Lee J, Robert JS, Atanasova KR, Chowdhury N, Han K, Yilmaz Ö. Human primary epithelial cells acquire an epithelial-mesenchymal-transition phenotype during long-term infection by the oral opportunistic pathogen, *Porphyromonas gingivalis*. Frontiers in Cellular and Infection Microbiology. 2017B;**7**:493. DOI: 10.3389/fcimb.2017.00493

[141] Ohshima J, Wang Q, Fitzsimonds ZR, Miller DP, Sztukowska MN, Jung YJ. *Streptococcus gordonii* programs epithelial cells to resist ZEB2 induction by *Porphyromonas gingivalis*. Proceedings of the National Academy of Sciences. 2019;**116**:8544-8553. DOI: 10.1073/pnas.1900101116

[142] Pudgar P, Povšič K, Cuk K, Seme K, Petelin M, Gašperšič R. Probiotic strains of lactobacillus brevis and lactobacillus plantarum as adjunct to non-surgical periodontal therapy: 3-month results of a randomized controlled clinical trial. Clinical Oral Investigations. 2021;**25**:1411-1422. DOI: 10.1007/s00784-020-03449-4

Chapter 8

The Use of Bacterial Lysates, an Alternative in the Prevention and Treatment of Periodontitis

Diana-Larisa Ancuța and Cristin Coman

Abstract

The chapter explores the potential of bacterial lysates as innovative biotherapeutics for preventing and treating periodontitis. These bacterial fragments, with immunomodulatory properties, may offer multiple therapeutic advantages by stimulating innate and adaptive immune responses in the oral cavity, having the ability to modulate oral microbiome dysbiosis, and may reduce the expression of proinflammatory cytokines involved in the destruction of periodontal tissue while regulating tissue protective factors. The experimental and clinical results presented in this chapter suggest that the oral application of specific bacterial lysates may reduce clinical parameters (probing depth, attachment loss, and bleeding on probing), inflammatory processes, and contribute to the establishment of a favorable host-microbiome balance that may prevent the occurrence of periodontitis. Current evidence supports the use of bacterial lysates in managing periodontitis, and controlled studies (*in vitro* and *in vivo*) contribute to establishing optimal formulation, dosing regimens, and long-term efficacy.

Keywords: periodontitis, bacterial lysate, oral microbiome, immunomodulatory activity, inflammatory response

1. Introduction

Bacterial lysates are substances obtained by mechanical or chemical lysis of bacterial cells, resulting in a complex mixture of bacterial components with immunomodulatory potential. These products were initially used with considerable success in the treatment and prevention of respiratory diseases, but their applications have gradually spread to other medical fields, including oral pathology [1].

Periodontitis is a chronic inflammatory condition caused by imbalances in the oral microbiome and aberrant host immune response, leading to progressive destruction of the supporting tissues of the teeth [2]. Despite significant advances in conventional therapies, including mechanical debridement, local or systemic antibiotic therapy, and surgical intervention, many cases remain refractory to treatment or frequently relapse [3]. This clinical reality emphasizes the need for the development of alternative therapeutic approaches, among which bacterial lysates represent a promising option.

The aim of this chapter is to analyze the potential use of bacterial lysates in the treatment of periodontitis, based on their demonstrated success in other conditions and exploring the mechanisms by which they could positively influence the course of periodontal disease.

The use of bacterial lysates in medical practice dates back to the first half of the twentieth century, when the first preparations were developed for the treatment of recurrent respiratory infections [4]. The concept was based on the observation that exposure to bacterial antigens may stimulate the immune system and confer protection against subsequent infections.

The first bacterial lysates were obtained from bacterial strains commonly implicated in respiratory tract infections, such as *Streptococcus pneumoniae*, *Haemophilus influenzae*, *Klebsiella pneumoniae*, and *Moraxella catarrhalis* [5]. These preparations were initially administered as oral or sublingual vaccines to stimulate local and systemic immunity.

Numerous clinical studies have demonstrated the efficacy of bacterial lysates in reducing the frequency, severity, and duration of respiratory infections in both children and adults [6, 7]. A meta-analysis published by Cazzola et al. [6] showed that the administration of bacterial lysates reduced the risk of recurrence of respiratory infections in children by approximately 40% [8].

OM-85 (Broncho-Vaxom®), one of the most studied bacterial lysates, has demonstrated efficacy in:

- Reducing the frequency of acute respiratory infections in children and adults [9],
- Decreasing the need for antibiotics [10],
- Reducing days of school absenteeism or work disability [11],
- Improved quality of life for patients with recurrent respiratory infections [1].

Bacterial lysates have also been shown to be useful in the management of chronic respiratory diseases such as chronic bronchitis, chronic obstructive pulmonary disease (COPD), and bronchial asthma. In patients with COPD, the administration of bacterial lysates has been associated with a reduction in the frequency of exacerbations and improvement in symptoms [12].

The beneficial effects of bacterial lysates in respiratory diseases are mediated by multiple immunomodulatory mechanisms and consist of:

- *Stimulation of innate immunity*: Activation of dendritic cells and macrophages through the interaction of bacterial components with molecular pattern recognition receptors (PRRs) such as Toll-like receptors (TLRs) [13].
- *Stimulation of acquired immunity*: Induction of T and B lymphocyte response, with production of specific antibodies, including secretory Immunoglobulin A (IgA) in mucosal mucosa [14].
- *Anti-inflammatory effects*: Modulation of pro-inflammatory and anti-inflammatory cytokine production, with restoration of a favorable balance [15].
- *Barrier effect*: Improve the barrier function of the respiratory mucosa and reduce bacterial adhesion [16].
- *Effects on microbiome*: Restoring a balanced microbiome in the airways [17].

The success of bacterial lysates in respiratory diseases has stimulated research into their applications in other medical applications.

Bacterial lysates have been studied in various *gastrointestinal disorders*, demonstrating beneficial effects in inflammatory bowel disease (IBD) where probiotic lysates have shown potential in reducing intestinal inflammation and improving the intestinal barrier in experimental models of colitis [18]. In irritable bowel syndrome, certain preparations have been shown to relieve symptoms and normalize the gut microbiome [19], and in enteropathogenic infections, bacterial lysates have been shown to reduce the duration of acute diarrhea and prevent recurrences [20].

In *dermatology*, bacterial lysates have shown promising results in atopic dermatitis by reducing the severity of lesions and the frequency of exacerbations [21], in acne, where these preparations modulated the immune response to *Propionibacterium acnes*, and in chronic inflammatory skin diseases, demonstrating anti-inflammatory and immunomodulatory effects [22, 23].

In *otorhinolaryngology*, bacterial lysates have been useful in ear diseases, especially in reducing the number of acute episodes and antibiotic administration in recurrent otitis media. In chronic rhinosinusitis, they helped to relieve symptoms and reduce the frequency of exacerbations, and in chronic tonsillitis, bacterial lysates modulated the local immune response and reduced infectious episodes [24].

In *oral pathology*, the use of bacterial lysates has been extended to various diseases such as recurrent aphthous stomatitis with a reducing effect on the frequency and severity of lesions [25], oral infections where bacterial lysates have acted as an adjuvant in the treatment of bacterial and fungal infections [26], and in patients with oral mucositis following chemotherapy, where it was possible to reduce the severity and accelerate healing [27].

2. Bacterial lysates methods of obtaining and processing

The process of obtaining bacterial lysates starts with the careful selection of the bacterial strains relevant to the targeted pathology. In the case of preparations for respiratory conditions, common pathogenic strains of the respiratory tract are used, whereas for oral conditions, including periodontitis, species associated with the oral microbiome are selected [28].

To obtain lysates for periodontal therapy, bacterial strains may include:

- Primary or "red complex" periodontopathogens: *Porphyromonas gingivalis, Aggregatibacter actinomycetemcomitans, Tannerella forsythia,*
- Secondary periodontopathogens ("orange complex"): *Prevotella intermedia, Fusobacterium nucleatum, Campylobacter rectus,*
- Commensal species with immunomodulatory potential: *Streptococcus salivarius, Streptococcus sanguinis, Veillonella spp.*, and so on.

There are several bacterial lysis methods for obtaining lysates, each with specific advantages and limitations.

Therefore, mechanical lysis can be achieved by ultrasonication of bacterial strains using ultrasonic waves that destroy cell walls. Other methods of mechanical lysis involve applying very high pressure to break the cell wall [29] or fragmenting the bacterial bodies using glass or ceramic beads [30].

Chemical lysis involves the use of detergents (surface-active substances that solubilize cell membranes), organic solvents (allowing the extraction of cellular components by selective solubilization), or alkaline or acidic agents, the latter method hydrolyzing cellular structures under extreme pH conditions [31, 32].

Enzymatic lysis of bacteria is a complex process of cellular degradation mediated by specific enzymes that act synergistically to destroy structural and functional components of the bacterial cell. This process involves three main mechanisms:

- Lysozyme attacks peptidoglycan, the essential structural component of the bacterial cell wall. This enzyme catalyzes the hydrolysis of the β-1,4 bonds between N-acetylglucosamine and N-acetylmuramic acid in peptidoglycan chains. Damage to the cell wall compromises the structural integrity of the bacteria, making it susceptible to osmotic lysis and exposing the plasma membrane to the action of other lytic agents [33].

- Nucleases attack bacterial genetic material, fragmenting deoxyribonucleic acid (DNA) and ribonucleic acid (RNA) by hydrolyzing phosphodiester bonds between nucleotides. This action compromises the bacterium's ability to replicate and synthesize essential proteins, leading to cessation of cellular functions and ultimately cell death [34].

- Together, these lytic enzymes create a cascade effect that compromises the structural integrity, metabolic functionality, and replicative capacity of bacteria, representing an important mechanism in the defense of host organisms against bacterial infections and being exploited in multiple biotechnological and therapeutic applications.

Of the methods described, the most used is the mechanical one, but combined methods can also be used to obtain these preparations, involving the application of osmotic shocks together with enzymatic treatments, correlation of freeze-thaw cycles combined with sonication or chemical treatments followed by mechanical lysis [35, 36].

After obtaining the crude lysate, it is subjected to processing steps to improve quality and stability. The first step is purification, which consists in the removal of undesirable components by centrifugation, filtration, or chromatographic techniques, followed by fractionation to separate the different components of the lysate according to their physicochemical properties [10] and standardization, which ensures a constant content of active products in the final preparation [37]. The last step involves the formulation of bacterial lysates into pharmaceutical forms suitable for the route of administration, currently available as tablets, suspensions, or gels [38].

Before being marketed, bacterial lysate preparation undergoes rigorous quality control tests that include microbiological (to verify the absence of viable microorganisms), biochemical (for protein content, nucleic acids, and other active components), immunological (to assess immunomodulatory activity in vitro), and stability (to assess the maintenance of properties during the shelf life) [39–42].

3. Mechanisms of action of bacterial lysates in periodontitis

As described in **Figure 1**, bacterial lysates have immunomodulatory, anti-inflammatory, and tissue regeneration actions, which together significantly improve clinical signs.

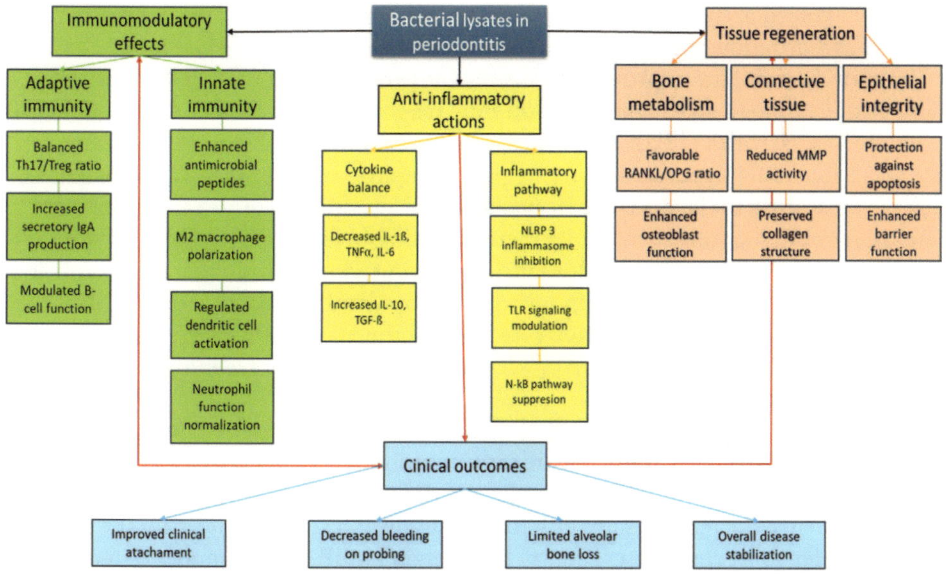

Figure 1.
A diagram of the mechanisms of bacterial lysis in periodontitis.

3.1 Modulation of the local immune response

Bacterial lysates are complex biological preparations obtained by mechanical, chemical, or enzymatic lysis of selected bacterial cultures to preserve intact antigenic structures and remove potentially toxic components. In the context of periodontal pathology, these preparations exert pleiotropic effects on the local immune system, helping to restore immune homeostasis disrupted during periodontitis.

3.1.1 Effects on innate immunity

Bacterial lysates interact with dendritic cells (DCs) and gingival macrophages *via* PRRs, inducing their modulated activation. In contrast to living bacteria that induce excessive and persistent activation of these cells, bacterial lysates promote a controlled activation phenotype characterized by:

- Moderate increase in the expression of co-stimulatory molecules (CD80, CD86) on the surface of dendritic cells, favoring efficient antigenic presentation,
- Induction of the production of Interlukin 10 (IL-10) and Transforming growth factor-beta (TGF-β) by gingival macrophages, mediators involved in limiting the excessive inflammatory response,
- Reduced secretion of pro-inflammatory mediators such as Interleukin 1β (IL-1β), and Tumoral Necrosis Factor α (TNF-α) involved in periodontal tissue destruction,
- Polarization of macrophages towards the regenerative and anti-inflammatory M2 phenotype at the expense of the pro-inflammatory M1 phenotype.

This balanced activation contributes to the elimination of periodontal pathogens without exacerbation of the destructive inflammatory response [43].

In periodontitis, the expression and sensitivity of TLR receptors is significantly increased, leading to an exaggerated immune response to bacterial components such as lipopolysaccharides (LPS). Bacterial lysates intervene in this process by reducing TLR2 and TLR4 hypersensitivity in gingival epithelial and myeloid epithelial cells, contributing to the decrease in the excessive production of pro-inflammatory cytokines, inducing tolerance to LPS by modulating Myeloid differentiation primary response 88 (MyD88) and (TIR-domain-containing adapter-inducing interferon-β (TRIF)-dependent intracellular signaling pathways, and downregulating TLR9 expression in gingival B cells, thereby decreasing the exaggerated response to bacterial DNA and rebalancing the ratio of activator and inhibitory receptors of the innate immune response.

These effects lead to interruption of the inflammatory vicious cycle characteristic of periodontitis without compromising antimicrobial defense capacity [44].

Gingival epithelial cells are the first line of defense against periodontopathogenic microorganisms. Bacterial lysates enhance their antimicrobial activity by the induction of β-defensins expression (Human β-defensin 2—hBD-2, Human β-defensin 3—hBD-3) in the gingival epithelium; the stimulation of LL-37 cathelicidin production, with direct bactericidal effect on periodontal pathogens; the increase of calprotectin and lipocalin secretion, with role in sequestering essential nutrients for bacteria (zinc, iron); and the amplification of bactericidal permeability-increasing protein (BPI) production, with specific effect on Gram-negative bacteria. All these mechanisms make bacterial lysates contribute to the control of the subgingival bacterial load, without inducing the bacterial resistance observed with conventional antibiotics [45].

3.1.2 Effects on acquired immunity

Bacterial lysates have an important role in inducing a balanced T lymphocyte response, so the imbalance between T lymphocyte subpopulations is essential in the pathogenesis of periodontitis. These changes contribute to the establishment of an immunologic microenvironment favorable to tissue regeneration and limit the progression of periodontal disease.

Secretory immunoglobulin A (sIgA) is the first line of humoral defense in the mucosa, including the gingival sulcus. Bacterial lysates amplify this protective mechanism by increasing the differentiation of IgA-producing plasma cells in gingival lymphoid follicles, stimulating the expression of the polymeric immunoglobulin receptor (pIgR) on epithelial cells (facilitating IgA transport into the gingival crevicular fluid), inducing isotype switching of B lymphocytes towards predominant IgA production (under the influence of TGF-β and IL-10), and increasing the specificity of IgA antibodies to surface antigens of key periodontal pathogens (*Porphyromonas gingivalis*, *Tannerella forsythia*, *Treponema denticola*). Thus, bacterial lysates help to neutralize pathogens and prevent their adhesion to epithelial surfaces, limiting tissue invasion and systemic activation of the immune response [46].

B lymphocytes participate in the pathogenesis of periodontitis not only by antibody production but also by cytokine secretion and antigenic presentation. Bacterial lysates influence these functions by reducing the differentiation of B lymphocytes into IgG-producing plasmablasts involved in hypersensitive reactions and immune complex formation, decreasing the secretion of receptor activator of nuclear factor kappa beta (RANKL) by activated B lymphocytes (thus limiting osteoclast activation), modulating the production of Interleukin 6 (IL-6) and TNF-α by B cells (cytokines with a central role in amplifying the local inflammatory response), inducing IL-10 expression by the regulatory B lymphocyte subset (contributing to the control of inflammation and promoting tissue regeneration), and limiting the formation of tertiary lymphoid structures in periodontal tissues, structures associated with severe forms of periodontitis. Through these complex effects, bacterial lysates contribute to restoring the local immune balance, facilitating the transition from a predominantly pro-inflammatory and destructive response to a regulated one, favorable to healing and tissue regeneration [47].

3.2 Molecular mechanisms of anti-inflammatory action in periodontitis

Periodontitis is a complex chronic inflammatory condition affecting the supporting structures of the teeth, characterized by an unbalanced immuno-inflammatory response to pathogens in the subgingival biofilm. Modern therapeutic approaches go beyond conventional mechanical treatment and focus on modulating the host response through targeted pharmacological interventions. Recent research has revealed multiple molecular mechanisms by which natural and synthetic therapeutic agents exert beneficial anti-inflammatory effects in the treatment of periodontitis. These mechanisms can be classified into three main categories: modulation of cytokine production, effects on immune cells, and effects on structural cells of periodontal tissues.

3.2.1 Modulation of cytokine production

3.2.1.1 Reduction of pro-inflammatory cytokines

An essential component of the anti-inflammatory effect in periodontitis is the ability of therapeutic agents to modulate the balance between pro- and anti-inflammatory cytokines. Numerous bioactive substances have been shown to significantly reduce the levels of pro-inflammatory cytokines such as IL-1β, IL-6, and TNF-α, which play central roles in the initiation and perpetuation of the periodontal inflammatory response [48]. These cytokines are predominantly produced by macrophages and other immune cells in response to microbial stimuli and cause amplification of the inflammatory cascade by activating transcription factors such as NF-κB and AP-1 [49].

Recent studies by Bunte et al. [50] have shown that curcumin derivatives reduce TNF-α and IL-1β expression in gingival epithelial cells stimulated with bacterial lipopolysaccharide, suggesting the potential of these compounds in the management of periodontitis.

3.2.1.2 Stimulation of anti-inflammatory cytokines

Concomitant with the suppression of pro-inflammatory cytokines, a stimulation of the production of anti-inflammatory cytokines, in particular IL-10 and TGF-β, is observed, which exert protective effects on periodontal tissues [51]. IL-10 limits the excessive inflammatory response and promotes resolution of inflammation, while TGF-β facilitates the healing and tissue regeneration processes through its effects on fibroblasts and other cells involved in tissue remodeling.

Research by Sima and Van Dyke [51] showed that omega-3 fatty acids stimulate IL-10 production in tissue macrophages, contributing to the restoration of immune homeostasis in periodontal tissues. Also, Kebschull and co-workers [52] demonstrated that some statins increase TGF-β expression in gingival fibroblasts and endothelial cells, suggesting beneficial effects beyond their known hypolipidemic action.

3.2.1.3 Inhibition of the NOD-like receptor protein 3 (NLRP3) inflammasome

A significant aspect of cytokine modulation is the inhibition of the activation of the NLRP3 inflammasome, a multi-protein complex involved in the pathogenesis of periodontitis [53]. Activation of the NLRP3 inflammasome leads to the processing and release of IL-1β and IL-18, amplifying the inflammatory response. Studies by Isola and co-workers [53] showed increased levels of NLRP3 inflammasome components in periodontal tissues of periodontitis patients compared to healthy subjects, emphasizing the role of this complex in the pathogenesis of the disease.

Huang et al. [54] demonstrated that *Ginkgo biloba* extracts inhibit NLRP3 inflammasome activation in lipopolysaccharide- and ATP-stimulated macrophages, suggesting a potential mechanism for the anti-inflammatory effects of these extracts in periodontitis. Similarly, Yamaguchi and co-workers [55] showed that resveratrol reduces NLRP3 inflammasome activation in gingival fibroblasts exposed to *Porphyromonas gingivalis*, contributing to attenuation of IL-1β release and limiting the destructive inflammatory response.

3.2.2 Effects on immune cells

3.2.2.1 Modulation of neutrophil activity

Imbalanced immune response is a defining feature of periodontitis. Anti-inflammatory therapeutic agents exert complex effects on the immune cells involved in this pathology. An important effect is the reduced recruitment and activation of neutrophils in periodontal tissues [56]. Although neutrophils are the first line of defense against pathogens, their excessive and persistent activation in periodontitis leads to the release of proteolytic enzymes and reactive oxygen species that contribute to tissue destruction.

Serhan and co-workers [56] demonstrated that resolvins and protectins, specialized lipid mediators derived from omega-3 fatty acids, reduce neutrophil infiltration into periodontal tissues and promote their efflux from inflammatory sites, facilitating resolution of inflammation. Studies by Hasturk et al. [57] on animal models of periodontitis showed that treatment with resolvin E1 significantly reduces neutrophil influx and prevents alveolar bone resorption, suggesting the therapeutic potential of these mediators in the management of periodontitis.

3.2.2.2 Macrophage polarization

It has also been observed that many anti-inflammatory agents promote macrophage polarization towards the M2 phenotype, with anti-inflammatory and regenerative properties [57]. M2 macrophages secrete anti-inflammatory growth factors and cytokines that facilitate resolution of inflammation and promote tissue regeneration, in contrast to pro-inflammatory M1 macrophages that amplify the inflammatory response and contribute to periodontal destruction.

Lam and co-workers [58] demonstrated that statin derivatives induce macrophage polarization towards the M2 phenotype in periodontal tissues, associated with reduced expression of pro-inflammatory mediators and increased levels of IL-10 and arginase-1, characteristic markers of M2 macrophages.

3.2.2.3 Inhibition of osteoclastic activity

A crucial aspect in the prevention of periodontitis-associated bone resorption is the inhibition of osteoclast activity mediated by the RANKL/RANK/OPG system [59]. By reducing the expression of RANKL (receptor activator receptor kappa B ligand) and/or increasing osteoprotegerin (OPG) levels, anti-inflammatory agents limit osteoclast formation and activation, thereby preventing alveolar bone resorption and maintaining the structural integrity of the dental supporting apparatus.

Graves and co-workers [59] demonstrated that bisphosphonates inhibit osteoclast differentiation and activity in experimental models of periodontitis, preventing alveolar bone resorption and tooth loss. Nakamura et al. [60] showed that probiotics reduce RANKL expression and increase OPG levels in periodontal tissues, helping to maintain the balance between bone resorption and bone formation. These findings emphasize the importance of modulating the RANKL/RANK/OPG system in the management of periodontitis and prevention of its complications.

3.2.3 Effects on structural cells

3.2.3.1 Modulation of matrix metalloproteinase production

In addition to modulating the immune response, anti-inflammatory agents exert direct effects on the structural cells of periodontal tissues, contributing to their protection and regeneration. An important action is to reduce the production of matrix metalloproteinases (MMPs) by gingival fibroblasts [61]. MMPs are proteolytic enzymes involved in the degradation of the extracellular matrix during periodontitis. By limiting the expression and activity of these enzymes, the degradation of collagen fibers and other extracellular matrix components is reduced, preventing loss of clinical attachment and progression of periodontitis.

Studies by Ebersole and coworkers [61] showed that subantimicrobial doses of doxycycline inhibited MMP-8 and MMP-9 activity in the gingival crevicular fluid of periodontitis patients, this effect being independent of its antimicrobial action.

3.2.3.2 Epithelial cell protection

Anti-inflammatory agents also exert cytoprotective effects on gingival epithelial cells, protecting them against apoptosis induced by bacterial factors [62]. Maintaining the integrity of the epithelial barrier is essential in limiting bacterial invasion and the subsequent inflammatory response. By protecting epithelial cells, the barrier function of the gingival epithelium is maintained, reducing the exposure of underlying tissues to pathogens and their products.

Martins et al. [62] demonstrated that resveratrol protects gingival epithelial cells against apoptosis induced by *Porphyromonas gingivalis* by inhibiting the JAK/STAT signaling pathway, contributing to the maintenance of epithelial integrity. Similarly, Lee et al. [63] showed that curcumin reduces apoptosis of gingival epithelial cells exposed to bacterial lipopolysaccharides by modulating the production of reactive oxygen species and activating cell survival pathways.

3.2.3.3 Stimulation of osteoblasts

Finally, numerous anti-inflammatory agents have been shown to stimulate the proliferation and differentiation of osteoblasts, the cells responsible for alveolar bone formation [59]. This effect, combined with the inhibition of osteoclastic activity, contributes to the rebalancing of bone remodeling processes in favor of new bone formation, facilitating the regeneration of lost bone tissue and the stabilization of teeth affected by periodontitis.

Chen et al. [64] demonstrated that vitamin D derivatives stimulate osteoblast differentiation and the expression of bone matrix proteins in cell cultures, suggesting a potential role in periodontal bone regeneration. Kobayashi et al. [65] also showed that statins increase the expression of vascular endothelial growth factor (VEGF) and bone morphogenetic protein-2 (BMP-2) in osteoblasts, promoting angiogenesis and osteogenesis in periodontal tissues.

4. The use of bacterial lysates in preclinical studies regarding periodontitis

Bacterial lysates are an emerging category of biologically active products with therapeutic potential in various inflammatory pathologies, including periodontal diseases. In preclinical studies, their use has been explored to reduce inflammation, combat oral dysbiosis, and support the regeneration of affected periodontal tissues.

Several *in vitro* and *in vivo* studies have demonstrated the ability of bacterial lysates to modulate the local immune response and influence the composition of the oral microbiota. For example, an *in vitro* study showed that lysates from *Lactobacillus plantarum* and *Lactobacillus rhamnosus* GG reduce the expression of inflammatory mediators induced by *Porphyromonas gingivalis* and inhibit the formation of *Streptococcus mutans* biofilm, thus supporting an anti-inflammatory and antibacterial action [66]. In another study on the toxicity of lysates of *Streptococcus oralis*, *Fusobacterium nucleatum*, and *Aggregatibcter actinomycetemcomitans*, the lack of negative effects on cell cultures and even inhibition of bacterial growth was proven when the cultures were contacted with the mentioned bacterial lysates [67].

In an animal model of experimental periodontitis, the administration of bacterial lysates was comparable in efficacy to antibiotic treatments, leading to a reduction in gingival inflammation and a decrease in leukocyte counts, as well as the elimination of some pathogenic bacterial strains [68]. Other research has indicated that lysates can protect oral epithelial cells by stimulating the secretion of proinflammatory cytokines and strengthening the integrity of the epithelial barrier, suggesting a role in maintaining oral mucosal homeostasis [69].

In addition, the administration of lyophilized probiotics in the form of lysates, such as *Lactobacillus paracasei* and *Bifidobacterium animalis*, has demonstrated the ability to modulate the subgingival microbiota by reducing the prevalence of pathogenic bacterial species involved in periodontitis, such as *Fusobacterium spp*. [70].

An important contribution to the literature is also the histological study conducted on rats with experimental periodontitis, in which the administration of bacterial lysates (Respibron) resulted in significant regeneration of periodontal tissues and a reduction in the severity of inflammation. Compared to a standard immunostimulatory agent (Imudon), the efficiency of the lysates was more than threefold superior in terms of the histological and morphometric parameters evaluated [71].

Preclinical data suggest that bacterial lysates may constitute a promising therapeutic strategy in the treatment of periodontitis, through immunomodulatory, anti-inflammatory and probiotic actions, with the potential to support the regeneration of affected tissues and restore the balance of the oral microbiome.

5. Research limitations and perspectives

The use of bacterial lysates in the treatment of periodontitis, although promising, faces several limitations that must be considered. First, the heterogeneity of the preparations represents a significant challenge. There is a great variety in the composition and methods of obtaining the lysates, which makes their standardization difficult. This variability may influence the effectiveness of the treatment and the comparability of the results between studies.

Second, the scientific evidence supporting the use of these preparations is still limited. The small number of long-term randomized clinical trials and the variability of the administration and evaluation protocols emphasize the need for further research. It is essential to conduct comparative studies with standard therapies to truly evaluate the effectiveness of bacterial lysates in the treatment of periodontitis.

Finally, biological limitations cannot be ignored. Individual response to treatment can vary significantly, and the immunogenic potential of lysates may depend on the patient's genetic profile. Also, the effectiveness of treatment may be reduced in severe or complicated cases, suggesting that not all individuals benefit equally from this therapeutic approach.

Although bacterial lysates are generally considered safe, it is important to consider certain safety aspects. Potential adverse reactions may include local irritation, discomfort, and taste changes, as well as rare systemic reactions such as transient fever or headache. In very rare cases, allergic reactions such as skin rash or bronchospasm may occur. There are also relative contraindications that must be observed. People with hypersensitivity to the components of the preparation, uncontrolled active autoimmune diseases, or severe immunodeficiencies should avoid the use of bacterial lysates. Special precautions are also necessary in case of pregnancy and lactation, as well as for children and adolescents, given that the available data are limited.

Future research will focus on improving bacterial lysates for periodontal applications. A promising direction is the targeted selection of bacterial strains, which could include the use of periodontal pathology-specific strains and optimized combinations of commensal and pathogenic species. Genetically modified strains with a superior immunogenic profile could also offer significant advantages. Advanced processing techniques will also play a crucial role. Lysis methods that preserve relevant antigenic determinants and fractionation of components with specific activity are essential for maximizing treatment efficacy. In addition, the use of nanotechnologies to improve the stability and bioavailability of preparations could revolutionize the way bacterial lysates are administered.

Personalized medicine represents a promising direction in periodontal therapy with bacterial lysates. Personalizing the treatment according to the patient's microbial profile, through metagenomic analyses, can help identify specific dysbiosis and select appropriate lysates. Monitoring changes in the microbiome during treatment will allow adjusting therapeutic strategies to maximize efficiency. Also, personalization according to the patient's immunological profile, including the determination of genetic polymorphisms and the evaluation of inflammatory biomarkers, will contribute to the adaptation of treatment protocols. Combination therapy, which associates bacterial lysates with probiotics or host response modulators, could provide synergistic and improved results. In addition to the treatment of periodontitis, bacterial lysates could have extensive clinical applications in the future. For example, their use in the prevention and treatment of peri-implant inflammation could improve the osteointegrity of dental implants. Also, as an adjuvant in guided tissue regeneration, bacterial lysates could be combined with biomaterials and growth factors to support the healing process. In addition, managing the oral manifestations of systemic diseases and reducing the impact of periodontitis on systemic conditions are other promising directions for the use of bacterial lysates in clinical practice.

6. Conclusions

Bacterial lysates represent a promising therapeutic approach in the management of periodontitis, offering a valuable alternative or adjunct to conventional treatments. These complex preparations, obtained by controlled lysis of bacterial cells, exert multiple effects on the pathogenetic factors involved in periodontitis: they modulate the local immune response, reduce chronic inflammation, favorably influence the composition of the oral microbiome, and stimulate regenerative processes.

The clinical experience accumulated in the use of bacterial lysates in respiratory diseases, where their efficacy and safety have been amply demonstrated, has paved the way for applications in oral pathology. Clinical studies conducted to date in the field of periodontology, although limited in number and scope, have shown promising results: improvement of clinical parameters, reduction of local and systemic inflammation, and potentiation of the effects of conventional therapy. Compared to antibiotic therapy, the use of bacterial lysates presents significant advantages: the absence of induction of bacterial resistance, a broad spectrum of action, a superior safety profile, and the potential for long-term use. These characteristics recommend them both for the active treatment of periodontitis and for the primary and secondary prevention of this condition. However, the full integration of bacterial lysates into periodontal therapeutic protocols requires overcoming some current limitations: the heterogeneity of available preparations, insufficient standardization, and the need for larger clinical studies with long-term follow-up. Future research should focus on optimizing the composition of lysates, developing innovative delivery systems and personalizing therapy according to individual patient characteristics. In conclusion, bacterial lysates represent a valuable therapeutic option in the complex approach to periodontitis, with significant potential to improve clinical outcomes and patients' quality of life. Their implementation in current clinical practice could mark an important step towards more effective, safer, and more tailored periodontal therapy to the specific needs of each patient.

Acknowledgements

This chapter is founded by the internal project entitled "Evaluation of tissue regeneration in periodontitis by using a bacterial lysate-based solution," acronym LIZATE, of the "Cantacuzino" National Military-Medical Institute for Research and Development, Bucharest, Romania.

Conflict of interest

The authors declare no conflict of interest.

Author details

Diana-Larisa Ancuța[1] and Cristin Coman[2,3]*

1 "Cantacuzino" National Military-Medical Institute for Research and Development, Bucharest, Romania

2 Faculty of Veterinary Medicine, University of Agronomic Sciences and Veterinary Medicine, Bucharest, Romania

3 Center of Excellence in Translational Medicine, "Fundeni" Clinical Institute, Bucharest, Romania

*Address all correspondence to: comancristin@yahoo.com

References

[1] Suárez N, Ferrara F, Rial A, Dee V, Chabalgoity JA. Bacterial lysates as immunotherapies for respiratory infections: Methods of preparation. Frontiers in Bioengineering and Biotechnology. 2020;**8**:545. DOI: 10.3389/fbioe.2020.00545

[2] Hajishengallis G. Periodontitis: From microbial immune subversion to systemic inflammation. Nature Reviews Immunology. 2015;**15**(1):30-44. DOI: 10.1038/nri3785

[3] Slots J. Periodontitis: Facts, fallacies and the future. Periodontology 2000. 2017;**75**(1):7-23. DOI: 10.1111/prd.12221

[4] De Benedetto F, Sevieri G. Prevention of respiratory tract infections with bacterial lysate OM-85 bronchomunal in children and adults: A state of the art. Multidisciplinary Respiratory Medicine. 2013;**8**(1):33. DOI: 10.1186/2049-6958-8-33

[5] Esposito S, Soto-Martinez ME, Feleszko W, Jones MH, Shen KL, SchaadUB.Nonspecificimmunomodulators for recurrent respiratory tract infections, wheezing and asthma in children: A systematic review of mechanistic and clinical evidence. Current Opinion in Allergy and Clinical Immunology. 2018;**18**(3):198-209. DOI: 10.1097/ACI.0000000000000433

[6] Cazzola M, Anapurapu S, Page CP. Polyvalent mechanical bacterial lysate for the prevention of recurrent respiratory infections: A meta-analysis. Pulmonary Pharmacology & Therapeutics. 2012;**25**(1):62-68. DOI: 10.1016/j.pupt.2011.11.002

[7] Del-Rio-Navarro BE, Espinosa Rosales F, Flenady V, Sienra-Monge JJ. Immunostimulants for preventing respiratory tract infection in children. Cochrane Database of Systematic Reviews. 2006;**2006**(4):CD004974. DOI: 10.1002/14651858.CD004974.pub2

[8] Cazzola M, Rogliani P, Curradi G. Bacterial extracts for the prevention of acute exacerbations in chronic obstructive pulmonary disease: A point of view. Respiratory Medicine. 2008;**102**(3):321-327. DOI: 10.1016/j.rmed.2007.11.002

[9] Schaad UB. OM-85 BV, an immunostimulant in pediatric recurrent respiratory tract infections: A systematic review. World Journal of Pediatrics. 2010;**6**(1):5-12. DOI: 10.1007/s12519-010-0001-x

[10] Braido F, Tarantini F, Ghiglione V, Melioli G, Canonica GW. Bacterial lysate in the prevention of acute exacerbation of COPD and in respiratory recurrent infections. International Journal of Chronic Obstructive Pulmonary Disease. 2007;**2**(3):335-345

[11] Huber M, Mossmann H, Bessler WG. Th1-orientated immunological properties of the bacterial extract OM-85-BV. European Journal of Medical Research. 2005;**10**(5):209-217

[12] Wang H, Zheng Y, He S. Induction of release and up-regulated gene expression of interleukin (IL)-8 in A549 cells by serine proteinases. BMC Cell Biology. 2006;**7**:22. DOI: 10.1186/1471-2121-7-22

[13] Dang AT, Pasquali C, Ludigs K, Guarda G. OM-85 is an immunomodulator of interferon-β production and inflammasome activity. Scientific Reports. 2017;**7**:43844. DOI: 10.1038/srep43844

[14] Pasquali C, Salami O, Taneja M, Gollwitzer ES, Trompette A, Pattaroni C, et al. Enhanced mucosal antibody production and protection against respiratory infections following an orally administered bacterial extract. Frontiers in Medicine (Lausanne). 2014;**1**:41. DOI: 10.3389/fmed.2014.00041

[15] Tang H, Fang Z, Saborío GP, Xiu Q. Efficacy and safety of OM-85 in patients with chronic bronchitis and/or chronic obstructive pulmonary disease. Lung. 2015;**193**(4):513-519. DOI: 10.1007/s00408-015-9737-3

[16] Parola C, Salogni L, Vaira X, Scutera S, Somma P, Salvi V, et al. Selective activation of human dendritic cells by OM-85 through a NF-kB and MAPK dependent pathway. PLoS One. 2013;**8**(12):e82867. DOI: 10.1371/journal.pone.0082867

[17] Zhu LL, Wang YH, Feng JH, Zhou Q. Oral bacterial lysate OM-85: Advances in pharmacology and therapeutics. Drug Design, Development and Therapy. 2024;**18**:4387-4399. DOI: 10.2147/DDDT

[18] Guéniche A, Bastien P, Ovigne JM, Kermici M, Courchay G, Chevalier V, et al. Bifidobacterium longum lysate, a new ingredient for reactive skin. Experimental Dermatology. 2010;**19**(8):e1-e8. DOI: 10.1111/j.1600-0625.2009.00932.x

[19] Vitetta L, Coulson S, Linnane AW, Butt H. The gastrointestinal microbiome and musculoskeletal diseases: A beneficial role for probiotics and prebiotics. Pathogens. 2013;**2**(4):606-626. DOI: 10.3390/pathogens2040606

[20] Guarino A, Guandalini S, Lo Vecchio A. Probiotics for prevention and treatment of diarrhea. Journal of Clinical Gastroenterology. 2015;**49**(Suppl. 1):S37-S45. DOI: 10.1097/MCG.0000000000000349

[21] Yeşilova Y, Çalka Ö, Akdeniz N, Berktaş M. Effect of probiotics on the treatment of children with atopic dermatitis. Annals of Dermatology. 2012;**24**(2):189-193. DOI: 10.5021/ad.2012.24.2.189

[22] Jung GW, Tse JE, Guiha I, Rao J. Prospective, randomized, open-label trial comparing the safety, efficacy, and tolerability of an acne treatment regimen with and without a probiotic supplement and minocycline in subjects with mild to moderate acne. Journal of Cutaneous Medicine and Surgery. 2013;**17**(2):114-122. DOI: 10.2310/7750.2012.12026

[23] Gueniche A, Knaudt B, Schuck E, Volz T, Bastien P, Martin R, et al. Effects of nonpathogenic gram-negative bacterium Vitreoscilla filiformis lysate on atopic dermatitis: A prospective, randomized, double-blind, placebo-controlled clinical study. The British Journal of Dermatology. 2008;**159**(6):1357-1363. DOI: 10.1111/j.1365-2133.2008.08836.x

[24] Heintz B, Schlenter WW, Kirsten R, Nelson K. Clinical efficacy of Broncho-Vaxom in adult patients with chronic purulent sinusitis--a multi-centric, placebo-controlled, double-blind study. International Journal of Clinical Pharmacology, Therapy, and Toxicology. 1989;**27**(11):530-534

[25] Koray M, Ak G, Kürklü E, Tanyeri H, Aydin F, Oguz FS, et al. The effect of beta-glucan on recurrent aphthous stomatitis. Journal of Alternative and Complementary Medicine. 2009;**15**(2):111-112. DOI: 10.1089/acm.2008.0118

[26] Villa A, Sonis S. Oral leukoplakia remains a challenging condition.

Oral Diseases. 2018;**24**(1-2):179-183. DOI: 10.1111/odi.12781

[27] Sonis ST. The pathobiology of mucositis. Nature Reviews Cancer. 2004;**4**(4):277-284. DOI: 10.1038/nrc1318

[28] Morath S, Stadelmaier A, Geyer A, Schmidt RR, Hartung T. Synthetic lipoteichoic acid from *Staphylococcus aureus* is a potent stimulus of cytokine release. The Journal of Experimental Medicine. 2002;**195**(12):1635-1640. DOI: 10.1084/jem.20020322

[29] Gérard HC, Mishra MK, Mao G, Wang S, Hali M, Whittum-Hudson JA, et al. Dendrimer-enabled DNA delivery and transformation of *Chlamydia pneumoniae*. Nanomedicine. 2013;**9**(7):996-1008. DOI: 10.1016/j.nano.2013.04.004

[30] Zagólski O, Stręk P, Kasprowicz A, Białecka A. Effectiveness of polyvalent bacterial lysate and autovaccines against upper respiratory tract bacterial colonization by potential pathogens: A randomized study. Medical Science Monitor. 2015;**21**:2997-3002. DOI: 10.12659/MSM.893779

[31] Rosadini CV, Kagan JC. Early innate immune responses to bacterial LPS. Current Opinion in Immunology. 2017;**44**:14-19. DOI: 10.1016/j.coi.2016.10.005

[32] Ho MH, Chen CH, Goodwin JS, Wang BY, Xie H. Functional advantages of *Porphyromonas gingivalis* vesicles. PLoS One. 2015;**10**(4):e0123448. DOI: 10.1371/journal.pone.0123448

[33] Caliot É, Dramsi S, Chapot-Chartier MP, Courtin P, Kulakauskas S, Péchoux C, et al. Role of the group B antigen of *Streptococcus agalactiae*: A peptidoglycan-anchored polysaccharide involved in cell wall biogenesis. PLoS Pathogens. 2012;**8**(6):e1002756. DOI: 10.1371/journal.ppat.1002756

[34] Kim W, Lee EJ, Bae IH, Myoung K, Kim ST, Park PJ, et al. *Lactobacillus plantarum*-derived extracellular vesicles induce anti-inflammatory M2 macrophage polarization in vitro. Journal of Extracellular Vesicles. 2020;**9**(1):1793514. DOI: 10.1080/20013078.2020.1793514

[35] Belkaid Y, Hand TW. Role of the microbiota in immunity and inflammation. Cell. 2014;**157**(1):121-141. DOI: 10.1016/j.cell.2014.03.011

[36] Jurkiewicz D, Zielnik-Jurkiewicz B. Bacterial lysates in the prevention of respiratory tract infections. Otolaryngologia Polska. 2018;**72**(5):1-8. DOI: 10.5604/01.3001.0012.7216

[37] Ricci R, Palmero C, Bazurro G, Riccio AM, Garelli V, Di Marco E, et al. The administration of a polyvalent mechanical bacterial lysate in elderly patients with COPD results in serological signs of an efficient immune response associated with a reduced number of acute episodes. Pulmonary Pharmacology & Therapeutics. 2014;**27**(1):109-113. DOI: 10.1016/j.pupt.2013.05.006

[38] Esposito S, Bianchini S, Bosis S, Tagliabue C, Coro I, Argentiero A, et al. A randomized, placebo-controlled, double-blinded, single-centre, phase IV trial to assess the efficacy and safety of OM-85 in children suffering from recurrent respiratory tract infections. Journal of Translational Medicine. 2019;**17**(1):284. DOI: 10.1186/s12967-019-2040-y

[39] Clua P, Kanmani P, Zelaya H, Fernández A, Villena J, Kitazawa H, et al. Peptidoglycan from immunobiotic *Lactobacillus rhamnosus* improves resistance of infant mice to respiratory

syncytial viral infection and secondary pneumococcal pneumonia. Frontiers in Immunology. 2017;**8**:948. DOI: 10.3389/fimmu.2017.00948

[40] Orcel B, Delclaux B, Baud M, Derenne JP. Oral immunization with bacterial extracts for protection against acute bronchitis in elderly institutionalized patients with chronic bronchitis. The European Respiratory Journal. 1994;**7**(3):446-452. DOI: 10.1183/09031936.94.07030446

[41] Emmerich B, Emslander HP, Pachmann K, Hallek M, Milatovic D, Busch R. Local immunity in patients with chronic bronchitis and the effects of a bacterial extract, Broncho-Vaxom, on T lymphocytes, macrophages, gamma-interferon and secretory immunoglobulin A in bronchoalveolar lavage fluid and other variables. Respiration. 1990;**57**(2):90-99. DOI: 10.1159/000195824

[42] Huber S, Schramm C, Lehr HA, Mann A, Schmitt S, Becker C, et al. Cutting edge: TGF-beta signaling is required for the in vivo expansion and immunosuppressive capacity of regulatory CD4+CD25+ T cells. Journal of Immunology. 2004;**173**(11):6526-6531. DOI: 10.4049/jimmunol.173.11.6526

[43] Gungor OE, Kirzioglu Z, Kivanc M. Probiotics: Can they be used to improve oral health? Beneficial Microbes. 2015;**6**(5):647-656. DOI: 10.3920/BM2014.0167

[44] Cazzola M, Capuano A, Rogliani P, Matera MG. Bacterial lysates as a potentially effective approach in preventing acute exacerbation of COPD. Current Opinion in Pharmacology. 2012;**12**(3):300-308. DOI: 10.1016/j.coph.2012.01.019

[45] Morandi B, Agazzi A, D'Agostino A, Antonini F, Costa G, Sabatini F, et al. A mixture of bacterial mechanical lysates is more efficient than single strain lysate and of bacterial-derived soluble products for the induction of an activating phenotype in human dendritic cells. Immunology Letters. 2011;**138**(1):86-91. DOI: 10.1016/j.imlet.2011.03.006

[46] Esposito S, Marchisio P, Prada E, Daleno C, Porretti L, Carsetti R, et al. Impact of a mixed bacterial lysate (OM-85 BV) on the immunogenicity, safety and tolerability of inactivated influenza vaccine in children with recurrent respiratory tract infection. Vaccine. 2014;**32**(22):2546-2552. DOI: 10.1016/j.vaccine.2014.03.055

[47] Georas SN, Wright RJ, Ivanova A, Israel E, LaVange LM, Akuthota P, et al. The Precision Interventions for Severe and/or Exacerbation-Prone (PrecISE) Asthma Network: An overview of network organization, procedures, and interventions. The Journal of Allergy and Clinical Immunology. 2022;**149**(2):488-516.e9. DOI: 10.1016/j.jaci.2021.10.035

[48] Didilescu AC, Chinthamani S, Scannapieco FA, Sharma A. NLRP3 inflammasome activity and periodontal disease pathogenesis-A bidirectional relationship. Oral Diseases. 2024;**30**(7):4069-4077. DOI: 10.1111/odi.15005

[49] Hajishengallis G, Lamont RJ. Breaking bad: Manipulation of the host response by *Porphyromonas gingivalis*. European Journal of Immunology. 2014;**44**(2):328-338. DOI: 10.1002/eji.201344202

[50] Bunte K, Hensel A, Beikler T. Polyphenols in the prevention and treatment of periodontal disease: A systematic review of in vivo, ex vivo and in vitro studies. Fitoterapia. 2019;**132**:30-39. DOI: 10.1016/j.fitote.2018.11.012

[51] Sima C, Van Dyke TE. Therapeutic targets for management of periodontitis and diabetes. Current Pharmaceutical Design. 2016;**22**(15):2216-2237. DOI: 10.2174/1381612822666160216150338

[52] Kebschull M, Demmer RT, Papapanou PN. "Gum bug, leave my heart alone!"–Epidemiologic and mechanistic evidence linking periodontal infections and atherosclerosis. Journal of Dental Research. 2010;**89**(9):879-902. DOI: 10.1177/0022034510375281

[53] Isola G, Polizzi A, Muraglie S, Leonardi R, Lo Giudice A. Assessment of vitamin C and antioxidant profiles in saliva and serum in patients with periodontitis and ischemic heart disease. Nutrients. 2019;**11**(12):2956. DOI: 10.3390/nu11122956

[54] Huang X, Yang X, Ni J, Xie B, Liu Y, Xuan D, et al. Hyperglucose contributes to periodontitis: Involvement of the NLRP3 pathway by engaging the innate immunity of oral gingival epithelium. Journal of Periodontology. 2015;**86**(2):327-335. DOI: 10.1902/jop.2014.140403

[55] Yamaguchi Y, Kurita-Ochiai T, Kobayashi R, Suzuki T, Ando T. Regulation of the NLRP3 inflammasome in *Porphyromonas gingivalis*-accelerated periodontal disease. Inflammation Research. 2017;**66**(1):59-65. DOI: 10.1007/s00011-016-0992-4

[56] Serhan CN, Chiang N, Dalli J, Levy BD. Lipid mediators in the resolution of inflammation. Cold Spring Harbor Perspectives in Biology. 2014;**7**(2):a016311. DOI: 10.1101/cshperspect.a016311

[57] Hasturk H, Kantarci A, Van Dyke TE. Paradigm shift in the pharmacological management of periodontal diseases. Frontiers of Oral Biology. 2012;**15**:160-176. DOI: 10.1159/000329678

[58] Lam RS, O'Brien-Simpson NM, Holden JA, Lenzo JC, Fong SB, Reynolds EC. Unprimed, M1 and M2 macrophages differentially interact with *Porphyromonas gingivalis*. PLoS One. 2016;**11**(7):e0158629. DOI: 10.1371/journal.pone.0158629

[59] Graves DT, Oates T, Garlet GP. Review of osteoimmunology and the host response in endodontic and periodontal lesions. Journal of Oral Microbiology. 2011;**3**(1). DOI: 10.3402/jom.v3i0.5304

[60] Nakamura H, Fukusaki Y, Yoshimura A, Shiraishi C, Kishimoto M, Kaneko T, et al. Lack of Toll-like receptor 4 decreases lipopolysaccharide-induced bone resorption in C3H/HeJ mice in vivo. Oral Microbiology and Immunology. 2008;**23**(3):190-195. DOI: 10.1111/j.1399-302X.2007.00410.x

[61] Ebersole JL, Kirakodu S, Novak MJ, Stromberg AJ, Shen S, Orraca L, et al. Cytokine gene expression profiles during initiation, progression and resolution of periodontitis. Journal of Clinical Periodontology. 2014;**41**(9):853-861. DOI: 10.1111/jcpe.12286

[62] Martins MD, Jiao Y, Larsson L, Almeida LO, Garaicoa-Pazmino C, Le JM, et al. Epigenetic modifications of histones in periodontal disease. Journal of Dental Research. 2016;**95**(2):215-222. DOI: 10.1177/0022034515611876

[63] Lee BS, Lee CC, Wang YP, Chen HJ, Lai CH, Hsieh WL, et al. Controlled-release of tetracycline and lovastatin by poly(D,L-lactide-co-glycolide acid)-chitosan nanoparticles enhances periodontal regeneration in dogs. International Journal of Nanomedicine. 2016;**11**:285-297. DOI: 10.2147/IJN.S94270

[64] Chen X, Liu Y, Miao L, Wang Y, Ren S, Yang X, et al. Controlled release of recombinant human cementum protein 1 from electrospun multiphasic scaffold for cementum regeneration. International Journal of Nanomedicine. 2016;**11**:3145-3158. DOI: 10.2147/IJN.S104324

[65] Kobayashi E, Flückiger L, Fujioka-Kobayashi M, Sawada K, Sculean A, Schaller B, et al. Comparative release of growth factors from PRP, PRF, and advanced-PRF. Clinical Oral Investigations. 2016;**20**(9):2353-2360

[66] Kim MY, Hyun IK, An S, Kim D, Kim KH, Kang SS. In vitro anti-inflammatory and antibiofilm activities of bacterial lysates from lactobacilli against oral pathogenic bacteria. Food & Function. 2022;**13**(24):12755-12765. DOI: 10.1039/d2fo00936f

[67] Ancuța DL, Vuță V, Șalgău C, Bărbuceanu F, Coman C. Innovative treatment against human periodontitis and periimplantitis—In vitro study. Farmácia. 2024;**72**:125-131

[68] Ancuța DL, Alexandru DM, Muselin F, Cristina RT, Coman C. Assessment of the effect on periodontitis of antibiotic therapy and bacterial lysate treatment. International Journal of Molecular Sciences. 2024;**25**(10):5432. DOI: 10.3390/ijms25105432

[69] Mercer SD, Doherty C, Singh G, Willmott T, Cheesapcharoen T, Teanpaisan R, et al. *Lactobacillus* lysates protect oral epithelial cells from pathogen-associated damage, increase secretion of pro-inflammatory cytokines and enhance barrier integrity. Scientific Reports. 2025;**15**(1):5894. DOI: 10.1038/s41598-025-86914-y

[70] Wu F, Fang B, Wuri G, Zhao L, Liu F, Zhang M. Metagenomic analysis reveals a mitigating role for *Lactobacillus paracasei* and *Bifidobacterium animalis* in experimental periodontitis. Nutrients. 2022;**14**(10):2125. DOI: 10.3390/nu14102125

[71] Ievtushenko M, Koshova O, Kryzhna S. Histological study of the effect of bacterial lysates on the state of periodontal tissue in experimental periodontitis in rats. ScienceRise: Medical Science. 2021;**5**(44):41-47. DOI: 10.15587/2519-4798.2021.241983

Section 3

Reviews

Chapter 9

Enhanced Osseointegration between Bone to Implant Featuring Super Hydrophilic Nanoscale Dental Implant Surface Roughness – Myth or Reality

Ofer Moses, Daniele Botticelli and Perry Raz

Abstract

The development of nanoscale hydrophilic surface roughness on dental implants arose from limitations observed with conventional sandblasted, large-grit, acid-etched (SLA) surfaces. SLA surfaces provide microroughness that enhances mechanical interlocking and osseointegration; however, they exhibit slower healing times and reduced performance in compromised bone conditions. Nanoscale modifications introduce surface topographies that influence polarization of key cells, promoting cell signaling at the implant interface. This nano-level structuring improves osteoblast differentiation and accelerates bone formation by influencing cell-protein interactions beyond the capabilities of microrough surfaces. Additionally, studies demonstrated that hydrophilicity significantly enhances early biological responses by increasing surface wettability, which facilitates blood clot formation, protein adhesion, and initial cell attachment, which are critical steps for rapid osseointegration. Studies have shown that hydrophilic nanoscale surfaces achieve higher bone-to-implant contact (BIC) in early healing phases compared to SLA surfaces, making them advantageous for immediate loading protocols and patients with poor bone quality or systemic conditions. By combining nanoscale roughness with super hydrophilic property, these surfaces aim to shorten osseointegration healing time seen with SLA implants and expand clinical indications, representing an evolutionary step toward biomimetic implant design for improved long-term outcomes.

Keywords: osseointegration, hydrophilic nano scale roughness, macrophage polarization, bone to implant contact, dental implants

1. Introduction

Osseointegration is the biological process by which a dental implant achieves a direct structural and functional connection with the surrounding bone tissue. This phenomenon ensures that the implant becomes a stable and permanent part of the oral environment, capable of supporting prosthetic restorations under normal functional loads. The concept was first introduced by Prof. Per-Ingvar Brånemark in the 1960s and remains the cornerstone of modern implant dentistry. Unlike natural teeth, which are anchored to alveolar bone by the periodontal ligament, dental implants rely on bone-to-implant contact for stability as demonstrated in light microscopy inspection. The implant surface, commonly titanium or titanium alloy, is biocompatible and designed to promote bone cell adhesion and growth. The absence of intervening soft tissue between the implant and bone is critical for achieving mechanical stability and long-term success.

1.1 Stages of osseointegration

Osseointegration is a dynamic, multi-stage process essential for the long-term success of dental implants. The initial healing phase (0–2 weeks) begins immediately after implant placement, characterized by blood clot formation and the initiation of angiogenesis, which provides nutrients for bone regeneration [1]. During the bone formation phase (2–6 weeks), osteoblasts migrate to the implant surface and deposit new bone matrix, facilitating the transition from primary mechanical stability to biological stability as bone integrates with the implant's micro-rough surface [2, 3].

Subsequently, bone remodeling and maturation occur between 6 weeks and 6 months, where woven bone is replaced by lamellar bone, enhancing strength and density and establishing secondary biological stability [4]. Once osseointegration is complete, the implant enters the functional loading phase, during which controlled occlusal forces are needed contributing to bone level maintenance [5]. Several factors influence the success of osseointegration. Implant material and surface properties play a critical role, with titanium and its alloys considered the gold standard due to their biocompatibility and ability to form a stable oxide layer [6]. Surface modifications such as sandblasting, acid-etching, and nanoscale hydrophilic coatings further enhance bone-to-implant adhesion [7]. Bone quality and quantity also significantly affect outcomes, as dense cortical bone provides superior initial stability compared to porous cancellous bone [8]. Surgical technique is another determinant, with minimally invasive procedures that preserve vascularization and prevent thermal damage during drilling being essential [9]. Healing time and loading protocols vary, with traditional recommendations favoring 3–6 months before loading, although immediate and early loading are feasible under optimal conditions [10]. Finally, patient-related factors such as systemic health, smoking habits, and oral hygiene critically influence osseointegration success [11].

1.2 Clinical significance

Achieving and maintaining osseointegration is essential for the longevity of dental implants. Failure of bone modeling and long-term remodeling process can lead to implant mobility, bone loss, and eventual implant failure. Advances in implant design, surface technology, and surgical protocols continue to improve predictability and success rates.

2. Macrophage interaction with hydrophobic sand blasted and acid etched titanium implant surface

Biomaterial implantation provokes an inflammatory response that controls integrative fate. Early in vivo work by Donath and colleagues (1984) was the first to clearly demonstrate the importance of macrophages in this response and their subsequent role in peri-implant endosseous healing. Macrophages, which are key early mediators of the host response, arrive at sites of inflammation following implant placement and become activated in response to signals present in the tissue [12]. These cells are described as mononuclear histocytes, today known as stationary form of connective tissue macrophages [13], on the surface of TPS-coated titanium screws, 3 days after implantation in the rat femur.

When a sandblasted and acid-etched (SLA) titanium implant is inserted into bone, macrophages are among the first immune cells to encounter the surface [14]. The implant's micro-rough topography and altered chemistry immediately influence macrophage adhesion and activation [14]. Upon contact, macrophages recognize the foreign material through pattern recognition receptors and integrins, triggering a cascade of signaling events [15]. This leads to the secretion of pro-inflammatory cytokines such as TNF-α, IL-1β, and IL-6, which recruit additional immune cells and initiate the early inflammatory phase. At the same time, the surface properties can modulate macrophage polarization, with hydrophobic SLA variants promoting a shift toward an anti-inflammatory M2 phenotype, characterized by IL-10 and TGF-β secretion. This dynamic interplay between inflammation and resolution sets the stage for subsequent tissue healing and osseointegration. Gudima et al. [16] mentioned that macrophages are major immune cells that control acceptance or failure of the implant.

2.1 Macrophage interaction with hydrophilic sand blasted and acid etched titanium surface

Increased titanium surface hydrophilicity accelerates osseointegration and modulates macrophage cytokine expression. Hydrophilic SLA (modSLA) surfaces down-regulated pro-inflammatory genes (TNF, IL-1β, and CCL chemokines) and reduced protein secretion compared to standard SLA surfaces, promoting a more reparative environment [17]. Another study explored how increasing titanium implant surface hydrophilicity through non-thermal atmospheric plasma (NTAP) treatment enhances osseointegration by modulating immune and osteogenic responses. Compared to hydrophobic surfaces, NTAP-modified hydrophilic titanium significantly promoted M2 macrophage polarization (three-fold increase in pro-healing markers) and improved osteogenic differentiation of mesenchymal stem cells. Mechanistically, these effects were mediated by integrin β1 and β2 signaling, activating downstream FAK-PI3K/Akt and NF-κB pathways, which regulate macrophage phenotype and osteo-immunomodulation. The study highlights the critical role of integrin-mediated immune modulation in creating a favorable microenvironment for bone healing and implant integration [18]. Changing a hydrophobic into hydrophilic titanium surface may induce a macrophage pro-osteogenic instead of proinflammatory response. Hamlet et al. [19] examined how titanium surface hydrophilicity influences macrophage phenotype and its downstream effect on osteogenic signaling. Rodent bone marrow-derived macrophages were polarized into M1 and M2 phenotypes and cultured on standard SLA (sandblasted, acid-etched) and hydrophilic-modified SLA (modSLA) titanium discs. Results showed that M1 macrophages on modSLA surfaces, shifted toward an M2-like phenotype, evidenced by increased CD163 protein and Arg1 gene expression. These macrophages secreted cytokines that significantly upregulated osteoblast genes associated with the TGF-β/BMP signaling pathway, promoting osteogenesis. Conversely, M2 macrophages on SLA hydrophobic surfaces exhibited a more inflammatory profile, which was not conducive to osteogenic gene expression. Their conclusions showed that hydrophilic micro-rough titanium surfaces can actively modulate macrophage behavior, reducing inflammation and promoting a pro-healing, pro-osteogenic environment. This immune-mediated mechanism highlights the importance of surface chemistry and topography in implant design, suggesting that hydrophilic modifications may accelerate osseointegration by leveraging macrophage-driven osteo-immunomodulation. A study performed by Hamlet et al. in 2012 [20] investigated how hydrophilic modification of microrough titanium surfaces influences macrophage cell line inflammatory cytokine gene expression. Macrophages were cultured for 24 hours on three titanium surface types: smooth polished titanium, sandblasted acid-etched (SLA), and hydrophilic-modified SLA (SLActive). While surface microroughness activated transcription of pro-inflammatory cytokines (e.g., TNF-α, IL-1α, and IL-1β), the hydrophilic SLActive surface significantly downregulated these key pro-inflammatory genes compared to SLA. Importantly, macrophage attachment and proliferation were similar across all surfaces, indicating that the observed differences were due to surface chemistry rather than cell density.

2.2 Macrophages and dental implants nanoscale surface roughness

As mentioned earlier, macrophages are among the first immune cells to interact with dental implant surfaces, and their response is strongly influenced by nanoscale topography. Surface nanostructures modulate protein adsorption and integrin-mediated signaling, which affects macrophage adhesion and morphology, ultimately shaping the inflammatory microenvironment [14, 21].

Nanoscale roughness can address direct macrophage polarization takes place: anodized nanoporous titanium surfaces and honeycomb-like TiO_2 nanostructures have been shown to promote an anti-inflammatory M2 phenotype, characterized by upregulation of CD206 and secretion of IL-10 and TGF-β, while reducing pro-inflammatory cytokines such as TNF-α and IL-1β [22–25].

This immunomodulatory effect enhances angiogenesis and osteogenesis, facilitating osseointegration and reducing the risk of chronic inflammation. Conversely, irregular or highly dense nanospike patterns may sustain M1 polarization, prolonging inflammation and impairing bone integration [26]. These findings emphasize the importance of rational design of implant surfaces with controlled nanoscale features to optimize immune compatibility consequences and clinical outcomes.

3. Osteoblast activity in hydrophobic titanium nanoscale level surface roughness

Hydrophobic surfaces tend to repel water, which influences the adsorption of plasma proteins (such as fibronectin and vitronectin) that are critical for cell adhesion. Osteoblasts require a surface that allows stable protein adsorption to initiate adhesion proliferation, and differentiation. Studies show that hydrophilic surfaces generally improve adhesion and osseointegration because they support the formation of a uniform protein layer and better integrin binding in osteoblasts [27].

During manufacturing, implants are treated with sand blasting with Al_2O_3, or TiO2 powder, followed by acid etching that increases surface area and provides roughened topography that promotes mechanical interlocking and cell adhesion. If the surface remains hydrophobic after these treatments, osseointegration may be slower because hydrophobicity hinders protein adsorption and stable water layer formation.

A study performed by Visalakshan et al. demonstrated that surface hydrophobicity strongly influences the amount and type of protein adsorbed on biomaterial surfaces, which in turn affects cellular responses. Hydrophobic surfaces tend to adsorb opsonins like IgG2, which can lead to pro-inflammatory signaling, whereas hydrophilic surfaces promote anti-inflammatory responses and better integration [28, 29].

In fact, osteoblasts can adhere to hydrophobic surfaces, but adhesion and proliferation rates are generally lower compared to hydrophilic surfaces.

Hydrophobicity can lead to a thin, unstable protein layer, resulting in weaker adhesion. For this reason, many manufacturers add treatments to increase hydrophilicity (e.g., SLA + water or UV treatment) to accelerate osseointegration [30].

3.1 Osteoblast activity in hydrophilic titanium nanoscale surface roughness

Hydrophilic titanium surfaces engineered with micro-/nanoscale roughness consistently enhance osteoblast attraction, maturation, and early matrix mineralization. Low water contact angle $\leq 15°$ increases protein adsorption and integrin engagement [31], thereby accelerating osteogenic responses (alkaline phosphatase and osteocalcin) relative to conventional SLA. In humans [32], hydrophilic, moderately rough implants (SLActive) yield superior early bone-to-implant contact at 2-4 weeks versus hydrophobic SLA, reflecting faster recruitment and apposition of new bone on debris-coated interfaces, while converging by 6 weeks as remodeling progresses. Clinically [33], randomized pilot data show that chemically modified hydrophilic SLA surfaces shift the stability curve earlier (transition from primary mechanical to biological secondary stability at 2 *vs*. 4 weeks for SLA). This fact is consistent with an accelerated osseointegration cascade mediated by wettability-driven protein assembly and osteoblast activation. Hydrophilic titanium surfaces with micro- and nanoscale roughness help implants bond to bone faster. These surfaces attract water and proteins, making it easier for bone-forming cells (osteoblasts) to stick, grow, and start building bone. Compared to traditional rough titanium, hydrophilic surfaces speed up early healing and improve implant stability in the first few weeks. This is because the combination of roughness and high surface energy creates a better [23, 33, 34] environment for cell attachment and bone formation. In a recent study, Shirazi et al. demonstrated that nanoscale surface features orchestrate also osteoprogenitor differentiation and macrophage-mediated immune signaling, thereby regulating bone formation in a surface-dependent manner. These findings emphasize the importance of nanoscale design in optimizing biomaterial performance for osteogenesis [35].

4. Effect of combining nanoscale super-hydrophilic titanium surface features on osteointegration

Super-hydrophilic titanium surfaces with nanoscale features significantly accelerate osseointegration by enhancing both biological and immunological responses at the implant interface [36]. The combination of nanoscale topography and high surface energy improves protein adsorption and integrin-mediated osteoblast adhesion, which promotes early cell spreading and differentiation [37]. Recent studies demonstrate that such surfaces not only stimulate osteogenic markers but also modulate macrophage polarization toward an M2 pro-healing phenotype, reducing inflammation and creating a favorable environment for bone formation [38]. This dual effect on osteoblast activation and immune modulation, shortens healing time and increases early implant stability compared to conventional hydrophobic or micron level rough surfaces. These features are linked to improved wettability, optimized nano-topography, and activation of integrin/FAK signaling pathways, which collectively drive osteogenesis and angiogenesis at the bone to implant interface [39] Buser et al. [40], performed a study evaluating bone apposition to modified sandblasted/acid-etched (modSLA/SLActive) titanium surface compared with standard SLA surface during early bone regeneration in miniature pigs. Test (SLActive) implants demonstrated significantly greater mean percentage of bone-implant contact compared with SLA controls at 2 weeks (49.30 vs. 29.42%; $p = 0.017$) and 4 weeks (81.91 vs. 66.57%; $p = 0.011$). At 8 weeks, similar results were observed. The test surface was created by submerging the implant in isotonic NaCl solution following acid-etching to avoid atmospheric contamination [40]. A 2024 systematic review of randomized controlled trials up to February 2023 [41] assessed implant stability through ISQ (Implant Stability Quotient) levels comparing SLA and SLActive implants over 12 weeks. Six RCTs comprising 326 implants (50.6% SLA, 49.4% SLActive) were analyzed. SLActive implants demonstrated comparable stability levels, as measured by ISQ, to SLA implants within the 12-week interval for implants placed in maxillary or mandibular regions. Studies showed that SLActive surfaces promote greater osseointegration compared to SLA surfaces in both animal and human studies, with animal experiments indicating faster osseointegration with SLActive implants within 4 weeks. Numerous studies demonstrated the advantage of such a combined surface during the creation of bone to implant contact, so we can agree about the fact that nanoscale superhydrophilic roughness is a factor contributing to speeding up osteointegration [42]. Wennerberg et al. (2011) published a comprehensive review summarizing 15 in vitro, 17 in vivo, and 16 clinical studies and concluded that SLActive surfaces demonstrate a stronger cell and bone tissue response than SLA surfaces during early healing. In most studies, however, this difference disappears after 6–8 weeks. The in vitro findings showed similar cell attachment on both surfaces within 3 hours, but a more differentiated phenotype of cells grown on SLActive was observed, with remarkable increases in alkaline phosphatase activity, osteocalcin, and osteoprotegerin production. Production of prostaglandin E_2 increased 10-fold and transforming growth factor-beta increased 2.5-fold on SLActive compared with SLA surfaces, emphasizing the advantage of super-hydrophilic nanoscale surface roughness on early osteointegration events [43]. An interesting issue deals with the potential of super-hydrophilic nanoscale roughness implant surface in a compromised systemic condition. Mardas et al. (2011) evaluated new bone formation using SLA and modSLA titanium domes in 36 New Zealand white rabbits comprising healthy, osteoporotic, and osteoporotic treated with bisphosphonates groups, sacrificed at 30 and 120 days. Newly formed total bone, newly formed mineralized bone, and bone to implant contact were higher at the modSLA-treated sites during all experimental periods, suggesting that modSLA may further promote bone formation and osseointegration in healthy and osteoporotic-like conditions [44].

A group of researchers [45] performed a study on SLA dental implants and diabetic pigs. Diabetes mellitus is recognized as a relative contraindication for dental implants, associated with increased failure rates. Using a domestic pig model mirroring human bone physiology, this study aimed to assess the impact of experimentally induced diabetes on peri-implant bone formation and mineralization during early and mid-term healing phase. Some of the findings indicated that collagen type I expression was elevated in diabetics at both timepoints, suggesting delayed remodeling and excessive matrix deposition and Osteocalcin levels were reduced in diabetic subjects, reflecting impaired maturation of the bone matrix and mineralization process. The main conclusion from this study was that controlled diabetes markedly impairs peri-implant bone formation by reducing bone-to-implant contact, decreasing mineral density, increasing immature collagen accumulation, and lowering mature osteocalcin levels. These alterations warrant careful consideration when planning implant therapy in diabetic patients [45]. Another study performed by Schlegel et al. (2013) aimed to assess the effects of diabetes mellitus on peri-implant osseointegration and to compare the performance of conventional SLA and chemically modified hydrophilic SLActive titanium implant surfaces in diabetic versus healthy domestic pigs. From results, we learn that diabetes significantly reduced BIC values at both 30 and 90 days versus controls. At 90 days, SLActive implants achieved higher BIC than SLA in diabetic pigs. From the conclusion of research studies, we can learn that untreated diabetes markedly impairs early osseointegration, as evidenced by significant reductions in bone-to-implant contact (BIC) and peri-implant bone density (BD). In contrast, implants featuring a hydrophilic SLActive® surface exhibited accelerated bone formation relative to conventional SLA® implants in diabetic subjects. These findings underscore the potential of hydrophilic implant surfaces to mitigate diabetes-associated deficits in osseointegration and enhance clinical outcomes in this patient population [46].

4.1 The way to develop a super-hydrophilic, nano-scale implant roughness

The scientific database showing the advantage of super-hydrophilic nanoscale implant surface roughness justify the attempt to apply it to a new implant surface. The development of a titanium implant (pure grade or alloy), featuring nanoscale super-hydrophilic surface roughness, is dependent and must be proved in three levels of analysis – in vitro osteoblast cell culture, pre-clinical in vivo (animal) and human clinical studies – that must show similar results that appear in the relevant published scientific articles. The first step was to develop a nanostructure surface roughness and turn it into a super-hydrophilic one.

During the development of the nanostructured surface, the resulting morphology was characterized and is presented below. The surface features were subsequently visually compared with those of a commercially available Roxolid® SLActive® surface (Straumann) using scanning electron microscopy (SEM) (**Figure 1**).

Surface roughness measurement of nanoABT mascale structure was performed using Atomic Force Microscopy, and the results are shown below (**Figure 2**).

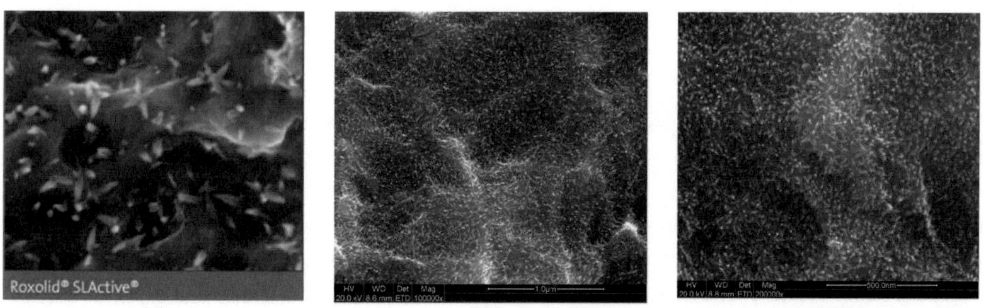

(a) (b) (c)

Figure 1.
Scanning electron microscopy demonstrating surface nanostructures: (a) Straumann SLA active, magnification 200 k, (b) AlphaBiotec magnification 100 k, and (c) Alpha Biotec magnification 200 k.

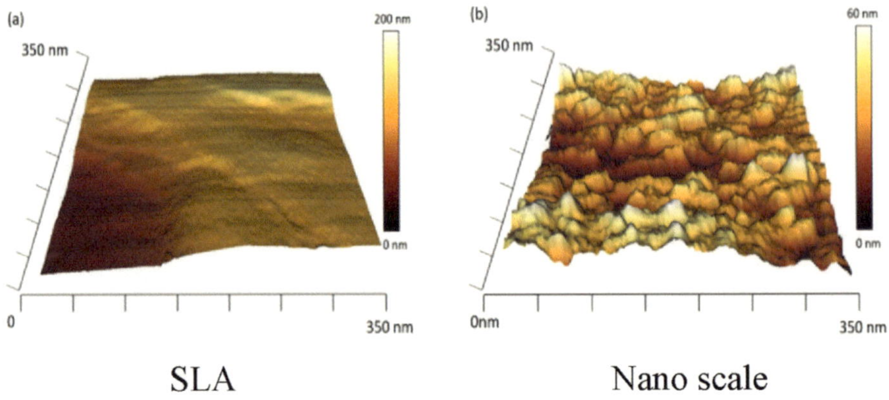

Figure 2.
3D registration following AFM roughness measurement.

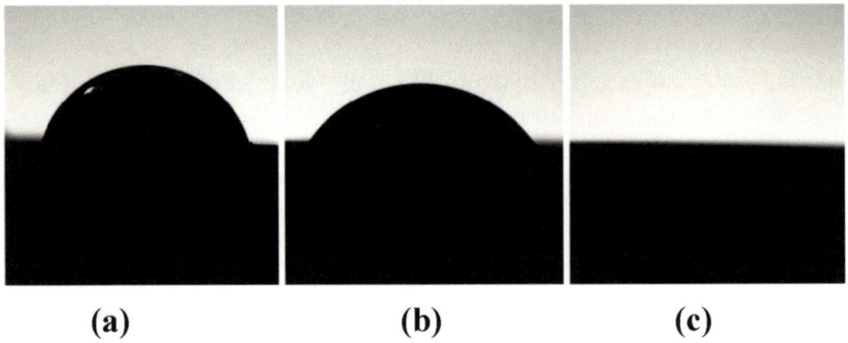

Figure 3.
Wettability of different disc samples: ABT (a), nano H_2O (b), and nanoscale (c). The contact angles are, respectively: 76.5; 55.3, and 0° (or not measurable).

AFM showed a major increase in average roughness of the surfaces of more than 400% increase for the nano-structured surface when compared to SLA. These features were studied by a third party and reported in a published article [47]. Superhydrophilicity was evaluated according to the method described by Duske et al. [48]. This was assessed by measuring the water contact angle on titanium alloy discs featuring a nanoscale, super-hydrophilic surface treatment (**Figure 3**).

4.2 Topographic analysis

In order to analyze the topographical features on the meso-, micro-, and nanoscale, the samples were inspected at different magnifications, varying from 1000× (horizontal field of view of 298 μm) to 500,000× (horizontal field of view of 597 nm) (**Figure 2**). For each disc, micrographs were acquired in randomly selected regions of the sample surface (excluding areas that were clearly non-commensurable) (**Figure 4**) [49].

According to the conclusion of this study, nanoscale surface topography of dental implants critically influences cell adhesion, proliferation, and differentiation. High-energy, hydrophilic surfaces enhance water molecule adsorption and subsequent protein-mediated cell attachment. This study characterizes a novel bioactivated surface produced via dry technology, emphasizing micrometric and nanometric features

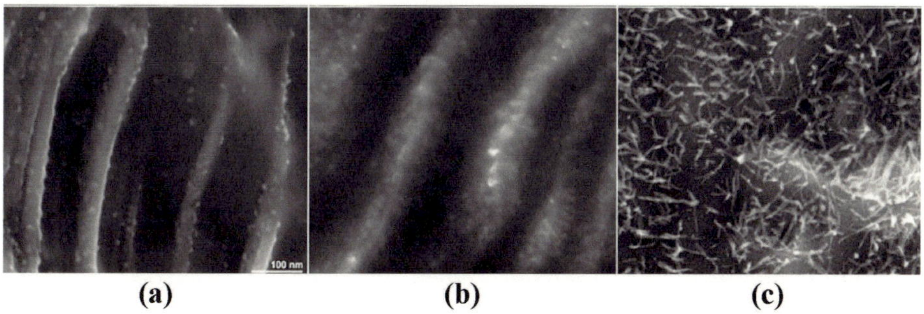

Figure 4.
High-magnification SEM micrographs showing the different appearance and density of the nanostructures (horizontal field widths of 2.98, 1.19 µm and 597 nm, respectively) of (a) AlphaBio Tec with dry salt maintaining hydrophilicity, (b) nano, and (c) nano-rinsed H_2O to remove salt maintaining hydrophilicity. The magnifications are 500,000x.

and wettability, with promising outcomes. The next step was confirming the innovative surface bioactivity of the developed surface and its influence in an osteoblast cell culture [50]. One of the aims of this study was to evaluate the osteogenic response of pre-osteoblast cell lines to dry bioactivated surface. MC3T3-E1 osteogenic cell lines [51] were cultured on SM (sandblasted and dual acid-etched surface) and HNS (SM surface with dry salts bioactive technology and nanoscale roughness). Among few

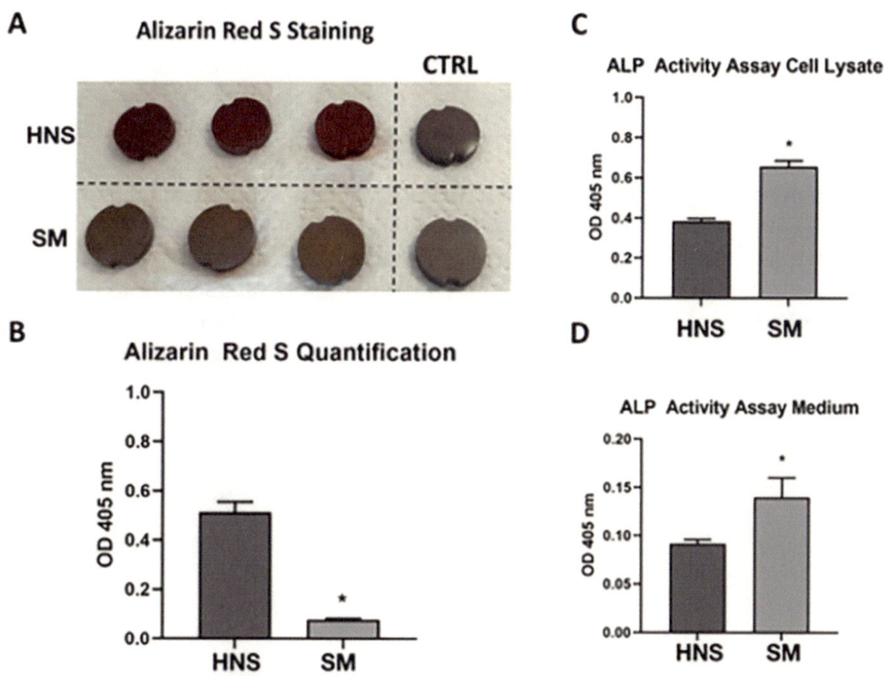

Figure 5.
Osteogenic activity of MC3T3-E1 cultured for 21 days in osteogenic medium on HNS or SM surfaces. Representative picture of staining of calcium deposit on titanium samples through Alizarin Red S (A). Quantification of optical density at 405 nm of solubilized Alizarin Red S staining with 10% acetic acid (B). Evaluation of ALP activity on cell lysate (C) and culture medium (D) of MC3T3-E1 by using ALP Activity Assay Kit ab83369 [Abcam]. Values represent mean ± SEM. The symbol (*) indicates the statistical significance vs. HNS surface, considering a p-value <0.05.

measured parameters, osteogenic activity was performed using Alizarin Red S and alkaline phosphatase (**Figure 5**).

Calcium deposition and alkaline phosphatase (ALP) activity, both established indicators of osteogenic differentiation, were evaluated in this study. Results demonstrated that the super-hydrophilic nanoscale (HNS) surface markedly enhanced calcium mineralization compared to the sandblasted and machined (SM) surface. Interestingly, ALP activity was higher in cells cultured on the SM surface. After 21 days, reduced ALP expression on HNS surfaces, coupled with increased calcified matrix formation, suggests that osteoblast-mediated bone apposition occurred earlier on bioactivated surfaces relative to SM surfaces.

The next step of concept proof, was a study, comparing four implant surfaces during immediate replacement procedure in the canine mandible: (1) ABT (SLA), a sandblasted and dual acid-etched standard control; (2) nano, a nanostructured surface alone, (3) hydro, an ultra-hydrophilic SLA surface, and (4) nano-active, which combines a nanostructured surface ultra-hydrophilic surface. Study Design included 12 dogs in a randomized split-mouth setup. In each dog: one implant of each type in healed mandibular molar sites (3 months post-extraction) one implant of each type placed immediately into fresh extraction sockets of premolars. Euthanasia was performed at 14 and 28 days post-op. Histological and histomorphometry following Stevenel's blue and alizarin red staining on non-decalcified sections.

All implant sites healed uneventfully. At 14 days, no significant differences in new bone formation were observed among the groups. By 28 days, the Nano-Active surface exhibited the highest bone formation at 51.0 ± 10.2%, significantly greater than the SLA surface at 36.0 ± 10.2%. The hydro surface also demonstrated enhanced performance, achieving 47.3 ± 10.7%, which was significantly higher than nano, indicating that bioactivated ultra-hydrophilic treatments promote accelerated early osseointegration compared to standard hydrophilic surfaces. From this study, we can conclude that combination of nanoscale ultra or super-hydrophilic roughness has an enhanced effect of bone healing following immediate implant replacement leading to higher BIC. This finding is with agreement with the literature following studies dealing with effect of implant nanoscale super-hydrophilic implant surface and BIC [52].

A clinical trial evaluated the transition from primary to secondary stability of nano-superhydrophilic, bioactive implant surfaces in patients with low-density (D3–D4) bone [53]. About 30 bioactive (MultiNeo NH, test) and 30 conventional

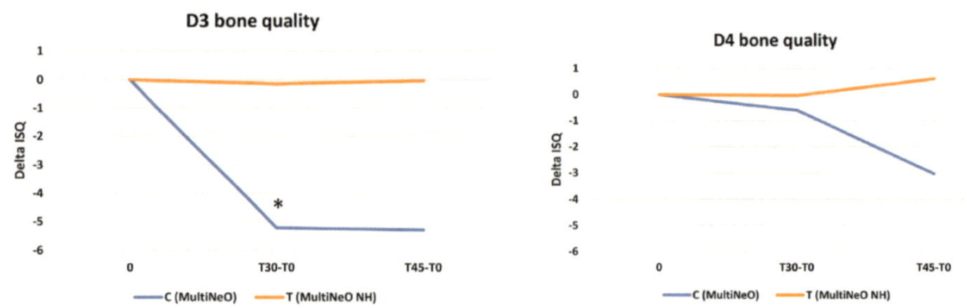

Figure 6.
T30 and T45 in D3 bone (left panel) and D4 bone (right panel). In the D3 bone, test implants with nanoscale superhydrophilic surface (T-MultiNeo NH) showed a small variation in ISQ, while control implants (MultiNeo) displayed a significant drop at 30 days. Non-significant changes in ISQ were recorded for implants placed in D4 bone. The findings in D3 bone likely reflect the complex molecular and cellular processes triggered by the placement of a bioactive surface implant in low-density bone, which appear to be more pronounced compared to those occurring with a conventional implant.

(MultiNeo, control) implants were placed in 36 patients, with primary stability assessed by insertion torque, cumulative torque, torque density, and Implant Stability Quotient (ISQ) at baseline (T0), 30 days (T30), and 45 days (T45).

At baseline, mean ISQ values were similar between groups (74.6 ± 7.9 vs. 77.1 ± 5.8). The test group maintained stable ISQ values over time [T0–T30, T30–T45], whereas the control group experienced significant reductions at both T30 ($p = 0.01$) and T45 ($p = 0.03$). Consequently, 26 test implants vs. 23 controls achieved ISQ ≥ 70 by day 45 and were loaded early; an additional four test and one control implant were loaded by day 90, while six control implants required loading at 180 days. Torque density correlated positively with baseline ISQ, especially in D3 bone in the test group at 30 and 45 days ($p < 0.01$), underscoring enhanced early biological stability. The authors concluded that bioactivated nano-superhydrophilic surfaces offer superior stabilization in low-density bone during the critical early healing phase (**Figure 6**).

5. Conclusion

The application of dental implants with bioactive surfaces warrants further investigation, particularly in systemically compromised conditions that impair bone healing, such as uncontrolled diabetes and severe osteoporosis. Establishing clinical evidence in such situations is essential to support informed surgical decision-making in high-risk cases. Despite the potential benefits, widespread adoption of bioactivated dental implants in patients with systemic disorders remains limited. Therefore, additional well-designed clinical studies are required to validate their efficacy and encourage clinician confidence in these challenging contexts.

Author details

Ofer Moses[1]*, Daniele Botticelli[2] and Perry Raz[3]

1 RND Department, AlphaBio Tec, Modiin, Israel

2 CEO and Scientific Director at ARDEC Academy, Rimini, Italy

3 Department of Periodontology and Dental Implantology, School of Dental Medicine, Tel Aviv University, Tel Aviv, Israel

*Address all correspondence to: mosesofer@gmail.com

References

[1] Brånemark PI, Hansson BO, Adell R, Breine U, Lindström J, Hallén O, et al. Osseointegrated implants in the treatment of the edentulous jaw. Scandinavian Journal of Plastic and Reconstructive Surgery. Supplementum. 1977;**16**:1-132

[2] Davies JE. Understanding peri-implant endosseous healing. Journal of Dental Education. 2003;**67**(8):932-949

[3] Albrektsson T, Tengvall P, Amengual L, Coli P, Kotsakis GA, Cochran D. Osteoimmune regulation underlies oral implant osseointegration and its perturbation. Frontiers in Immunology. 2023;**13**:1056914

[4] Albrektsson T, Zarb G, Worthington P, Eriksson AR. The long-term efficacy of currently used dental implants: A review and proposed criteria of success. The International Journal of Oral & Maxillofacial Implants. 1986;**1**(1):11-25

[5] Cochran DL, Zarb G, Worthington P, Eriksson AR. Biologic width around titanium implants. Clinical Oral Implants Research. 1997;**8**(2):97-102

[6] Elias CN, Lima JHC, Valiev R, Meyers MA. Biomedical applications of titanium and its alloys. Journal of Materials Research and Technology. 2019;**8**(1):1060-1067

[7] Wennerberg A, Albrektsson T. Effects of titanium surface topography on bone integration: A systematic review. Clinical Oral Implants Research. 2009;**20**(Suppl. 4):172-184

[8] Lekholm U, Zarb GA. Patient selection and preparation. In: Brånemark PI, Zarb GA, Albrektsson T, editors. Tissue-Integrated Prostheses: Osseointegration in Clinical Dentistry. Chicago: Quintessence; 1985. pp. 199-209

[9] Eriksson AR, Albrektsson T. Temperature threshold levels for heat-induced bone tissue injury: A vital-microscopic study in the rabbit. The Journal of Prosthetic Dentistry. 1983;**50**(1):101-107

[10] Vogl S, Stopper M, Hof M, Wegscheider WA, Lorenzoni M. Immediate occlusal versus non-occlusal loading of implants: A randomized clinical pilot study. Clinical Implant Dentistry and Related Research. 2015;**17**(3):589-597

[11] Staedt H, Rossa M, Lehmann KM, Al-Nawas B, Kämmerer PW, Heimes D. Potential risk factors for early and late dental implant failure: A retrospective clinical study on 9080 implants. International Journal of Implant Dentistry. 2020;**6**(1):81

[12] Donath K, Kirsch A, Osborn JF. Zelluläre Dynamik um enossale Titanimplantate. Fortschritte der Zahnärztlichen Implantologie. 1984;**1**:55-58

[13] Galli SJ, Borregaard N, Wynn TA. Phenotypic and functional plasticity of cells of innate immunity: Macrophages, mast cells and neutrophils. Nature Immunology. 2011;**12**:1035-1044

[14] Pitchai M, Ipe D, Tadakamadla S, Hamlet S. Titanium implant surface effects on adherent macrophage phenotype: A systematic review. Materials. 2022;**15**(20):7314

[15] Donohoe E, Kahatab R, Barrak F. A systematic review comparing the

macrophage inflammatory response to hydrophobic and hydrophilic sandblasted large grit, acid-etched titanium or titanium–zirconium surfaces during in vitro studies. Clinical and Experimental Dental Research. 2023;**9**(3):437-448

[16] Gudima A et al. Titanium induces proinflammatory and tissue-destructive responses in primary human macrophages. Journal of Leukocyte Biology. 2024;**116**(4):706-725

[17] Alfarsi MA, Hamlet SM, Ivanovski S. Titanium surface hydrophilicity modulates the human macrophage inflammatory cytokine response. Journal of Biomedical Materials Research Part A. 2013;**102**(1):60-67

[18] Zheng Z, Gan S, Yang S, Hou C, Zhu Z, Wang H, et al. Enhanced surface hydrophilicity improves osseointegration of titanium implants via integrin-mediated osteoimmunomodulation. Journal of Materials Chemistry B. 2025;**13**(2):496-451

[19] Hamlet SM, Lee RSB, Moon HJ, Alfarsi M, Ivanovski S. Hydrophilic titanium surface-induced macrophage modulation promotes pro-osteogenic signaling. Clinical Oral Implants Research. 2019;**30**(11):1085-1096

[20] Hamlet S, Alfarsi M, George R, Ivanovski S. The effect of hydrophilic titanium surface modification on macrophage inflammatory cytokine gene expression. Clinical Oral Implants Research. 2012;**23**(5):584-590

[21] Souza JCM, Sordi MB, Kanazawa M, Ravindran S, Henriques B, Silva FS, et al. Nano-scale modification of titanium implant surfaces to enhance osseointegration. Acta Biomaterialia. 2019;**94**:112-131

[22] Moon HJ, Gulati K, Li T, Moran CS, Ivanovski S. Inflammatory or reparative? Tuning macrophage polarization using anodized anisotropic nanoporous titanium implant surfaces. Small Science. 2024;**4**(10):2400211

[23] Zhu Y, Liang H, Liu X, Wu J, Yang C, Wong TM, et al. Regulation of macrophage polarization through surface topography design to facilitate implant-to-bone osteointegration. Science Advances. 2021;**7**:eabf6654

[24] Karazisis D, Sarunas Petronis S, Hossein Agheli H, Emanuelsson L, Norlindh B, Johansson A, et al. The influence of controlled surface nanotopography on the early biological events of osseointegration. Acta Biomaterialia. 2017;**53**:559-571

[25] Shi X, Xu C, Chen Z, Li M, Yin Z, Wang B, et al. Biomaterial-mediated macrophage polarization remodeling and sequential regulation: A potential strategy in bone infections treatment. Bone Research. 2025;**13**(1):11

[26] Kartikasari N, Yamada M, Watanabe J, He TW, X, Kamano Y, Egusa H. Titanium surface with nanospikes tunes macrophage polarization to produce inhibitory factors for osteo-clastogenesis through nanotopographic cues. Acta Biomaterialia. 2022;**137**:316-330

[27] Cruz M. Effects of implant surface modifications on osteogenic cell behavior. Molecular Biology. 2024;**13**:473. DOI: 10.4172/2168-9547.1000473

[28] Visalakshan RM, MacGregor MN, Sasidharan S, et al. Biomaterial surface hydrophobicity-mediated serum protein adsorption and immune responses. ACS Applied Materials & Interfaces. 2019;**11**(31):28641-28653

[29] Tuikampee S, Tuikampee S, Chaijareenont P, Rungsiyakull P,

Yavirach A. Titanium surface modification techniques to enhance osteoblasts and bone formation for dental implants: A narrative review on current advances. Meta. 2024;**14**(5):515

[30] Sánchez-Puetate JC, Graciliano Silva BL, Pinotti FE, Marcantonio CC, Pimentel Lopes de Oliveira GJ, Marcantonio Junior E. Assessing bone formation on hydrophilic and hydrophobic implant surfaces in a murine model treated with bisphosphonates. Clinical Oral Investigations. 2024;**28**(1):89

[31] Rupp F, Scheideler L, Rehbein D, Axmann D, Geis-Gerstorfer J. Roughness induced dynamic changes of wettability of acid etched titanium implant modifications. Biomaterials. 2004;**25**(7-8):1429-1438

[32] Lang NP, Salvi GE, Huynh-Ba G, Ivanovski S, Donos N, Bosshardt DD. Early osseointegration to hydrophilic and hydrophobic implant surfaces in humans. Clinical Oral Implants Research. 2011;**22**(4):349-356

[33] Oates T, Valderrama P, Bischof M, Nedir R, Jones A, Simpson J, et al. Enhanced implant stability with a chemically modified SLA surface: A randomized pilot study. The International Journal of Oral & Maxillofacial Implants. 2007;**22**(5):755-760

[34] Rausch-Fan X, Qu Z, Wieland M, Matejka M, Schedle A. Differentiation and cytokine synthesis of human osteoblasts on hydrophilic and hydrophobic titanium surfaces. Clinical Oral Implants Research. 2008;**19**(4):381-386

[35] Shirazi S, Huang CC, Kang M, Lu Y, Leung KS, Pitol-Palin L, et al. Evaluation of nanoscale versus hybrid micro/nano surface topographies for endosseous implants. Acta Biomaterialia. 2020;**173**:199-216

[36] Illing B, Mohammadnejad L, Theurer A, Schultheiss J, Kimmerle-Mueller E, Rupp F, et al. Biological performance of titanium surfaces with different hydrophilic and nanotopographical features. Materials (Basel). 2023;**16**(23):7307

[37] Zheng Z, Gan S, Yang S, Hou C, Zhu Z, Wang H, et al. Enhanced surface hydrophilicity improves osseointegration of titanium implants via integrin-mediated osteo-immunomodulation. Journal of Materials Chemistry B. 2025;**13**(2):456-468

[38] Chen L, Ma Q, Fang L, Wang Y, Liu R, Zhang Y, et al. Super-hydrophilic nanostructured titanium surface improves implant osseointegration by mediating macrophage polarization. Journal of Immunology. 2014;**192**(Suppl. 1):180.4

[39] Li Q, Wang Z. Involvement of FAK/P38 signaling pathways in mediating the enhanced osteogenesis induced by nano-graphene oxide modification on titanium implant surface. International Journal of Nanomedicine. 2020;**15**:4659-4676

[40] Buser D, Broggini N, Wieland M, Schenk RK, Denzer AJ, Cochran DL, et al. Enhanced bone apposition to a chemically modified SLA titanium surface. Journal of Dental Research. 2004;**83**(7):529-533

[41] Patel R, Patel S, S, Girgis W, Ahmed W, Barrak F. A systematic assessment of the stability of SLA® vs. SLActive® implant surfaces over 12 weeks. Evidence-Based Dentistry. 2025;**26**(1):67-68

[42] Lai HC, Zhuang LF, Liu X, Wieland M, Zhang ZY, Zhang ZY.

The influence of surface energy on early adherent events of osteoblast on titanium substrates. Journal of Biomedical Materials Research. Part A. 2010;**93**(1):289-296

[43] Wennerberg A, Galli S, Albrektsson T. Current knowledge about the hydrophilic and nanostructured SLActive surface. Clinical, Cosmetic and Investigational Dentistry. 2011;**3**:59-67

[44] Mardas N, Schwarz F, Petrie A, Hakimi AR, Donos N. The effect of SLActive surface in guided bone formation in osteoporotic-like conditions. Clinical Oral Implants Research. 2011;**22**(4):406-415

[45] von Wilmowsky C, Stockmann P, Harsch I, Amann K, Metzler P, Lutz R, et al. Diabetes mellitus negatively affects peri-implant bone formation in the diabetic domestic pig. Journal of Clinical Periodontology. 2011;**38**(8):771-779

[46] Schlegel KA, Precht C, Möst T, Seidl C, Lutz R, von Wilmowsky C. Osseointegration of SLActive implants in diabetic pigs. Clinical Oral Implants Research. 2013;**24**(2):128-134

[47] Gianfreda F, Antonacci D, Raffone C, Muzzi M, Pistilli V, Patrizio BP. Microscopic characterization of bioactivate implant surfaces: Increasing wettability using salts and dry technology. Materials (Basel). 2021;**14**(10):2608

[48] Duske K, Koban I, Kindel E, Schroeder K, Nebe B, Holtfreter B, et al. Atmospheric plasma enhances wettability and cell spreading on dental implant metals. Journal of Clinical Periodontology. 2012;**39**:400-407

[49] Wennerberg A, Albrektsson T. Suggested guidelines for the topographic evaluation of implant surfaces. The International Journal of Oral & Maxillofacial Implants. 2000;**15**:331-344

[50] Gianfreda F, Raffone C, Antonacci D, Mussano F, Genova T, C hinigò G, Canullo L, Bollero P. Early biological response of an ultra-hydrophilic implant surface activated by salts and dry technology: An in-vitro study. Applied Sciences. 2021;**11**(13):6120

[51] Mussano F, Genova T, Petrillo S, Roato I, Ferracini R, Munaron L. Osteogenic differentiation modulates the cytokine, chemokine, and growth factor profile of ASCs and SHED. International Journal of Molecular Sciences. 2018;**19**:1454

[52] Moses O, Bengazi F, Ferri M, Gianfreda F, Urbizo Velez J, Botticelli D, et al. Bioactivated implant surfaces placed in healed sites or extraction sockets: A preliminary experimental study in dogs. The International Journal of Oral & Maxillofacial Implants. 2022;**37**(5):963-970

[53] Canullo L, Menini M, Pesce P, Iacono R, Sculean A, Del Fabbro M. Nano-superhydrophilic and bioactive surface in poor bone environment. Part 1: Transition from primary to secondary stability. A controlled clinical trial: Bioactive implant surfaces in poor density bone. Clinical Oral Investigations. 2024;**28**(7):372

Chapter 10

Biological Mechanisms of Oral Mucosal Keratinization: A Comprehensive Review

Evgeny Weinberg and Haim Tal

Abstract

Oral mucosal keratinization is a finely regulated biological process essential for maintaining masticatory function, barrier integrity, and periodontal stability. This comprehensive review traces the evolution of our understanding of oral epithelial phenotype determination, from pioneering transplantation studies conducted in the 1970s that established the stromal connective tissue as the key determinant of epithelial fate, to recent molecular and transcriptomic discoveries. Modern research reveals that extracellular matrix components, basement membrane proteins such as COL4A6 and COL18A1, and soluble mediators including TGFβ-binding proteins, retinoic acid, and BMP2 orchestrate keratinization through dynamic epithelial-stromal interactions. Single-cell and bulk transcriptomic analyses further uncover cellular heterogeneity within gingival and lining mucosa, highlighting mesenchymal stem cell-rich niches in keratinized tissues. Clinically, these insights redefine strategies for managing soft-tissue deficiencies around teeth and implants, emphasizing biologically guided rather than purely surgical approaches. Emerging spatial transcriptomic technologies now enable high-resolution mapping of gene expression within intact oral tissues, bridging histology and molecular biology. Together, these advances lay the groundwork for next-generation regenerative therapies aimed at inducing keratinized mucosa through the targeted modulation of stromal signaling networks and epithelial differentiation pathways.

Keywords: oral mucosal keratinization, epithelial-stromal interactions, basement membrane, extracellular matrix, mesenchymal stromal cells

1. Introduction

The oral mucosa is one of the most intricate barrier systems in the human body, playing a crucial role in various functions, such as mastication and speech, while also serving as a key site for immune interactions [1]. The proper functioning of this tissue relies on the presence of diverse cell types and the complex interplay between them. Failure in the mucosal barrier mechanisms may lead to pathogen invasion and to the onset of chronic inflammatory conditions, such as gingival inflammation and periodontal disease. Moreover, healthy oral mucosa is vital for maintaining functional masticatory stability and esthetic appearance [2–4]. Consequently, the oral mucosa must rapidly adapt to support tissue regeneration and healing following injury. A comprehensive studying of mucosal anatomy, physiology, and cellular function *in situ* is essential for understanding the dynamics of health and disease, thereby supporting the preservation of oral health.

2. Classification and characteristics of oral mucous membranes

There are three types of mucous membranes lining the oral cavity that are anatomically, histologically, and functionally distinct: a. *masticatory mucosa*, covered by a layer of protective keratin, located in the areas subjected to mechanical forces of mastication (gingiva and hard palate); b. *lining* (non-keratinized) mucosa, covering most of the rest of the oral cavity; and c. *specialized* (mix of the other two) mucosa on the dorsum of the tongue (**Figure 1**) [5].

Whether keratinized (resembling the epidermis of the skin) or non-keratinized, all types of oral mucous membranes are lined with stratified squamous epithelium (**Figure 2**) [6–8]. The underlying connective tissue layer of the oral mucosa, called the *lamina propria*, is analogous to the dermis in the skin. Located between the

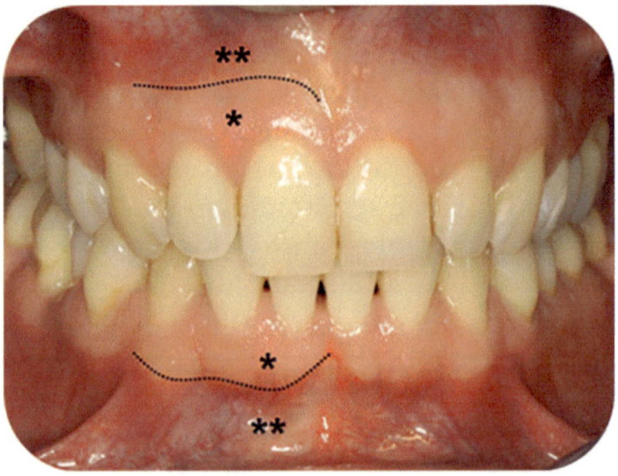

Figure 1.
Labial view of oral mucosa: (*) Gingiva = masticatory keratinized mucosa; (**) non-keratinized lining mucosa. All images are original and were obtained from the authors' own database, unless otherwise stated.

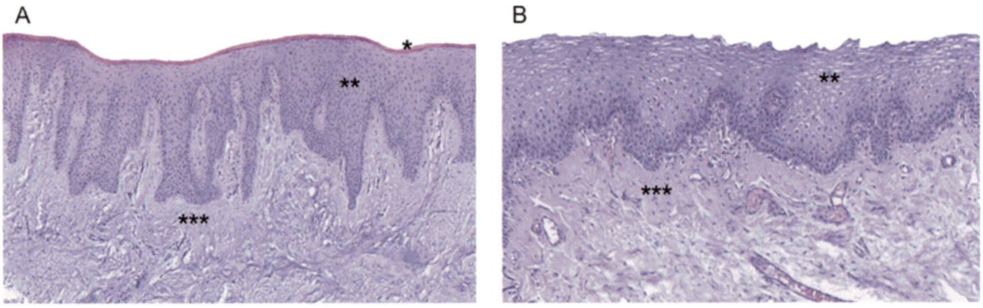

Figure 2.
Histological view of oral mucosae: (A) masticatory keratinized mucosa; (B) non-keratinized lining mucosa. (*) Keratinized layer; (**) stratified squamous epithelium; (***) lamina propria.

epithelium and the lamina propria is a sheet-like extracellular matrix (ECM), known as the basement membrane, which plays an important role in maintaining tissue homeostasis [9].

Besides the differences in keratinization of the overlying epithelium, the lining and masticatory mucosae differ also in their healing pattern, barrier functions, immune responsiveness, and proneness to drug-induced overgrowth [10–13].

3. Gingival health and soft tissue management: Clinical importance

In periodontics and dental implantology, interest in the management and care of soft tissues in the oral cavity is continuously rising. The presence of healthy, attached keratinized mucosa adjacent to teeth (gingiva) and implants (peri-implant mucosa) contributes to stability in function, improved plaque control, and optimized esthetic outcomes [2, 3].

When gingival tissue, a part of the masticatory keratinized mucosa, is thin and delicate, recession defects may develop, exposing the cemento-enamel junction (CEJ) and the root surface (**Figure 3A**) [14, 15]. Such defects can result in esthetic impairment, dentin hypersensitivity, difficulty in maintaining oral hygiene, and other adverse conditions of concern to both patients and clinicians.

Clinically, soft tissue management comprises gingival augmentation procedures aimed at expanding the width of keratinized tissue around teeth and dental implants [16, 17]. These procedures are typically surgical, involving both a donor site (usually the hard palate or edentulous alveolar ridges) and a recipient site (**Figure 3**) [18, 19]. As a result, they are highly invasive and may be quite traumatic for patients [20, 21].

A better understanding of the molecular mechanisms behind oral mucosa keratinization could enable the development of less invasive procedures to augment keratinized gingiva. Advanced molecular insights may enable targeted therapies that stimulate oral mucosa keratinization, such as growth factors, cell therapies, or gene regulation techniques, thus minimizing the need for surgical procedures [22].

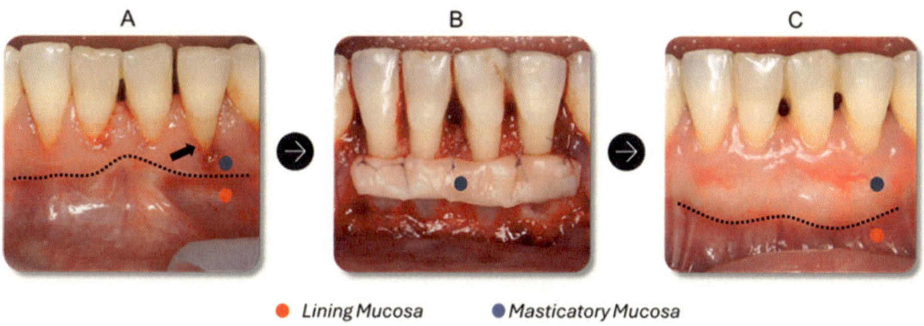

Figure 3.
Case presentation of a surgical procedure to increase gingival width and cover a buccal recession defect. (A) Preoperative view of a 6-mm buccal gingival recession defect (black arrow), classified as Miller Class III (Cairo RT2), affecting tooth 32, with reduced width of keratinized mucosa; (B) surgical intervention using a coronally advanced flap combined with a connective tissue graft harvested from the masticatory mucosa of hard palate and fixated at the recipient site, aimed at increasing keratinized tissue and promoting epithelial transition from lining to keratinized masticatory epithelium; (C) twelve-month postoperative follow-up demonstrating a significant gain in gingival width with successful recession coverage. All clinical photographs originate from the authors' own database; the surgical procedure was performed by one of the authors (EW).

4. A paradigm shift: From environmental stimuli to genetic and stromal control of keratinization

Throughout much of the twentieth century, structural and morphological changes in tissues were widely attributed to environmental stimuli. For instance, it was proposed that the epithelium responds to mechanical abrasion from mastication by increasing the thickness of its keratinized layer [23].

This paradigm was decisively overturned more than 50 years ago by two foundational studies from Karring and colleagues, who demonstrated that oral epithelial phenotype is determined by the identity of the underlying connective tissue rather than by functional adaptation or mechanical wear. Their landmark experiments established principles that remain central to oral biology, periodontology, and regenerative surgery [6, 7].

In the first of these studies (1971), Karring et al. transplanted full-thickness mucosal tissue segments containing both epithelium and lamina propria between keratinized gingiva and non-keratinized alveolar mucosa in non-human primates [6]. Importantly, most grafts were not disconnected from the host bed but intertwined with the recipient site, maintaining vascularization and close stromal integration, while additional free palatal grafts were independently placed on the alveolar mucosa. Clinical and histological evaluation over a 12-month period demonstrated that the epithelial phenotype was preserved according to the donor tissue: Keratinized mucosa remained keratinized even when transplanted into lining mucosal zones, whereas lining mucosa maintained its non-keratinized epithelium when relocated to gingival sites. A particularly striking observation was that when non-keratinized mucosa was transplanted adjacent to teeth, a narrow strip of keratinized epithelium reappeared next to the tooth, suggesting that gingival and periodontal connective tissue, likely derived from the most coronal periodontal ligament and supra-alveolar gingiva, induced keratinization in the root-associated environment.

The second study (1975) provided a direct test of this hypothesis [7]. Here, de-epithelialized connective tissue grafts were transplanted into alveolar mucosa. Crucially, after healing, the overlying epithelium was surgically removed to allow re-epithelialization from surrounding non-keratinized mucosa. This procedural step is often overlooked, yet it is essential: Transmucosal connective tissue grafts covered by intact lining epithelium do not themselves induce keratinization. Only after surgical exposure of the grafted connective tissue was the epithelium able to regenerate under the influence of the stromal environment. The results were definitive: When non-keratinized lining epithelium migrated over exposed gingival connective tissue, it converted into a keratinized gingival phenotype. In contrast, migration over exposed alveolar connective tissue preserved the non-keratinized epithelial character. The epithelial transition line mapped precisely to the underlying stromal boundary between collagen-rich, non-elastic gingival connective tissue and the more elastic alveolar connective tissue.

Together, these studies established a durable conceptual and clinical framework. Connective tissue identity dictates epithelial fate. Gingival connective tissue drives keratinization, whereas alveolar connective tissue enforces a lining phenotype. Clinically, this explains why palatal or gingival grafts reliably establish keratinized mucosa in recipient sites, while alveolar connective tissue cannot substitute. These insights established more than half a century ago continue to guide periodontal surgical approaches and inspire tissue engineering strategies aimed at regenerating or inducing keratinized mucosa.

The relevance of these principles has been further tested in modern experimental models, particularly in relation to dental implants, where peri-implant mucosa frequently differs from gingiva in both structure and function. Liñares et al., using a dog model, excised all keratinized tissue around both teeth and implants [24]. Approximately 2 mm of keratinized tissue regenerated around natural teeth within 1 month and remained stable thereafter, whereas no keratinized mucosa developed around implants in the same animals. Placement of a transmucosal connective tissue graft reduced recession around implants but did not reliably generate new keratinized tissue in sites where it was absent. These findings underscore a fundamental biological divergence: The periodontium possesses an inherent capacity to re-establish keratinization, whereas peri-implant tissues lack this potential.

Further evidence came from Imber et al., who performed heterotopic transpositions of keratinized into non-keratinized tissue and vice versa using a Z-plasty design in dogs [25]. At tooth sites, keratinization reappeared at the gingival margin even when initially displaced, confirming the inductive influence of gingival connective tissue. At implant sites, however, keratinization failed to extend coronally toward the margin. Instead, the transposed keratinized band retained its phenotype but remained apical to the implant margin, resulting in a clinical presentation of zero millimeters of keratinized mucosa coronally. Histological mapping of elastic fibers reinforced the parallel with earlier transplantation studies, showing that connective tissue beneath keratinized and non-keratinized epithelia retained distinctive features consistent with gingival versus alveolar connective tissue identity.

Taken together, both the foundational transplantation studies and these modern implant investigations converge on a central theme: Keratinization is not an adaptive response to environmental wear but a stromally programmed epithelial phenotype. Around teeth, gingival connective tissue is both necessary and sufficient to impose a keratinized program, enabling regeneration and stability of keratinized zones. Around implants, the absence of periodontal ligament and supra-alveolar gingival connective tissue precludes this capacity, limiting grafting procedures to improving tissue volume and reducing recession without reliably re-establishing keratinized mucosa. This divergence in biology has critical implications for periodontal and peri-implant therapy, as well as for the design of regenerative strategies in oral medicine.

5. Biological regulators of oral epithelial keratinization

Recent research has uncovered multiple stromal and molecular regulators that contribute to the induction or suppression of epithelial keratinization in the oral cavity. A central theme emerging from these studies is that keratinization results from a tightly regulated interplay between extracellular matrix (ECM) components, basement membrane (BM) structures, soluble morphogens, and signaling molecules within the connective tissue. Many factors, including vitamin D_3, calcium ions, interferon γ, transforming growth factors, integrins, and retinoids in the supporting connective tissue, are known to influence the gene expression programs responsible for the heterogeneity of epithelial tissues [26]. The following section integrates insights from key mechanistic studies investigating how specific biological factors modulate oral mucosal keratinization.

One important line of investigation has focused on the role of elastin-rich ECM in suppressing keratinization. In a foundational study by Hsieh et al., the authors examined how the composition of the underlying connective tissue influences epithelial phenotype [26]. Using a bioengineered three-dimensional (3D) oral mucosa model, they showed that both the native and the engineered keratinized gingiva changed phenotypes and expressed keratins 4 and 13 (the markers of non-keratinized oral mucosa) when treated with exogenous elastin. Conversely, enzymatic degradation of endogenous elastin in non-keratinized mucosa by elastase induced a keratinized phenotype, marked by the expression of keratins 1 and 10. These findings provided compelling evidence that stromal elastin supports the maintenance of the non-keratinized epithelial phenotype in the oral mucosa.

Another important finding concerns the modulation of keratinization through latent transforming growth factor beta (TGF-β) binding proteins (LTBPs), specifically LTBP-1 and LTBP-2. Chiang et al. demonstrated that TGF-β–mediated regulation of keratinization is governed by opposing roles of latent TGF-β binding proteins, with LTBP-1 promoting keratinization and LTBP-2 exerting an inhibitory effect [27].

Additional evidence for BM regulation comes from the work of Komori et al., who investigated the α6 chain of type IV collagen (COL4A6) [28]. This protein is abundant in the BM underlying keratinized gingiva but absent in non-keratinized regions. In COL4A6-knockout newborn mice, epithelial development was delayed and keratin 10 expression was markedly reduced. Additionally, siRNA-mediated down-regulation of COL4A6 in human gingival epithelial cells suppressed epithelial keratinization. Collectively, these findings indicate that the type IV collagen α6 chain plays a key role in regulating keratin 10 expression and the keratinization of oral mucosal epithelium.

In a related study, Nguyen et al. investigated type XVIII collagen (COL18A1), a basement membrane-associated heparan sulfate proteoglycan highly expressed in keratinized oral mucosa [29]. In COL18A1-knockout mice, the absence of type XVIII collagen caused a marked reduction in keratin 10 expression and a decrease in both the number and size of keratohyalin granules in the granular layer of the epithelium. Moreover, *in vitro* down-regulation of COL18A1 suppressed epithelial keratinization. Collectively, these findings indicate that type XVIII collagen functions as a key modulator of oral epithelial keratinization.

Mu et al. suggested that soluble growth factors contribute to the regulation of epithelial keratinization [30]. They demonstrated that bone morphogenetic protein 2 (BMP-2) enhances the expression of the keratinization markers in monocultured epithelial cells. However, when epithelial cells were co-cultured with fibroblasts at the air-liquid interface (ALI), BMP-2 exerted little to no effect on keratinization.

A complementary mechanism of soluble regulation involves vitamin A derivatives (retinoids), which act through retinoic acid receptor (RAR)-mediated signaling. Miyazono et al. demonstrated that all-trans retinoic acid (atRA) suppresses oral epithelial keratinization by inhibiting the expression of loricrin while inducing keratin 4 [31]. Using 3D air-liquid interface cultures of human, porcine, and murine keratinocytes, they found that mouse cells required significantly higher atRA concentrations to achieve suppression of keratinization compared with human or porcine cells, suggesting species-specific differences in retinoid sensitivity. Inhibition of RAR signaling reversed the atRA-induced changes, restoring keratin 10 and loricrin expression and normal barrier function. These findings position retinoic acid as a potent soluble morphogen that counteracts epithelial keratinization, and they highlight that the lower susceptibility of mouse keratinocytes to retinoic acid may underlie the keratinized nature of rodent oral mucosa.

Collectively, these studies reveal that oral epithelial keratinization is governed by a complex, multilayered network of stromal cues and epithelial responses. Structural ECM components such as elastin and collagen chains, basement membrane proteins like COL4A6 and COL18A1, and regulatory molecules including LTBPs, retinoic acid, and soluble morphogens (e.g., BMP-2) cooperate to determine the keratinization state of the oral epithelium. Rather than being dictated by epithelial cells alone, keratinization emerges as a tissue-level phenomenon shaped by reciprocal stromal-epithelial interactions, where the biochemical composition and signaling activity of the connective tissue define epithelial phenotype and function. Understanding this finely tuned regulation provides a conceptual and mechanistic foundation for future therapeutic approaches aimed at restoring or inducing keratinized mucosa in health and disease.

6. Transcriptomic insights into the cellular and molecular heterogeneity of oral mucosae

In our previous studies, we first demonstrated, using Next Generation bulk RNA sequencing [32], and later through large-scale single-cell transcriptomic profiling [33], that *ex vivo*-expanded cells derived from the lamina propria of either the lining (non-keratinized) or masticatory oral mucosa are phenotypically heterogeneous, exhibiting distinct biological and molecular characteristics. Cluster analysis revealed 11 distinct cell clusters or subpopulations, some of which were identified as fibroblasts and others as smooth muscle cells [33]. Notably, one of the clusters, located at the intersection of the plots of the lining and masticatory mucosa-derived cells, was annotated as mesenchymal stem cells (MSCs). Most members of this cluster (78%) were cells derived from the lamina propria of the masticatory mucosa, indicating that this tissue contains many more MSCs than the lining mucosa, which supports our previous conclusions that masticatory mucosa is a more attractive donor site for cell therapy [32].

Our research also revealed that stromal cells originating from the lining oral mucosa are highly enriched in biological processes associated with the positive regulation of epithelial cell proliferation [32, 33], which may partly explain the increased turnover rate of the lining oral mucosa epithelium [5]. Furthermore, we proposed that the distinct gene expression profiles observed in these stromal cells [32, 33] contribute to the modulation of keratinization in the overlying epithelium. This modulation, for example, may be related to the distinct turnover rates of the extracellular matrix in the connective tissues of the lining versus the masticatory oral mucosae [32]. Given that connective tissues play a pivotal role in directing epithelial differentiation and regulating keratin expression, it is crucial to identify the specific components within the connective tissues of gingiva and non-keratinized lining mucosa that drive these differences.

7. Implications and future perspectives

Understanding the molecular and stromal regulation of oral mucosal keratinization offers significant clinical and translational potential. As keratinized mucosa plays a vital role in maintaining oral health, particularly in periodontal therapy and implantology, insights into its regulatory mechanisms could guide the development of novel strategies to enhance tissue resilience and regeneration.

Recent advances in spatial transcriptomics (ST) now allow high-resolution mapping of gene expression within intact tissue architecture while preserving the native relationships between epithelial and stromal compartments. This technology bridges a critical gap left by single-cell RNA sequencing, which, although powerful, loses the spatial context essential for interpreting epithelial-mesenchymal interactions. Applying ST to the oral mucosa provides an unprecedented opportunity to decode how regional stromal cues, basement membrane components, and extracellular matrix dynamics shape epithelial keratinization patterns.

In the near future, the integration of spatially resolved omics with proteomics, three-dimensional tissue models, and bioengineered scaffolds is expected to deepen our understanding of the molecular microenvironments that determine keratinized versus non-keratinized phenotypes. Such insights could be harnessed to design biomaterial-based or cell-guided therapies that activate keratinization pathways in desired oral regions. Furthermore, identifying spatially organized signaling networks, such as those involving collagen, desmosomal proteins, or growth factor gradients, may enable targeted pharmacological modulation of epithelial differentiation.

Ultimately, these advances may transform the management of mucogingival and peri-implant conditions by enabling precision regeneration of keratinized mucosa tailored to each patient's biological context.

Author details

Evgeny Weinberg[1,2]* and Haim Tal[1]

1 Department of Periodontology and Oral Implantology, Goldschleger School of Dental Medicine, Gray Faculty of Medical and Health Sciences, Tel Aviv University, Tel Aviv, Israel

2 Department of Oral Biology, Goldschleger School of Dental Medicine, Gray Faculty of Medical and Health Sciences, Tel Aviv University, Tel-Aviv, Israel

*Address all correspondence to: evgenywein@gmail.com

References

[1] Caetano AJ, Sharpe PT. Redefining mucosal inflammation with spatial genomics. Journal of Dental Research. 2024;**103**(2):129-137

[2] Thoma DS, Benić GI, Zwahlen M, Hämmerle CHF, Jung RE. A systematic review assessing soft tissue augmentation techniques. Clinical Oral Implants Research. 2009;**20**:146-165

[3] Imber JC, Roccuzzo A, Stähli A, Bosshardt DD, Muñoz F, Ramseier CA, et al. Spontaneous regeneration of keratinized tissue at implants and teeth. Journal of Clinical Periodontology. 2023;**50**(8):1064-1074

[4] Zigdon H, Machtei EE. The dimensions of keratinized mucosa around implants affect clinical and immunological parameters. Clinical Oral Implants Research. 2008;**19**(4):387-392

[5] Squier CA, Kremer MJ. Biology of oral mucosa and esophagus. JNCI Monographs. 2001;**2001**(29):7-15

[6] Karring T, Ostergaard E, Löe H. Conservation of tissue specificity after heterotopic transplantation of gingiva and alveolar mucosa. Journal of Periodontal Research. 1971;**6**(4):282-293

[7] Karring T, Lang NP, Löe H. The role of gingival connective tissue in determining epithelial differentiation. Journal of Periodontal Research. 1975;**10**(1):1-11

[8] Koren N, Zubeidat K, Saba Y, Horev Y, Barel O, Wilharm A, et al. Maturation of the neonatal oral mucosa involves unique epithelium-microbiota interactions. Cell Host & Microbe. 2021;**29**(2):197-209.e5

[9] Tsutsui K, Machida H, Nakagawa A, Ahn K, Morita R, Sekiguchi K, et al. Mapping the molecular and structural specialization of the skin basement membrane for inter-tissue interactions. Nature Communications. 2021;**12**(1):2577

[10] Nakasone N, Kubota T, Hoshino C, Nohno K, Itagaki M, Shimizu T, et al. Differential gene and protein expression of tissue inhibitors of metalloproteinases (TIMP)-3 and TIMP-4 in gingival tissues from drug induced gingival overgrowth. Archives of Oral Biology. 2009;**54**(7):634-641

[11] Zhang QZ, Nguyen AL, Yu WH, Le AD. Human oral mucosa and gingiva: A unique reservoir for mesenchymal stem cells. Journal of Dental Research. 2012;**91**(11):1011-1018

[12] Moutsopoulos NM, Konkel JE. Tissue-specific immunity at the oral mucosal barrier. Trends in Immunology. 2018;**39**(4):276-287

[13] Heyman O, Koren N, Mizraji G, Capucha T, Wald S, Nassar M, et al. Impaired differentiation of Langerhans cells in the murine Oral epithelium adjacent to titanium dental implants. Frontiers in Immunology. 2018;**9**:1712

[14] Di Domenico GL, Di Martino M, Arrigoni G, Aroca S, de Sanctis M. Multiple coronally advanced flap with a selective use of connective tissue graft: A 3-year prospective clinical and histological study. Journal of Periodontology. 2023;**94**(10):1200-1209

[15] Galli F, Deflorian M, Zucchelli G, Del Fabbro M, Testori T. The biologically oriented preparation technique (BOPT) approach for preventing gingival recessions in fixed prosthodontics. A 5- to 13-year follow-up retrospective

study. The International Journal of Esthetic Dentistry. 2024;**19**(2):112-124

[16] Aroca S, Di Domenico GL, Darnaud C, de Sanctis M. Modified coronally advanced tunnel technique with site-specific application of connective tissue graft for the treatment of multiple adjacent maxillary gingival recessions: A case series. The International Journal of Periodontics & Restorative Dentistry. 2021;**41**(2):253-259

[17] Tavelli L, McGuire MK, Zucchelli G, Rasperini G, Feinberg SE, Wang HL, et al. Biologics-based regenerative technologies for periodontal soft tissue engineering. Journal of Periodontology. 2020;**91**(2):147-154

[18] Zucchelli G, Tavelli L, McGuire MK, Rasperini G, Feinberg SE, Wang HL, et al. Autogenous soft tissue grafting for periodontal and peri-implant plastic surgical reconstruction. Journal of Periodontology. 2020;**91**(1):9-16

[19] González-Febles J, Romandini M, Laciar-Oudshoorn F, Noguerol F, Marruganti C, Bujaldón-Daza A, et al. Tunnel vs. coronally advanced flap in combination with a connective tissue graft for the treatment of multiple gingival recessions: A multi-center randomized clinical trial. Clinical Oral Investigations. 2023;**27**(7):3627-3638

[20] Tavelli L, Barootchi S, Stefanini M, Zucchelli G, Giannobile WV, Wang HL. Wound healing dynamics, morbidity, and complications of palatal soft-tissue harvesting. Periodontology 2000. 2023;**92**(1):90-119

[21] McGuire MK, Tavelli L, Feinberg SE, Rasperini G, Zucchelli G, Wang HL, et al. Living cell-based regenerative medicine technologies for periodontal soft tissue augmentation. Journal of Periodontology. 2020;**91**(2):155-164

[22] Sanchez N, Vignoletti F, Sanz-Martin I, Coca A, Nuñez J, Maldonado E, et al. Cell therapy based on gingiva-derived mesenchymal stem cells seeded in a xenogeneic collagen matrix for root coverage of RT1 gingival lesions: An in vivo experimental study. International Journal of Molecular Sciences. 2022;**23**(6):1-17

[23] Mackenzie IC, Hill MW. Connective tissue influences on patterns of epithelial architecture and keratinization in skin and oral mucosa of the adult mouse. Cell and Tissue Research. 1984;**235**(3):551-559

[24] Liñares A, Rubinos A, Puñal A, Muñoz F, Blanco J. Regeneration of keratinized tissue around teeth and implants following coronal repositioning of alveolar mucosa with and without a connective tissue graft: An experimental study in dogs: Fifty years after Karring's landmark study: Fifty years after Karring's 71 landmark study. Journal of Clinical Periodontology. 2022;**49**(11):1133-1144

[25] Imber JC, Roccuzzo A, Stähli A, Bosshardt DD, Muñoz F, Ramseier CA, et al. Clinical and histologic evaluation of heterotopic mucosa transpositioning at teeth and dental implants. Clinical Oral Implants Research. 2023;**34**(12):1395-1405

[26] Hsieh PC, Jin YT, Chang CW, Huang CC, Liao SC, Yuan K. Elastin in oral connective tissue modulates the keratinization of overlying epithelium. Journal of Clinical Periodontology. 2010;**37**(8):705-711

[27] Chiang MS, Yang JR, Liao SC, Hsu CC, Hsu CW, Yuan K. Latent transforming growth factor-β binding proteins (LTBP-1 and LTBP-2) and gingiva keratinization. Oral Diseases. 2015;**21**(6):762-769

[28] Komori T, Ono M, Hara ES, Ueda J, Nguyen HTT, Nguyen HT, et al. Type IV collagen α6 chain is a regulator of keratin 10 in keratinization of oral mucosal epithelium. Scientific Reports. 2018;**8**(1):2612

[29] Nguyen HTT, Ono M, Hara ES, Komori T, Edamatsu M, Yonezawa T, et al. Type XVIII collagen modulates keratohyalin granule formation and keratinization in oral mucosa. International Journal of Molecular Sciences. 2019;**20**(19):1-14

[30] Mu X, Ono M, Nguyen HTT, Wang Z, Zhao K, Komori T, et al. Exploring the regulators of keratinization: Role of BMP-2 in oral mucosa. Cells. 2024;**13**(10):807

[31] Miyazono S, Otani T, Ogata K, Kitagawa N, Iida H, Inai Y, et al. The reduced susceptibility of mouse keratinocytes to retinoic acid may be involved in the keratinization of oral and esophageal mucosal epithelium. Histochemistry and Cell Biology. 2020;**153**(4):225-237

[32] Kabakov L, Nemcovsky CE, Plasmanik-Chor M, Meir H, Bar DZ, Weinberg E. Fibroblasts from the oral masticatory and lining mucosa have different gene expression profiles and proliferation rates. Journal of Clinical Periodontology. 2021;**48**(10):1393-1401

[33] Pinkhasov I, Kabakov L, Nemcovsky CE, Weinreb M, Schlesinger P, Bender O, et al. Single-cell transcriptomic analysis of oral masticatory and lining mucosa-derived mesenchymal stromal cells. Journal of Clinical Periodontology. 2023;**50**(60):807-818

Chapter 11

Frontiers in the Understanding of Peri-Implant Disease

Alexandre Perez and Tommaso Lombardi

Abstract

Peri-implant diseases are plaque-associated pathologic condition characterized by the inflammatory process affecting hard and soft tissues around endosseous dental implants. These frequent complications are the result of an imbalance between the host response and bacterial challenge, which may affect the peri-implant mucosa "mucositis" or also involve the supporting bone "peri-implantitis". Clinical aspects/signs of peri-implant diseases should be detected at each recall visit as well as swelling, erythema, bleeding on probing and suppuration. Moreover, many risk factors are involved in the development of peri-implant disease and most patients may have multiple risk factors including smoking, substance use disorders, socio-economic status, mental health disorders, old age and poor home dental care. In addition, iatrogenic, local, systemic, type of prosthesis and implant site-specific factors have been involved in the development of such complication. Clinicians must be aware of and recognizes the importance of such risk factors in order to manage them appropriately. This chapter aims to provide clinicians with an up-to-date understanding of peri-implant disease.

Keywords: peri-implantitis, peri-implant mucositis, dental implants, periodontal disease, treatment

1. Introduction

1.1 The growing penetration of dental implant therapy

Dental implant therapy has been established as a predictable and effective treatment option for replacing missing teeth. Cumulative survival rates of implant-borne restorations range from 90.5–100% after 5 years and 85.5–100% after 10 years, reflecting remarkably low failure rates—as low as 0 to 1.56 or 2 per 100 placed implants, respectively [1–6]. Recent systematic reviews have estimated a total survival rate of 96.4% [6]. Furthermore, by carefully adopting patient and case selection criteria, immediate implant protocols—traditionally considered challenging—may today be realized with the comparable survival rates to those of conventional delayed approaches [7–9]. Encouraging long-term success rates and evolving treatment strategies have contributed to the rapid growth and global acceptance of dental implant therapy, with an estimated 12–15 million implants placed worldwide in 2023 [10]. Similarly, the prevalence of U.S. citizens rehabilitated with dental implants has increased at an annual rate of approximately 14%, rising from 5.7% in 2016 to a projected 23% by 2026 [11]. This substantial and growing proportion of the population rehabilitated with dental implants underscores the significance of implant therapy as a topic of increasing epidemiological and public health relevance.

The growing adoption of dental implant therapy has prompted an evolution in its evaluation criteria. Early success benchmarks, as defined by Albrektsson et al. in 1986, primarily focused on functional outcomes such as implant survival, prosthetic stability, radiographic bone loss and absence of peri-implant infection [12]. More recently, these criteria have expanded to include peri-implant soft tissue health, natural esthetics, prosthodontic performance and patient-centred outcomes such as satisfaction—reflecting a modern, multidimensional approach to assessing long-term implant success [13–16].

1.2 Dental implant complications, biological complications and their interplay

Despite their established long-term success, dental implant restorations are not complications-free. Dental implant complications are commonly classified into biological, technical and esthetic complications [5, 17, 18]. They may arise at any stage of treatment—whether during planning, surgery or implant function—and are influenced by various factors, including material and prosthetic design, anatomical constraints, unforeseen treatment plan deviations and patient-related systemic or behavioral aspects [17, 19–22]. For example, implant positioning and prosthetic design factors have been associated with long-term biological complications, suggesting a causal interplay between different types of implant-related complications [21–23].

Biological complications, that is peri-implant disease, represent the most common type of implant-related complication resulting in implant loss, followed by implant fracture and prosthetic overload. Notably, a potential association—regardless of causal direction—between mechanical and biological complications cannot be excluded [24].

1.3 Understanding and defining the clinical picture and diagnostic criteria of peri-implant disease

Peri-implant disease encompasses a spectrum of progressive inflammatory conditions of the peri-implant soft and/or hard tissues [25, 26]. Notably, the disease often progresses silently, remaining asymptomatic and undetectable by the patient [27]. Compounding this issue, many implant patients remain largely uneducated about potential complications, limiting early self-recognition outside of clinical examinations [28]. Despite the lack of overt symptoms, peri-implant disease is characterized by gradual and progressive tissue deterioration that can lead to esthetic and functional impairments up to the complete loss of the restoration [26].

Peri-implant disease is classified into two stages: peri-implant mucositis and peri-implantitis. Peri-implant mucositis is characterized by reversible inflammation of the peri-implant soft tissues. Peri-implantitis, on the other hand, involves inflammation of both soft and hard tissues accompanied by progressive and accelerating loss of supporting bone [25, 29].

Over the past decades, the scientific community has made the repeated efforts to standardize and refine the diagnostic criteria for peri-implant diseases.

Albrektsson and Isidor defined peri-implant mucositis as a reversible inflammation of the soft tissues as opposed to peri-implantitis being diagnosed by the irreversible and progressive loss of supporting bone [30]. Subsequent consensus reports, including those by Linde and Meyle and Zitzmann and Berglundh in 2008, defined peri-implant disease based on clinical indicators such as bleeding on probing (BoP) and radiographic bone loss [31, 32]. Lang and Berglundh extended these definitions within the broader context of tissue-level changes [33]. The 2017 World Workshop on the Classification of Periodontal and Peri-implant Diseases provided the most recent and potentially most comprehensive and clinically applicable criteria to date differentiating Peri-Implant Mucositis and Peri-Implantitis from Peri-Implant Health (**Figure 1**, **Table 1**) [14, 33, 34].

In clinical practice, it is important to recognize that a certain degree of marginal bone remodeling after implant placement and prosthetic loading is part of the normal physiological adaptation and should be expected [12, 35]. Seminal reports on crestal bone changes following prosthetic restoration in two-stage surgical protocols with delayed loading established that up to 1.5 mm of bone loss in the first year after loading and less than 0.2 mm annually thereafter may be considered within the range of physiological remodeling [12, 14, 36]. While these thresholds prevail as general clinical indicators, contemporary consensus emphasizes the importance of temporal stability in peri-implant bone levels rather than strict adherence to absolute values [14]. Progressive bone loss beyond initial remodeling, particularly when associated

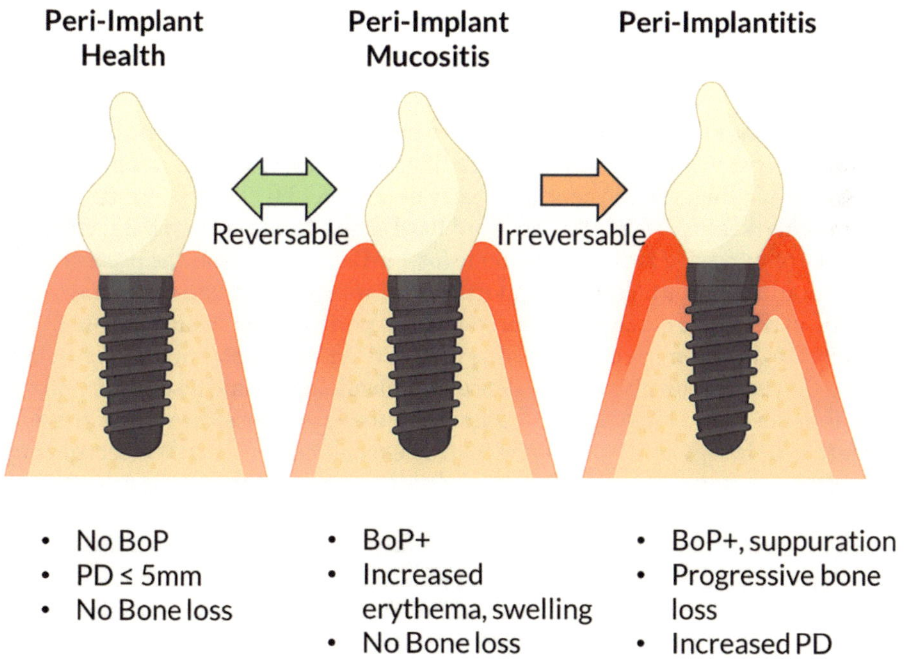

Figure 1.
Schematic illustration comparing peri-implant health, peri-implant mucositis, and peri-implantitis. Healthy peri-implant tissues characterize peri-implant health, no bleeding on probing (BoP), normal probing depth within normal ranges, and no radiographic bone loss. Peri-implant mucositis presents with BoP, increased erythema, and swelling of the soft tissues but without bone loss; this condition is considered reversible upon appropriate intervention. In contrast, peri-implantitis is associated with BoP and/or suppuration, progressive marginal bone loss, and increased probing depths; this condition is considered irreversible and requires surgical intervention.

Authors	Peri-implant mucositis		Peri-implantitis	
	Key features	Clinical parameters	Key features	Clinical parameters
Albrektsson & Isidor [30]	Reversible; only soft tissues	Soft tissue inflammation only	Irreversible inflammation and progressive bone loss	Mobility, radiographic bone loss, inflammation
Lindhe & Meyle [31]	BoP+; inflammation	No radiographic bone loss; BoP+	Inflammation with bone loss	BoP+/ suppuration; radiographic bone loss
Zitzmann & Berglundh [32]	BoP without bone loss beyond normal remodeling	BoP+, stable bone level	Bone loss beyond expected remodeling	Probing depth increase; radiographic bone loss
Lang & Berglundh [33]	Inflammation; reversible upon therapy	BoP+, no additional bone loss; inflammation present	Inflammation of both soft and hard tissues with bone loss	Increased probing depth, recession, bone loss
World Workshop / Berglundh & Armitage [14]	BoP+ and/or suppuration without bone loss beyond normal remodeling	BoP+, Probing depth may increase, but bone levels remain stable	BoP+ / suppuration, increased probing depth, and bone loss ≥3 mm	BoP+, PD ≥ 5 mm, bone level ≥ 3 mm apical of implant shoulder

BoP+: positive bleeding on probing, PD: probing depth.

Table 1.
Key features and clinical parameters of peri-implant mucositis and peri-implantitis.

with clinical signs of inflammation, indicates peri-implant disease. Regular diagnostic follow-ups, including clinical and radiographic examinations compared to baseline post-loading, remain central to early detection [33]. The maintenance of stable, unremarkable peri-implant soft and hard tissue conditions—characterized by the absence of excessive radiographic bone loss, inflammation and the presence of healthy, keratinized epithelium—supports peri-implant health and can be regarded as a leitmotif in the clinical diagnostic for long-term peri-implant health (**Table 2**) [37].

Despite the development of refined diagnostic criteria and their importance in standardizing the research on disease prevalence in epidemiological and disease surveillance studies, the clinical and biological heterogeneity in tissue response, disease progression and defect morphology continues to present challenges—not necessarily in recognizing peri-implant disease itself, but in adequately classifying its severity, progression and clinical therapeutic approaches [38–41]. Unlike, for example periodontitis and other pathological conditions that benefit from established staging systems, current definitions of peri-implant diseases remain largely binary [42, 43]. Future research efforts may contribute to developing more differentiated grading systems, enabling improved prognostic accuracy and refined therapeutic approaches (**Figure 2**).

1.4 Epidemiology of peri-implant disease

In epidemiology, two fundamental metrics are used to characterize disease patterns: prevalence and incidence. Prevalence describes the proportion of individuals affected by a condition at a specific point or over a defined period, while incidence refers to the number of new cases that arise within a specified timeframe. Together, these measures

Time after implant loading	Expected bone level changes
First-year	≤1.5 mm
After the first year	≤ 0.2 mm per year

Table 2.
Time after implant loading and expected level changes.

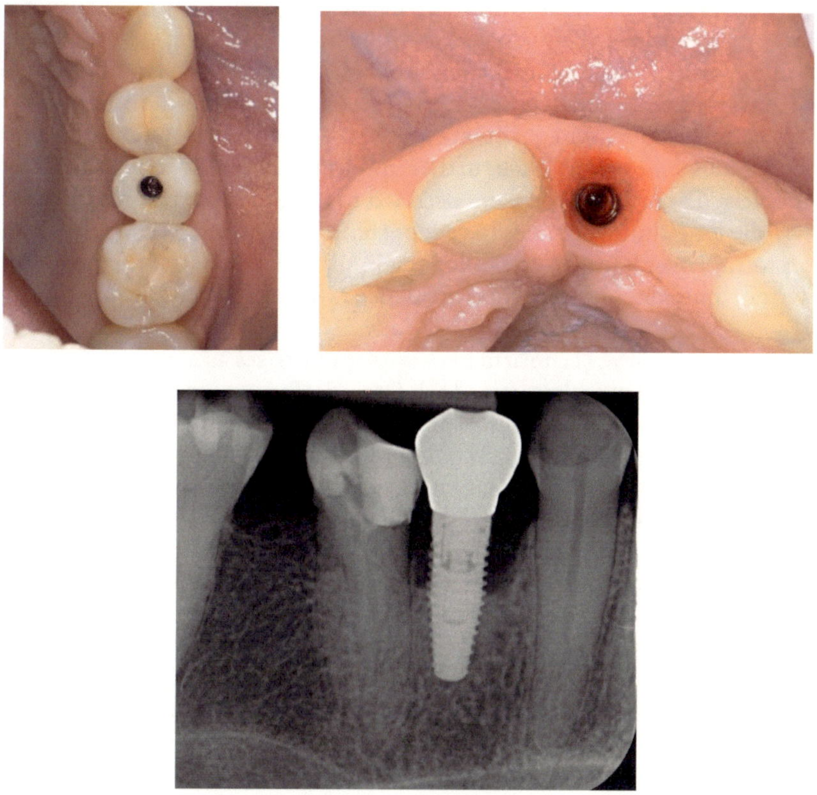

Figure 2.
Screw-retained single-unit crown placement site 25 showing good peri-implant health (top left), peri-implant mucositis highlighted after removal of a crown site 21 (top right) and peri-implantitis site 44 on intraoral radiography.

provide insight into the burden and dynamics of peri-implant disease within a given population. They may be assessed at the implant level (implant-based) or at the patient level (subject-based), offering a more nuanced understanding of both peri-implantitis and peri-implant mucositis across diverse clinical and patient-centred contexts.

The reported prevalence of peri-implant diseases varies considerably across clinical studies. Comprehensive systematic reviews published in 2015 and 2017 reported that the patient-level prevalence of peri-implant mucositis ranges from 19 to 65% and that of peri-implantitis from 1 to 47% [44]. Calculated average and weighted prevalence estimates derived from meta-analytical approaches may offer a more tangible indication of the overall epidemiological burden of peri-implant diseases. Based on aggregated data from multiple cross-sectional studies, peri-implant mucositis affects approximately 1 in 2 patients (43–47%), while peri-implantitis is observed in about 1 in 5 patients (20–22%) [44, 45].

The weighted mean prevalence of peri-implantitis at the implant level is estimated at 9.3%, compared to 19.8% at the patient level [45]. This discrepancy highlights the greater clinical impact of subject-based prevalence, as individual patients often present with multiple implants.

The considerable variability in the reported prevalence rates of peri-implant diseases can be attributed to several methodological and clinical factors. One of the most critical sources of inconsistency is the lack of standardized case definitions and diagnostic criteria across studies—particularly regarding parameters such as marginal bone levels [46]. This gap was rectified by the 2017 World Workshop on the Classification of Periodontal and Peri-Implant Diseases and Conditions, which introduced consensus-based diagnostic criteria for both disease entities [14, 34].

Incidence data of peri-implantitis are less well documented but indicate a relatively consistent trend [47–52]. It is further important to consider that the incidence of peri-implant disease has been demonstrated to increase with time in function [48, 50, 52]. While longitudinal studies have reported a patient-level cumulative incidence from 14.5 to 22% over 9 to 10 years following implant placement, other investigations have documented higher annual incidence rates of up to 16% per patient-year [50–52].

Finally, clinician surveys confirm peri-implant diseases as a frequently encountered complication in clinical practice [41]. Specifically, surveys among US periodontologists indicated that up to 10% of implants required to be removed due to peri-implantitis. This finding highlights a significant unmet need for effective, evidence-based treatment protocols, underscoring the ongoing clinical challenge of managing peri-implant disease.

1.5 Plaque and biofilm association of peri-implant disease and differences between implant-associated and tooth-associated biofilm

Strong evidence suggests that bacterial biofilms represent the most important etiological factor for the onset and progression of peri-implant disease [14, 33]. Clinical studies have demonstrated a direct causal effect of biofilm accumulation on triggering a peri-implant inflammatory tissue response, with a significant dose-dependent association [53–56]. Full mouth plaque scores above 25% have, for example, correlated with a greater prevalence of peri-implantitis in patients with a history of periodontitis [57]. In contrast, anti-infective therapy has demonstrated efficacious in reducing peri-implant soft tissue inflammation and arresting disease progression [58]. In addition, ligature-induced preclinical models have advanced the understanding of peri-implantitis by clearly demonstrating the role of infectious bacterial biofilms in driving the progressive inflammatory breakdown of peri-implant soft tissues and alveolar bone, specifically on a histological level [59].

Compared to orthopedic implants, osseointegrated dental implants feature a transmucosal design penetrating the oral mucosa, establishing a direct interface between the peri-implant tissues—particularly the alveolar bone—and the bacteria-rich oral environment. This anatomical configuration increases their susceptibility to biofilm accumulation and subsequent inflammatory complications [60]. Like natural teeth, implants are surrounded by a soft tissue seal that protects the underlying bone from microbial challenges. Specifically, the oral, sulcular, and junctional (or junctional-like) epithelium around implants forms a biological barrier against the external environment [33, 61]. However, unlike natural teeth—where gingival connective tissue fibers insert perpendicularly into the cementum—dental implants lack a true connective tissue attachment [61]. Instead, circumferential collagen fibers aligned parallel to the implant surface stabilize the peri-implant soft tissue seal without, however, inserting into the implant material, thereby reducing the mechanical resilience of the seal to disruption [61].

Despite both bearing effective soft-tissue seals, the biofilm-associated inflammatory response between teeth and implants differs markedly. Specifically, implants show significantly faster tissue breakdown and a markedly faster progression into bone loss upon infection. This difference might be associated with the potential weakening of the epithelial barrier due to ulceration and edematous swelling [29, 33, 62]. Comparative analyses of soft tissue biopsies from teeth and implants revealed notable histopathological differences between peri-implantitis and periodontitis. Specifically, lesions associated with peri-implantitis compared to periodontitis are characterized by a larger inflammatory infiltrate and greater density of immune cells, that is plasma cells, macrophages and neutrophils. Peri-implant inflammatory infiltrates tend furthermore to extend more apically beyond the pocket epithelium compared to those in periodontitis and are not contained by a surrounding capsule of healthy connective tissue, arresting its progression (**Figure 3**) [29, 63].

These observed differences in the inflammatory response may be attributed to the lower vascularisation of peri-implant soft tissues. Specifically, soft tissue blood supply in peri-implant tissues is primarily derived from the periosteum of the crestal bone as opposed to natural teeth, where the richly vascularised periodontal ligament contributes to blood supply significantly [64]. Over time, bone remodeling and recession around implants can further compromise the limited blood supply, affecting the ability of peri-implant tissues to respond to inflammatory challenges further [61].

Despite advances in understanding peri-implant disease, the transition from health to peri-implantitis appears to be driven by a complex and partly self-reinforcing interplay between biofilm maturation on the implant surface and the host's inflammatory response [29]. A key event in disease progression is the shift from a symbiotic to a dysbiotic implant-associated biofilm, which has been described to be lower in quality and less diverse, with a higher accumulation of specific bacteria

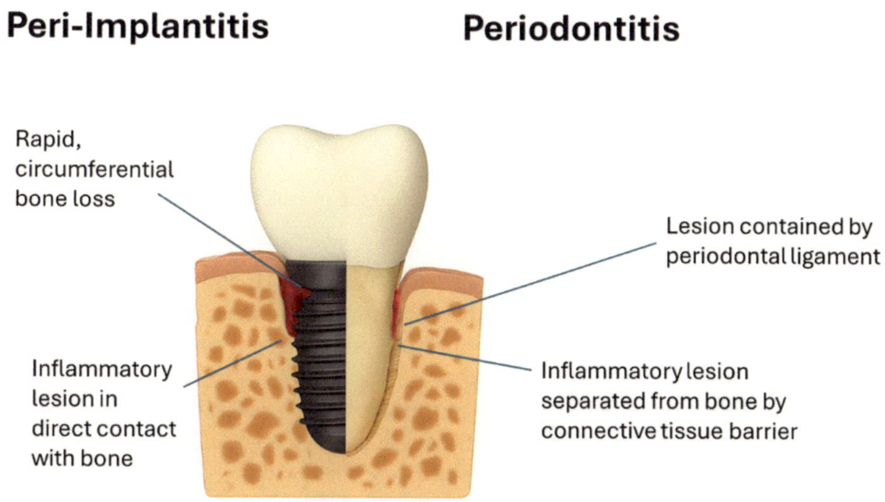

Figure 3.
Anatomical and inflammatory differences between peri-implantitis (left) and periodontitis (right).

compared to periodontal biofilms [60, 65]. This shift is promoted by changes in nutrient availability, pH alterations, oxygen depletion and the emergence of pathobionts, all fueled by sustained chronic inflammation [66]. As the disease progresses, biofilms mature and become increasingly resistant to host immune responses and chemotherapeutic agents [65]. Notably, mature biofilms are less responsive to antiseptic and antibiotic treatments as opposed to, for example planktonic bacteria and early, immature biofilm communities, which have proven well controllable through established preventive antibiotic protocols during, for example implant provision [66, 67].

1.6 Novel concepts in the understanding of dental implant integration and rejection

Recent research has highlighted the role of immunological factors in implant osseointegration, giving rise to the emerging field of osteoimmunology [68–70]. Within this framework, implant placement induces a transient, acute inflammatory response which—when involving an inert biomaterial such as titanium—may result in a favorable regenerative healing response, that is osseointegration. This process contrasts a situation in which chronic inflammation may lead to fibrous encapsulation of the biomaterial and eventual implant rejection [71].

Unlike natural teeth, dental implants trigger a controlled foreign body reaction that leads to the formation of a cortical bone capsule—commonly referred to as osseointegration. This structure reflects a state of tissue homeostasis, maintained by a balance between osteoclastic and osteoblastic activities [69]. The evolving understanding of osseointegration has been propelled, in part, by insights into macrophage behavior—specifically, their polarization from a pro-inflammatory M1 into a pro-regenerative M2 phenotype [72–74]. Conversely, M1 macrophages play a critical role in the pathogenesis of peri-implant disease by releasing pro-inflammatory cytokines such as interleukin-1 (IL-1) and tumor necrosis factor-alpha (TNF-α), both of which are the potent mediators of osteolysis and inflammatory tissue degradation [75].

Disruption of peri-implant tissue homeostasis—whether by plaque accumulation or other factors—can trigger an inflammatory response leading to peri-implant osteolysis and a reduced capacity for tissue repair. The onset and progression of peri-implantitis may be influenced by a combination of local, systemic and patient-related behavioral factors, rendering it a clinically complex and challenging condition to manage [29].

2. Risk factors

The susceptibility of dental implants to peri-implantitis is shaped by a range of systemic, local, and iatrogenic factors. Accurate prognostic assessment is essential for effective risk management and implementing preventive strategies throughout implant therapy.

From an academic perspective, the determinants of disease development are typically classified as either risk indicators or risk factors. Risk indicators are characteristics or exposures associated with disease presence, primarily identified through cross-sectional studies and denote correlation rather than causation. In contrast, risk factors are established through longitudinal research and imply a temporal and potentially causal relationship with disease onset.

Importantly, most studies on peri-implant disease are observational in nature and do not meet the methodological criteria required to establish the true risk factors. Nevertheless, to provide clinicians with a practical framework for evaluating patient-specific risks during implant placement and maintenance, this chapter will use the term risk factors in a broad sense—encompassing both evidence-based risk factors and strongly associated risk indicators.

In clinical practice, it is often useful to distinguish between risk factors that are intrinsic to the patient and those that are treatment-related or behaviourally driven—and therefore potentially modifiable. A more nuanced classification differentiates among patient-related systemic and local factors, iatrogenic influences, behavioral risks and implant- or site-specific conditions. It is also important to acknowledge that while some risk factors are well-established, others remain under investigation, with current evidence insufficient to confirm a definitive causal relationship (**Table 3**).

Patient-related systemic and local factors constitute the foundational determinants of an individual's susceptibility to peri-implantitis. These factors are often non-modifiable or only marginally amenable to change. In contrast, iatrogenic and behavioral factors represent key opportunities for risk mitigation through appropriate clinical decision-making, patient education and reinforcement of compliance—ideally initiated prior to implant placement as part of primordial prevention concepts [76]. Finally, implant- and site-specific variables, such as implant design and bone quality, must be carefully assessed for their potential influence on case-specific outcomes and long-term treatment success (**Figure 4**).

2.1 Patient-related risk factors

2.1.1 History of periodontitis

Both longitudinal and cross-sectional studies evidence that patients with a history of periodontitis are more susceptible to peri-implantitis [50, 52, 77–79]. Meta-analysis has indicated that a history of periodontitis exposes patients to a 2.2 to 9.2 elevated risk for peri-implantitis [29]. From an epidemiological point of view, it is important to note that the global prevalence of periodontitis, particularly its moderate to severe forms, is high and consistent across populations, with estimates showing that severe

Category	Description	Examples
Systemic	Factors related to the patient's general health influencing susceptibility to inflammation and healing.	Smoking, diabetes mellitus, genetic predisposition, osteoporosis, immunodeficiency
Local factor-related	Conditions in the oral environment affecting plaque control and tissue response.	History of periodontitis, poor oral hygiene, keratinized mucosa deficiency
Behavioral	Patient habits and compliance affecting disease control	Poor plaque control, irregular maintenance visits, smoking
Iatrogenic	Factors related to clinical procedures, surgical techniques and prosthetic design.	Residual cement, implant malposition, inadequate prosthetic emergence profile, overloading
Implant- and site-specific	Implant or anatomical site-related factors affecting peri-implant tissue health.	Implant surface characteristics, bone quality, soft tissue thickness

Table 3.
Risk factors.

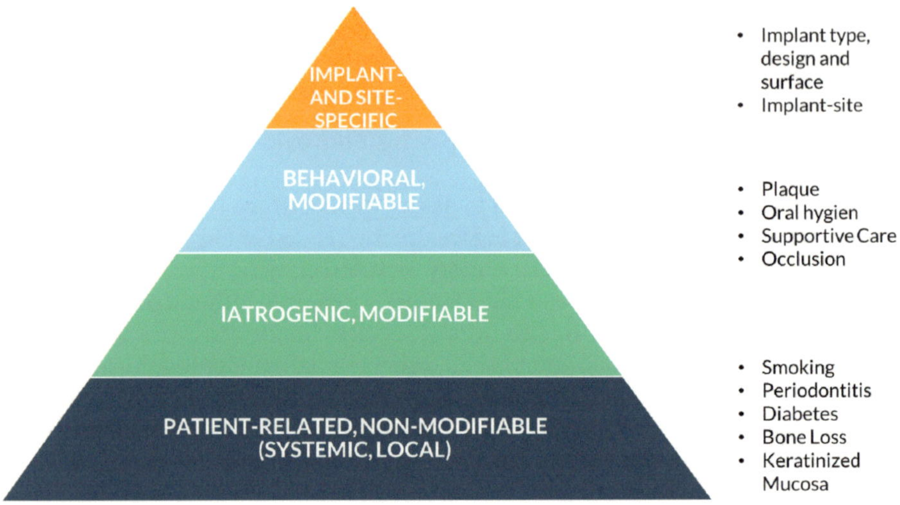

Figure 4.
Hierarchical classification of peri-implantitis risk factors. The pyramid illustrates the layered influence of risk factors, from fundamental patient-related systemic and local factors at the base to implant- and site-specific factors at the top.

periodontitis affects 10–15% of adults worldwide and overall periodontitis (including mild and moderate) affects more than 50% of adults [80–82]. Clinicians planning implant therapy are therefore advised to assess patients for signs of periodontal disease and to identify the indicators of current or past disease activity, such as a history of periodontitis-related tooth loss. Identifying affected patients may necessitate adjustments to the treatment and follow-up plan, such as periodontal treatment prior to commencing implant therapy and implementing supportive periodontal care protocols [78, 83, 84]. Although some studies suggest that implant placement into previously infected periodontal sites may be feasible—provided that extraction sockets are thoroughly debrided and meticulously disinfected—there is currently limited evidence supporting the long-term prognosis of such approaches [85]. There is also currently insufficient evidence to support the notion that only severe forms of periodontitis significantly increase the risk of peri-implantitis [78].

2.1.2 Smoking

Smoking, as well as electronic cigarette use, has been reported to significantly affect implant failure rates, the risk of postoperative infection as well as marginal bone loss [81–83]. In addition, several studies have reported smoking to affect osteogenesis, angiogenesis and plaque accumulation, essential for implant integration and health [83–85]. Individual studies have evidenced that smokers may exhibit a 2.7 to 31.6 times elevated risk for peri-implantitis [29, 86–93] Although numerous studies have demonstrated a strong association between smoking and peri-implantitis, methodological limitations—particularly the inability to control for confounding factors adequately—have so far omitted a consensus on the relation between smoking and peri-implantitis [14, 29]. Clinicians may consider this important factor during treatment provision as a modifiable patient-behavioral factor with relatively high potential importance for treatment prognosis.

2.1.3 Diabetes

With a global prevalence of 8%, type I and insulin-deficient type II (accounting for 90–95% of cases) diabetes comprises a group of metabolic disorders characterized by impaired glycemic control. Evidence supports a causal relationship between diabetes and a moderately elevated 1.9- to 3-fold risk for peri-implantitis and peri-implant bone loss [54, 94, 95]. Specifically, poor glycemic control has been reported to significantly increase the risk of peri-implantitis and implant failure [54, 95–97].

Elevated HbA1c levels exert multiple detrimental effects on peri-implant health, including impairing bone metabolism and osseointegration, compromising the quality and resilience of the peri-implant soft tissue seal and impairing neutrophil function, thereby weakening the host's ability to control biofilm-induced inflammation [98–100]. Importantly, evidence also suggests that patients with adequate glycemic control (HbA1c $\leq$7%) do not exhibit an increased risk of peri-implantitis compared to non-diabetic individuals [101–104].

However, study inconsistencies remain, particularly regarding the heterogeneous use of diagnostic parameters (e.g. HbA1c levels, fasting blood glucose, or self-reported diabetes status). For example, as opposed to type type 1, only type 2 diabetes has been associated with a higher incidence of peri-implant disease [105–107]. These discrepancies may explain why current consensus reports have not yet recognized diabetes as a definitive risk factor for peri-implantitis or implant loss [14, 29]. In conclusion, the detrimental effect of poorly controlled diabetes on peri-implant health is relatively well established and should be carefully considered during both the planning and maintenance phases of implant therapy.

2.1.4 Other systemic conditions

A whole series of other systemic conditions that may be associated with an elevated risk for peri-implantitis comprising, for example cardiovascular disease, rheumatoid arthritis, osteoporosis, specifically when medicated with bisphosphonates, obesity, as well as age and gender, have been researched and discussed throughout the literature [29, 108–112]. Compared to other systemic risk factors, these conditions remain insufficiently studied, and a conclusive association with peri-implantitis has yet to be established [14, 29]. However, certain conditions—such as obesity—may serve as surrogate indicators of other well-established risk factors and could, therefore, contribute to the overall assessment of a patient's risk profile for peri-implantitis. Other conditions, such as osteoporosis, have been associated with increased peri-implant bone loss and may, therefore, be considered modifying factors in the onset and progression of peri-implantitis [112].. Finally, patients may also exhibit a genetic predisposition to peri-implantitis, involving polymorphisms in genes related to immune regulation and inflammatory response—such as interleukin-1 (IL-1), interleukin-6 (IL-6), interleukin-10 (IL-10) and tumor necrosis factor-alpha (TNF-α) [113]. While some evidence suggests a potential role of these genetic factors in the pathogenesis of peri-implantitis, they are not yet considered clinically actionable [29].

2.1.5 Keratinized mucosa

There is growing interest in the role of keratinized mucosa (KM) in maintaining peri-implant health and ensuring a stable peri-implant soft tissue seal [61]. Clinical studies and systematic reviews suggest that implant sites with a limited width of KM (≤ 2 mm) are more prone to plaque accumulation and present higher plaque and bleeding on probing scores, indicative of increased peri-implant mucosal inflammation [114–117]. Notably, the absence of KM has been associated with patient-reported brushing discomfort and reduced oral hygiene effectiveness, potentially contributing to plaque accumulation and inflammation [118]. Conversely, implants surrounded by an adequate band of KM appear to respond more favorably to peri-implant mucositis treatment, underlining the role of KM in supporting disease resolution [119].

A recent systematic review reported that implants lacking KM have a 2.78-fold higher risk of developing peri-implantitis than those with sufficient KM [120]. However, it should be noted that much of the current evidence stems from observational studies with inherent limitations, and a direct causal relationship remains under debate. Nonetheless, these findings underscore the importance of ensuring an adequate peri-implant soft tissue phenotype—including both KM width and mucosal thickness—as part of comprehensive strategies to promote long-term peri-implant health.

2.2 Iatrogenic and behavioral factors

2.2.1 Plaque control, oral hygiene and professional supportive peri-implant care

Given the plaque-associated nature of peri-implant disease, poor plaque control remains one of the most significant risk factors and predictors for peri-implantitis, with studies reporting a 3- to 14-fold increased risk in patients with inadequate plaque control [54, 57, 121–124]. While plaque scores indicate an elevated microbial burden, the progression to peri-implantitis depends on the host's inflammatory response, highlighting the importance of clinical indicators such as bleeding on probing to assess the individual susceptibility [125]. Plaque accumulation is closely linked to oral hygiene practices but also to factors affecting accessibility for self-care and the provision of regular professional maintenance therapy. Clinical studies have demonstrated that peri-implantitis occurs more frequently at sites with limited accessibility for cleaning compared to well-accessible areas, underscoring the importance of accessibility in prosthetic planning and design [126, 127].

Furthermore, supportive peri-implant care (SPIC) has been shown to significantly reduce peri-implantitis incidence from 44 to 18% over 5 years and the necessity for associated treatment intervention from 41 to 27% over a ten-year period [78, 128]. Importantly, patients adhering to regular SPIC exhibited a sevenfold lower risk of developing peri-implantitis compared to non-compliant individuals, underscoring the dual benefit of professional biofilm removal and early diagnosis of biological complications during recall visits [129]. Likewise, early marginal bone loss around implants has been identified as a significant risk indicator for peri-implantitis development, making its early detection during maintenance visits crucial for preventive intervention [50, 78]. Although not exclusively related to iatrogenic factors or patient behavior, effective plaque control remains crucial for reducing the risk of peri-implantitis. This requires attention from a restorative design, patient education and compliance and clinician awareness standpoint [130].

2.2.2 Occlusal overload

Clinical studies indicate a potential correlation between clinical signs of occlusal overload and an increased incidence of peri-implantitis [123, 131]. Furthermore, occlusal overload has also been reported to potentially cause peri-implant bone loss increasing the susceptibility for peri-implantits [132]. Likewise, bruxism, although not directly related to peri-implantitis, has been correlated to a significantly higher risk of failure [133, 134].

Systematic reviews remain inconclusive regarding a direct causal relationship between occlusal overload and peri-implantitis, as occlusal overload alone does not appear to induce peri-implantitis but, conversely, may accelerate bone loss in the presence of plaque-induced inflammation [135]. As a result, occlusal overload is potentially best considered a modifying rather than a causative factor in peri-implant tissue breakdown. In the context of primary prevention, clinicians are advised to routinely assess and manage potential malocclusion in implant patients, particularly in those displaying elevated risk profiles.

2.3 Implant- and site-specific factors

Implant- and site-specific factors refer to anatomical, surgical and implant-design-related aspects that may influence a patient's susceptibility to peri-implantitis or modulate the disease's progression. These factors typically indirectly affect plaque accumulation, soft tissue resilience or access for maintenance. Certain aspects—such as implant positioning or the emergence profile—originate from clinical decisions and may, therefore, be considered iatrogenic. Nevertheless, once established, these factors define the long-term anatomical and biomechanical environment in which peri-implant disease may develop or progress.

Material- and design-related aspects of implant-borne restorations vary widely and include factors such as implant type, surface characteristics, the implant–prosthetic connection type, and the contour and type of the prosthetic restoration, all potentially having a direct causal or potentially modifying effect on the risk of peri-implantitis (**Figures** 5 and **6**).

The implant–abutment microcap has long been discussed as a potential reservoir for bacterial colonization and a potentially contributing factor to peri-implant inflammation and marginal bone loss (**Figure** 7) [136].

Tissue-level implants and platform-switching concepts relocate the microgap away from the marginal bone, thereby reducing or eliminating its direct impact on peri-implant tissues [137–141]. Both designs have been demonstrated to reduce crestal bone loss compared to platform-matched variants significantly [142, 143].

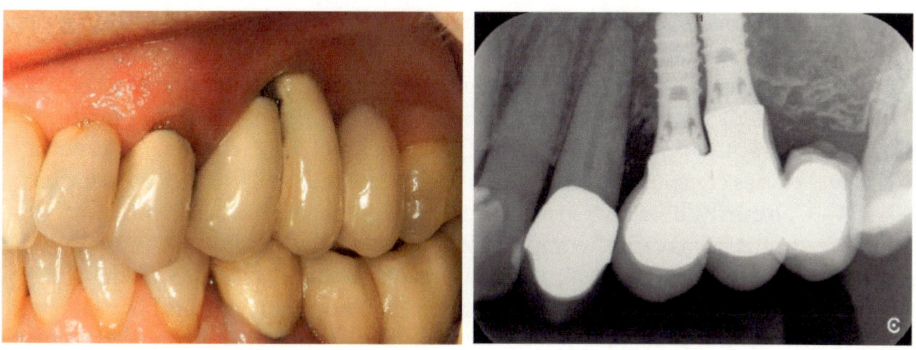

Figure 5.
Iatrogenic peri-implantitis sites 24 and 25 resulting from inadequate inter-implant distances and prosthetic design (on the left clinical image, on the right intraoral radiograph).

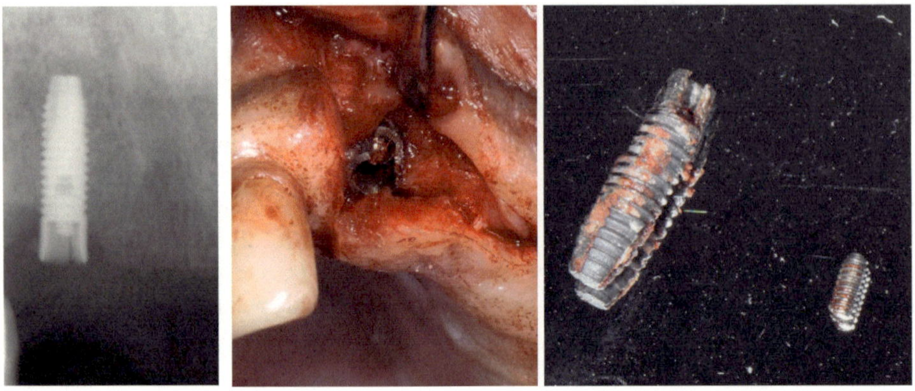

Figure 6.
Peri-implantitis following implant fracture resulting from insufficient implant diameter as a bridge abutment.

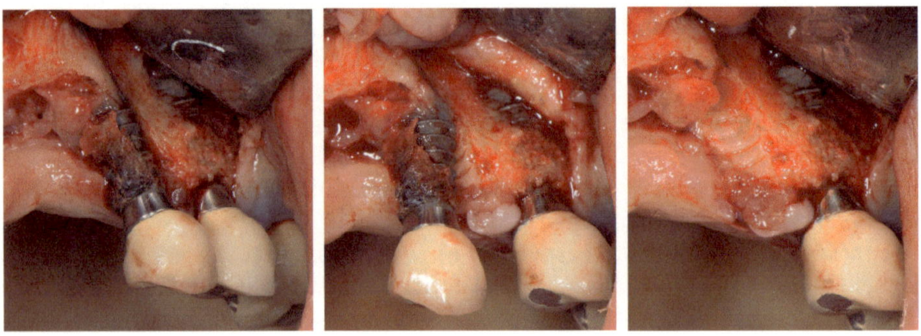

Figure 7.
Severe peri-implantitis: site 24, risk factor is poor fit between abutment and crown; site 25, presence of fenestration. Implant 24 failed: explantation.

Observational studies have further indicated that tissue-level implants may be less prone to peri-implantitis [29, 44, 142]. Nevertheless, the influence of implant or implant abutment connection types on peri-implantitis, irrespective of subcrestal or crestal placement modalities, remains inconclusive [144–147]. Irrespective of the current level of evidence, the biological plausibility of certain implant designs—such as tissue-level implants—in promoting peri-implant tissue stability remains strong. This may justify their preferential use in patients at elevated risk for peri-implant disease despite the lack of conclusive supporting data.

The retention mechanism, that is cement as opposed to screw retention, as a potential risk factor for peri-implantitis, has also recently gained increasing attention [148, 149]. Literature indicates a direct causal association of peri-implantitis with subgingival excess cement resulting from incomplete removal during cementation [150–154]. Contrarily, literature also appears to suggest that both cement and screw-retained restorations may yield comparable alveolar bone stability and implant loss in the absence of excess cement [146, 155]. Clinicians should carefully consider the type and specific design of the retention mechanism depending on various factors, comprising the extension, type, location of the cementation margin and any requirements for potential future maintenance and removal [152].

Lastly, the type of prosthesis and its contouring are critical determinants of oral hygiene accessibility and plaque retention, thereby influencing the risk of developing peri-implantitis. Full-arch restorations, for example, have been associated with a 16.1-fold increased risk of peri-implantitis compared to single crowns, possibly due to, for example, reduced inter-implant spacing compromising cleanability [131, 156]. Prosthetic designs that promote plaque accumulation and limit access for hygiene with convex emergence profiles and bulky contours in splinted restorations have been shown to elevate the risk of peri-implant disease significantly [126, 157, 158]. In some cases, over-contoured or bulky restorations may result from suboptimal implant positioning, thus representing iatrogenic factors [29, 130]. Clinicians are therefore encouraged to implement appropriate measures in anatomically or prosthetically challenging cases to prevent the delivery of restorations that may increase the risk for future biological complications.

Author details

Alexandre Perez[1]* and Tommaso Lombardi[2]

1 Unit of Oral Surgery and Implantology, Division of Oral and Maxillofacial Surgery, Department of Surgery, University of Geneva and University Hospitals of Geneva, Faculty of Medicine, Geneva, Switzerland

2 Unit of Oral Medicine and Oral Maxillofacial Pathology, Division of Oral and Maxillofacial Surgery, Department of Surgery, Geneva University Hospitals, Faculty of Medicine, University of Geneva, Geneva, Switzerland

*Address all correspondence to: alexandre.perez@hug.ch

References

[1] Buser D, Janner SFM, Wittneben J-G, Brägger U, Ramseier CA, Salvi GE. 10-year survival and success rates of 511 titanium implants with a sandblasted and acid-etched surface: A retrospective study in 303 partially edentulous patients. Clinical Implant Dentistry and Related Research. 2012;**14**:839-851

[2] Francetti L, Cavalli N, Taschieri S, Corbella S. Ten years follow-up retrospective study on implant survival rates and prevalence of peri-implantitis in implant-supported full-arch rehabilitations. Clinical Oral Implants Research. 2019;**30**:252-260

[3] Adell R, Lekholm U, Rockler B. A 15-year study of osseointegrated implants in the treatment of the edentulous jaw. International Journal of Oral Surgery. 1981;**10**:387-416

[4] Jung RE, Pjetursson BE, Glauser R, Zembic A, Zwahlen M, Lang NP. A systematic review of the 5-year survival and complication rates of implant-supported single crowns. Clinical Oral Implants Research. 2008;**19**:119-130

[5] Pjetursson BE, Thoma D, Jung R, Zwahlen M, Zembic A. A systematic review of the survival and complication rates of implant-supported fixed dental prostheses (FDP s) after a mean observation period of at least 5 years. Clinical Oral Implants Research. 2012;**23**:22-38

[6] Howe M-S, Keys W, Richards D. Long-term (10-year) dental implant survival: A systematic review and sensitivity meta-analysis. Journal of Dentistry. 2019;**84**:9-21

[7] Hamilton A, Gonzaga L, Amorim K, Wittneben J, Martig L, Morton D, et al. Selection criteria for immediate implant placement and immediate loading for single tooth replacement in the maxillary esthetic zone: A systematic review and meta-analysis. Clinical Oral Implants Research. 2023;**34**:304-348

[8] Buser D, Chappuis V, Belser UC, Chen S. Implant placement post extraction in esthetic single tooth sites: When immediate, when early, when late? Periodontology 2000. 2017;**73**:84-102

[9] Patel R, Ucer C, Wright S, Khan RS. Differences in dental implant survival between immediate vs. delayed placement: A systematic review and meta-analysis. Dentistry Journal. 2023;**11**:218

[10] Bentour E, Papamanoli E, Karoussis IK. The decision between tooth retention or replacement with implants: A continuing dilemma. Dentistry Journal. 2025;**13**:99

[11] Elani HW, Starr JR, Da Silva JD, Gallucci GO. Trends in dental implant use in the U.S., 1999-2016, and projections to 2026. Journal of Dental Research. 2018;**97**:1424-1430

[12] Albrektsson T, Zarb G, Worthington P, Eriksson AR. The long-term efficacy of currently used dental implants: A review and proposed criteria of success. The International Journal of Oral & Maxillofacial Implants. 1986;**1**:11-25

[13] Wittneben J, Wismeijer D, Brägger U, Joda T, Abou-Ayash S. Patient-reported outcome measures focusing on aesthetics of implant- and tooth-supported fixed dental prostheses: A systematic review and meta-analysis. Clinical Oral Implants Research. 2018;**29**:224-240

[14] Berglundh T, Armitage G, Araujo MG, Avila-Ortiz G, Blanco J, Camargo PM, et al. Peri-implant diseases and conditions: Consensus report of workgroup 4 of the 2017 world workshop on the classification of periodontal and Peri-implant diseases and conditions. Journal of Periodontology. 2018;**89**:S313-S318

[15] Misch CE, Perel ML, Wang H-L, Sammartino G, Galindo-Moreno P, Trisi P, et al. Implant success, survival, and failure: The International Congress of Oral Implantologists (ICOI) Pisa Consensus conference. Implant Dentistry. 2008;**17**:5-15

[16] Papaspyridakos P, Chen C-J, Singh M, Weber H-P, Gallucci GO. Success criteria in implant dentistry: A systematic review. Journal of Dental Research. 2012;**91**:242-248

[17] Pjetursson BE, Heimisdottir K. Dental implants – Are they better than natural teeth? European Journal of Oral Sciences. 2018;**126**:81-87

[18] Chackartchi T, Romanos GE, Sculean A. Soft tissue-related complications and management around dental implants. Periodontology 2000. 2019;**81**:124-138

[19] Al-Sabbagh M, Bhavsar I. Key local and surgical factors related to implant failure. Dental Clinics of North America. 2015;**59**:1-23

[20] Sakka S, Baroudi K, Nassani MZ. Factors associated with early and late failure of dental implants. Journal of Investigative and Clinical Dentistry. 2012;**3**:258-261

[21] Safi Y, Amid R, Zadbin F, Ghazizadeh Ahsaie M, Mortazavi H. The occurrence of dental implant malpositioning and related factors: A cross-sectional cone-beam computed tomography survey. Imaging Science in Dentistry. 2021;**51**:251

[22] Chen ST, Buser D, Sculean A, Belser UC. Complications and treatment errors in implant positioning in the aesthetic zone: Diagnosis and possible solutions. Periodontology 2000. 2023;**92**:220-234

[23] Canullo L, Bignozzi I, Cocchetto R, Cristalli MP, Iannello G. Immediate positioning of a definitive abutment versus repeated abutment replacements in post-extractive implants: 3-year follow-up of a randomised multicentre clinical trial. European Journal of Oral Implantology. 2010;**3**:285-296

[24] Tomasi C, Derks J. Etiology, occurrence, and consequences of implant loss. Periodontology 2000. 2022;**88**:13-35

[25] Ting M, Suzuki JB. Peri-Implantitis. Dentistry Journal. 2024;**12**:251

[26] Scarano A, Khater AGA, Gehrke SA, Serra P, Francesco I, Di Carmine M, et al. Current status of peri-implant diseases: A clinical review for evidence-based decision making. Journal of Periodontal & Implant Science. 2023;**14**:210

[27] Romandini M, Lima C, Pedrinaci I, Araoz A, Costanza Soldini M, Sanz M. Clinical signs, symptoms, perceptions, and impact on quality of life in patients suffering from peri-implant diseases: A university-representative cross-sectional study. Clinical Oral Implants Research. 2021;**32**:100-111

[28] Insua A, Monje A, Wang H, Inglehart M. Patient-Centered perspectives and understanding of Peri-Implantitis. Journal of Periodontology. 2017;**88**:1153-1162

[29] Schwarz F, Derks J, Monje A, Wang H-L. Peri-implantitis. Journal of Periodontology. 2018;**89**(Suppl. 1):S267-S290

[30] Albrekstsson T, Isidor F. Consensus report of session IV. In: Proceedings of the 1st European Workshop on Periodontology. Quintessence Publishing Co Ltd; 1994. pp. 365-369

[31] Lindhe J, Meyle J, On behalf of Group D of the European Workshop on Periodontology. Peri-implant diseases: Consensus report of the sixth European workshop on periodontology. Journal of Clinical Periodontology. 2008;**35**:282-285

[32] Zitzmann NU, Berglundh T. Definition and prevalence of peri-implant diseases. Journal of Clinical Periodontology. 2008;**35**:286-291

[33] Lang NP, Berglundh T. On behalf of working group 4 of the seventh European workshop on periodontology. Periimplant diseases: Where are we now? – Consensus of the seventh European workshop on periodontology. Journal of Clinical Periodontology. 2011;**38**:178-181

[34] Renvert S, Persson GR, Pirih FQ, Camargo PM. Peri-implant health, peri-implant mucositis, and peri-implantitis: Case definitions and diagnostic considerations: Diagnostic criteria of peri-implant health and diseases. Journal of Periodontology. 2018;**89**:S304-S312

[35] Zheng Z, Ao X, Xie P, Jiang F, Chen W. The biological width around implant. Journal of Prosthodontic Research. 2021;**65**:11-18

[36] Smith DE, Zarb GA. Criteria for success of osseointegrated endosseous implants. The Journal of Prosthetic Dentistry. 1989;**62**:567-572

[37] Araujo MG, Lindhe J. Peri-implant health. Journal of Periodontology. 2018;**89**:S249-S256

[38] Wehner C, Bertl K, Durstberger G, Arnhart C, Rausch-Fan X, Stavropoulos A. Characteristics and frequency distribution of bone defect configurations in peri-implantitis lesions—A series of 193 cases. Clinical Implant Dentistry and Related Research. 2021;**23**:178-188

[39] Monje A, Pons R, Insua A, Nart J, Wang H, Schwarz F. Morphology and severity of peri-implantitis bone defects. Clinical Implant Dentistry and Related Research. Aug 2019;**21**(4):635-643

[40] Schwarz F, Sahm N, Schwarz K, Becker J. Impact of defect configuration on the clinical outcome following surgical regenerative therapy of peri-implantitis. Journal of Clinical Periodontology. 2010;**37**:449-455

[41] Papathanasiou E, Finkelman M, Hanley J, Parashis AO. Prevalence, etiology and treatment of peri-implant mucositis and peri-implantitis: A survey of periodontists in the United States. Journal of Periodontology. 2016;**87**:493-501

[42] Papapanou PN, Sanz M, Buduneli N, Dietrich T, Feres M, Fine DH, et al. Periodontitis: Consensus report of workgroup 2 of the 2017 world workshop on the classification of periodontal and peri-implant diseases and conditions. Journal of Periodontology. Jun 2018;**89**(Suppl. 1):S173-S182. DOI: 10.1002/JPER.17-0721

[43] Caton JG, Armitage G, Berglundh T, Chapple ILC, Jepsen S, Kornman KS, et al. A new classification scheme for periodontal and peri-implant diseases and conditions - Introduction and key changes from the 1999 classification. Journal of Clinical Periodontology. 2018;**45**:S1-S8

[44] Derks J, Tomasi C. Peri-implant health and disease. A systematic review of current epidemiology. Journal of Clinical Periodontology. 2015;**42**:S158-S171

[45] Lee C-T, Huang Y-W, Zhu L, Weltman R. Prevalences of peri-implantitis and peri-implant mucositis: Systematic review and meta-analysis. Journal of Dentistry. 2017;**62**:1-12

[46] Tomasi C, Derks J. Clinical research of peri-implant diseases - quality of reporting, case definitions and methods to study incidence, prevalence and risk factors of peri-implant diseases. Journal of Clinical Periodontology. 2012;**39**:207-223

[47] Mombelli A, Müller N, Cionca N. The epidemiology of peri-implantitis. Clinical Oral Implants Research. 2012;**23**:67-76

[48] Roos-Jansåker A, Lindahl C, Renvert H, Renvert S. Nine- to fourteen-year follow-up of implant treatment. Part II: Presence of peri-implant lesions. Journal of Clinical Periodontology. 2006;**33**:290-295

[49] Koldsland OC, Scheie AA, Aass AM. Prevalence of Peri-Implantitis related to severity of the disease with different degrees of bone loss. Journal of Periodontology. 2010;**81**:231-238

[50] Derks J, Schaller D, Håkansson J, Wennström JL, Tomasi C, Berglundh T. Effectiveness of implant therapy analyzed in a Swedish population: Prevalence of Peri-implantitis. Journal of Dental Research. 2016;**95**:43-49

[51] Roccuzzo M, Layton DM, Roccuzzo A, Heitz-Mayfield LJ. Clinical outcomes of peri-implantitis treatment and supportive care: A systematic review. Clinical Oral Implants Research. 2018;**29**:331-350

[52] Kordbacheh Changi K, Finkelstein J, Papapanou PN. Peri-implantitis prevalence, incidence rate, and risk factors: A study of electronic health records at a U.S. dental school. Clinical Oral Implants Research. 2019;**30**:306-314

[53] Salvi GE, Aglietta M, Eick S, Sculean A, Lang NP, Ramseier CA. Reversibility of experimental peri-implant mucositis compared with experimental gingivitis in humans. Clinical Oral Implants Research. 2012;**23**:182-190

[54] Ferreira SD, Silva GLM, Cortelli JR, Costa JE, Costa FO. Prevalence and risk variables for peri-implant disease in Brazilian subjects. Journal of Clinical Periodontology. 2006;**33**:929-935

[55] Zitzmann NU, Berglundh T, Marinello CP, Lindhe J. Experimental peri-implant mucositis in man. Journal of Clinical Periodontology. 2001;**28**:517-523

[56] Pontoriero R, Tonelli MP, Carnevale G, Mombelli A, Nyman SR, Lang NP. Experimentally induced peri-implant mucositis. A clinical study in humans. Clinical Oral Implants Research. 1994;**5**:254-259

[57] Aguirre-Zorzano LA, Estefanía-Fresco R, Telletxea O, Bravo M. Prevalence of peri-implant inflammatory disease in patients with a history of periodontal disease who receive supportive periodontal therapy. Clinical Oral Implants Research. 2015;**26**:1338-1344

[58] Berglundh T, Wennström JL, Lindhe J. Long-term outcome of surgical treatment of peri-implantitis. A 2-11-year retrospective study. Clinical Oral Implants Research. 2018;**29**:404-410

[59] Schwarz F, Sculean A, Engebretson SP, Becker J, Sager M.

Animal models for peri-implant mucositis and peri-implantitis. Periodontology 2000. 2015;(68):168-181

[60] Subramani K, Jung RE, Molenberg A, Hammerle CHF. Biofilm on dental implants: A review of the literature. The International Journal of Oral & Maxillofacial Implants. 2009;**24**:616-626

[61] Atsuta I, Ayukawa Y, Kondo R, Oshiro W, Matsuura Y, Furuhashi A, et al. Soft tissue sealing around dental implants based on histological interpretation. Journal of Prosthodontic Research. 2016;**60**:3-11

[62] Schwarz F, Mihatovic I, Golubovic V, Eick S, Iglhaut T, Becker J. Experimental peri-implant mucositis at different implant surfaces. Journal of Clinical Periodontology. 2014;**41**:513-520

[63] Salvi GE, Stähli A, Imber J, Sculean A, Roccuzzo A. Physiopathology of peri-implant diseases. Clinical Implant Dentistry and Related Research. 2023;**25**:629-639

[64] Berglundh T, Lindhe J, Jonsson K, Ericsson I. The topography of the vascular systems in the periodontal and peri-implant tissues in the dog. Journal of Clinical Periodontology. 1994;**21**:189-193

[65] Butera A, Pascadopoli M, Pellegrini M, Gallo S, Zampetti P, Scribante A. Oral microbiota in patients with Peri-implant disease: A narrative review. Applied Sciences. 2022;**12**:3250

[66] Hall-Stoodley L, Costerton JW, Stoodley P. Bacterial biofilms: From the natural environment to infectious diseases. Nature Reviews. Microbiology. 2004;**2**:95-108

[67] Kashani H, Hilon J, Rasoul MH, Friberg B. Influence of a single preoperative dose of antibiotics on the early implant failure rate. A randomized clinical trial. Clinical Implant Dentistry and Related Research. 2019;**21**:278-283

[68] Shirazi S, Ravindran S, Cooper LF. Topography-mediated immunomodulation in osseointegration; ally or enemy. Biomaterials. 2022;**291**:121903

[69] Albrektsson T, Becker W, Coli P, Jemt T, Mölne J, Sennerby L. Bone loss around oral and orthopedic implants: An immunologically based condition. Clinical Implant Dentistry and Related Research. 2019;**21**:786-795

[70] Baseri M, Radmand F, Hamedi R, Yousefi M, Kafil HS. Immunological aspects of dental implant rejection. BioMed Research International. 2020;**2020**:7279509

[71] Ratner BD, Bryant SJ. Biomaterials: Where we have been and where we are going. Annual Review of Biomedical Engineering. 2004;**6**:41-75

[72] Murray PJ. Macrophage polarization. Annual Review of Physiology. 2017;**79**:541-566

[73] Pitchai M, Ipe D, Tadakamadla S, Hamlet S. Titanium implant surface effects on adherent macrophage phenotype: A systematic review. Materials. 2022;**15**:7314

[74] Fretwurst T, Buzanich G, Nahles S, Woelber JP, Riesemeier H, Nelson K. Metal elements in tissue with dental peri-implantitis: A pilot study. Clinical Oral Implants Research. 2016;**27**:1178-1186

[75] Jacobi-Gresser E, Huesker K, Schütt S. Genetic and immunological markers predict titanium implant failure: A retrospective study. International Journal of Oral and Maxillofacial Surgery. 2013;**42**:537-543

[76] Jepsen S, Berglundh T, Genco R, Aass AM, Demirel K, Derks J, et al. Primary prevention of peri-implantitis: Managing peri-implant mucositis. Journal of Clinical Periodontology. 2015;**42**(Suppl. 16):S152-S157

[77] Karoussis IK, Muller S, Salvi GE, Heitz-mayfield LJA, Bragger U, Lang NP. Association between periodontal and peri-implant conditions: A 10-year prospective study. Clinical Oral Implants Research. 2004;**15**:1-7

[78] Roccuzzo M, De Angelis N, Bonino L, Aglietta M. Ten-year results of a three-arm prospective cohort study on implants in periodontally compromised patients. Part 1: Implant loss and radiographic bone loss. Clinical Oral Implants Research. 2010;**21**:490-496

[79] Chrcanovic BR, Albrektsson T, Wennerberg A. Periodontally compromised vs. periodontally healthy patients and dental implants: A systematic review and meta-analysis. Journal of Dentistry. 2014;**42**:1509-1527

[80] Eke PI, Dye BA, Wei L, Thornton-Evans GO, Genco RJ. Prevalence of periodontitis in adults in the United States: 2009 and 2010. Journal of Dental Research. 2012;**91**:914-920

[81] Eke PI, Borgnakke WS, Genco RJ. Recent epidemiologic trends in periodontitis in the USA. Periodontology 2000. 2000;**2020**(82):257-267

[82] Nazir M, Al-Ansari A, Al-Khalifa K, Alhareky M, Gaffar B, Almas K. Global prevalence of periodontal disease and lack of its surveillance. The Scientific World Journal. 2020;**2020**:1-8

[83] Kaldahl WB, Kalkwarf KL, Patil KD, Dyer JK, Bates RE. Evaluation of four modalities of periodontal therapy. Mean probing depth, probing attachment level and recession changes. Journal of Periodontology. 1988;**59**:783-793

[84] Cho-Yan Lee J, Mattheos N, Nixon KC, Ivanovski S. Residual periodontal pockets are a risk indicator for peri-implantitis in patients treated for periodontitis. Clinical Oral Implants Research. 2012;**23**:325-333

[85] Chrcanovic BR, Martins MD, Wennerberg A. Immediate placement of implants into infected sites: A systematic review: Immediate implants in infected sites. Clinical Implant Dentistry and Related Research. 2015;**17**:e1-e16

[86] Chrcanovic BR, Albrektsson T, Wennerberg A. Smoking and dental implants: A systematic review and meta-analysis. Journal of Dentistry. 2015;**43**:487-498

[87] Guney Z, Altingoz SM, Has H, Serdar MA, Kurgan S. The impact of electronic cigarettes on peri-implant health: A systematic review and meta-analysis. Journal of Dentistry. 2024;**143**:104883

[88] Heitz-Mayfield LJA, Huynh-Ba G. History of treated periodontitis and smoking as risks for implant therapy. The International Journal of Oral & Maxillofacial Implants. 2009;**24**(Suppl.):39-68

[89] Ma L, Zheng LW, Sham MH, Cheung LK. Uncoupled angiogenesis and osteogenesis in nicotine-compromised bone healing. Journal of Bone and Mineral Research. 2010;**25**:1305-1313

[90] Ma L, Zwahlen RA, Zheng LW, Sham MH. Influence of nicotine on the biological activity of rabbit osteoblasts: Influence of nicotine on gene expression in osteoblasts. Clinical Oral Implants Research. 2011;**22**:338-342

[91] Rinke S, Ohl S, Ziebolz D, Lange K, Eickholz P. Prevalence of periimplant disease in partially edentulous patients: A practice-based cross-sectional study: Cross-sectional study on the prevalence of periimplant disease. Clinical Oral Implants Research. 2011;**22**:826-833

[92] Roos-Jansåker AM, Lindahl C, Renvert H, Renvert S. Nine-to fourteen-year follow-up of implant treatment. Part I: Implant loss and associations to various factors. Journal of Clinical Periodontology. 2006;**33**:283-289

[93] Romandini M, Lima C, Pedrinaci I, Araoz A, Soldini MC, Sanz M. Prevalence and risk/protective indicators of peri-implant diseases: A university-representative cross-sectional study. Clinical Oral Implants Research. 2021;**32**:112-122

[94] Chrcanovic BR, Albrektsson T, Wennerberg A. Diabetes and Oral implant failure: A systematic review. Journal of Dental Research. 2014;**93**:859-867

[95] Daubert DM, Weinstein BF, Bordin S, Leroux BG, Flemmig TF. Prevalence and predictive factors for Peri-implant disease and implant failure: A cross-sectional analysis. Journal of Periodontology. 2015;**86**:337-347

[96] Moy PK, Medina D, Shetty V. Dental implant failure rates and associated risk factors. The International Journal of Oral & Maxillofacial Implants. 2005;**20**:569-577

[97] Monje A, Catena A, Borgnakke WS. Association between diabetes mellitus/hyperglycaemia and peri-implant diseases: Systematic review and meta-analysis. Journal of Clinical Periodontology. 2017;**44**:636-648

[98] Aguilar-Salvatierra A, Calvo-Guirado JL, González-Jaranay M, Moreu G, Delgado-Ruiz RA, Gómez-Moreno G. Peri-implant evaluation of immediately loaded implants placed in esthetic zone in patients with diabetes mellitus type 2: A two-year study. Clinical Oral Implants Research. 2016;**27**:156-161

[99] Zhang Z, Ji C, Wang D, Wang M, Song D, Xu X, et al. The burden of diabetes on the soft tissue seal surrounding the dental implants. Frontiers in Physiology. 2023;**14**:1136973

[100] Preshaw PM, Alba AL, Herrera D, Jepsen S, Konstantinidis A, Makrilakis K, et al. Periodontitis and diabetes: A two-way relationship. Diabetologia. 2012;**55**:21-31

[101] Tawil G, Od D, Younan R. Conventional and advanced implant treatment in the type II diabetic patient: Surgical protocol and long-term clinical results. The International Journal of Oral & Maxillofacial Implants. 2007;**23**:744-752

[102] Eskow CC, Oates TW. Dental implant survival and complication rate over 2 years for individuals with poorly controlled type 2 diabetes mellitus. Clinical Implant Dentistry and Related Research. 2017;**19**:423-431

[103] Javed F, Romanos GE. Impact of diabetes mellitus and Glycemic control on the Osseointegration of dental implants: A systematic literature review. Journal of Periodontology. 2009;**80**:1719-1730

[104] Naujokat H, Kunzendorf B, Wiltfang J. Dental implants and diabetes mellitus—A systematic review. International Journal of Implant Dentistry. 2016;**2**:5

[105] Sannino G, Montemezzi P, Pantaleo G, Agliardi E. Dental implants

survival rate in controlled type I diabetic patients: A prospective longitudinal study with a 2-year follow-up. Journal of Biological Regulators and Homeostatic Agents. 2020;**34**:37-45

[106] Alrabiah M, Al-Aali KA, Al-Sowygh ZH, Binmahfooz AM, Mokeem SA, Abduljabbar T. Association of advanced glycation end products with peri-implant inflammation in prediabetes and type 2 diabetes mellitus patients. Clinical Implant Dentistry and Related Research. 2018;**20**:535-540

[107] Mokeem S, Alfadda SA, Al-Shibani N, Alrabiah M, Al-Hamdan RS, Vohra F, et al. Clinical and radiographic peri-implant variables around short dental implants in type 2 diabetic, prediabetic, and non-diabetic patients. Clinical Implant Dentistry and Related Research. 2019;**21**:60-65

[108] Dreyer H, Grischke J, Tiede C, Eberhard J, Schweitzer A, Toikkanen SE, et al. Epidemiology and risk factors of peri-implantitis: A systematic review. Journal of Periodontal Research. 2018;**53**:657-681

[109] Máximo MB, De Mendonça AC, Alves JF, Cortelli SC, Peruzzo DC, Duarte PM. Peri-implant diseases may Be associated with increased time loading and generalized periodontal bone loss: Preliminary results. Journal of Oral Implantology. 2008;**34**:268-273

[110] Dvorak G, Arnhart C, Heuberer S, Huber CD, Watzek G, Gruber R. Peri-implantitis and late implant failures in postmenopausal women: A cross-sectional study: Peri-implantitis in postmenopausal women. Journal of Clinical Periodontology. 2011;**38**:950-955

[111] Renvert S, Aghazadeh A, Hallström H, Persson GR. Factors related to peri-implantitis - a retrospective study. Clinical Oral Implants Research. 2014;**25**:522-529

[112] De Medeiros FCFL, Kudo GAH, Leme BG, Saraiva PP, Verri FR, Honório HM, et al. Dental implants in patients with osteoporosis: A systematic review with meta-analysis. International Journal of Oral and Maxillofacial Surgery. 2018;**47**:480-491

[113] Lafuente-Ibáñez De Mendoza I, Setien-Olarra A, García-De La Fuente AM, Aguirre-Urizar JM, Marichalar-Mendia X. Role of proinflammatory mutations in peri-implantitis: Systematic review and meta-analysis. International Journal of Implant Dentistry. 2022;**8**:2

[114] Wennström JL, Derks J. Is there a need for keratinized mucosa around implants to maintain health and tissue stability? Clinical Oral Implants Research. 2012;**23**:136-146

[115] Gobbato L, Avila-Ortiz G, Sohrabi K, Wang C-W, Karimbux N. The effect of keratinized mucosa width on peri-implant health: A systematic review. The International Journal of Oral & Maxillofacial Implants. 2013;**28**:1536-1545

[116] Lin G, Chan H, Wang H. The significance of keratinized mucosa on implant health: A systematic review. Journal of Periodontology. 2013;**84**:1755-1767

[117] Roccuzzo M, Grasso G, Dalmasso P. Keratinized mucosa around implants in partially edentulous posterior mandible: 10-year results of a prospective comparative study. Clinical Oral Implants Research. 2016;**27**:491-496

[118] Souza AB, Tormena M, Matarazzo F, Araújo MG. The influence of peri-implant keratinized mucosa on

brushing discomfort and peri-implant tissue health. Clinical Oral Implants Research. 2016;**27**:650-655

[119] Fons-Badal C, Agustín-Panadero R, Labaig-Rueda C, Solá-Ruiz M, García-Selva M, Fons FA. The influence of keratinized mucosa on the nonsurgical therapeutic treatment of peri-implantitis. Journal of Clinical Medicine. 2022;**11**:4118

[120] Mahardawi B, Jiaranuchart S, Damrongsirirat N, Arunjaroensuk S, Mattheos N, Somboonsavatdee A, et al. The lack of keratinized mucosa as a risk factor for peri-implantitis: A systematic review and meta-analysis. Scientific Reports. 2023;**13**:3778

[121] Schwarz F, Becker K, Sahm N, Horstkemper T, Rousi K, Becker J. The prevalence of peri-implant diseases for two-piece implants with an internal tube-in-tube connection: A cross-sectional analysis of 512 implants. Clinical Oral Implants Research. 2017;**28**:24-28

[122] Rokn A, Aslroosta H, Akbari S, Najafi H, Zayeri F, Hashemi K. Prevalence of peri-implantitis in patients not participating in well-designed supportive periodontal treatments: A cross-sectional study. Clinical Oral Implants Research. 2017;**28**:314-319

[123] Canullo L, Peñarrocha-Oltra D, Covani U, Botticelli D, Serino G, Penarrocha M. Clinical and microbiological findings in patients with peri-implantitis: A cross-sectional study. Clinical Oral Implants Research. 2016;**27**:376-382

[124] De Araújo NM, Mano Azul A, Rocha E, Maló P. Risk factors of peri-implant pathology. European Journal of Oral Sciences. 2015;**123**:131-139

[125] Heitz-Mayfield LJA, Heitz F, Lang NP. Implant disease risk assessment IDRA–a tool for preventing peri-implant disease. Clinical Oral Implants Research. 2020;**31**:397-403

[126] Serino G, Ström C. Peri-implantitis in partially edentulous patients: Association with inadequate plaque control. Clinical Oral Implants Research. 2009;**20**:169-174

[127] Tormena M, Matarazzo F, De Oliveira BM, Pereira O, Previdelli I, Araújo MG. The effect of inadequate access to peri-implant hygiene on marginal bone level. A 4-year cohort prospective study. Clinical Oral Implants Research. 2020;**31**:836-845

[128] Costa FO, Takenaka-Martinez S, Cota LOM, Ferreira SD, Silva GLM, Costa JE. Peri-implant disease in subjects with and without preventive maintenance: A 5-year follow-up. Journal of Clinical Periodontology. 2012;**39**:173-181

[129] Monje A, Wang H-L, Nart J. Association of Preventive Maintenance Therapy Compliance and Peri-Implant Diseases: A cross-sectional study. Journal of Periodontology. 2017;**88**:1030-1041

[130] Cortellini S, Favril C, De Nutte M, Teughels W, Quirynen M. Patient compliance as a risk factor for the outcome of implant treatment. Periodontology 2000. 2019;**81**:209-225

[131] Dalago HR, Schuldt Filho G, Rodrigues MAP, Renvert S, Bianchini MA. Risk indicators for Peri-implantitis. A cross-sectional study with 916 implants. Clinical Oral Implants Research. 2017;**28**:144-150

[132] Misch CE, Suzuki JB, Misch-Dietsh FM, Bidez MW. A positive correlation between occlusal trauma and Peri-implant bone loss: Literature support. Implant Dentistry. 2005;**14**:108-116

[133] Häggman-Henrikson B, Ali D, Aljamal M, Chrcanovic BR. Bruxism and dental implants: A systematic review and meta-analysis. Journal of Oral Rehabilitation. 2024;**51**:202-217

[134] Ionfrida JA, Stiller HL, Kämmerer PW, Walter C. Dental implant failure risk in patients with bruxism—A systematic review and meta-analysis of the literature. Dentistry Journal. 2024;**13**:11

[135] Isidor F. Influence of forces on peri-implant bone. Clinical Oral Implants Research. 2006;**17**:8-18

[136] Hermann JS, Schoolfield JD, Schenk RK, Buser D, Cochran DL. Influence of the size of the microgap on Crestal bone changes around titanium implants. A Histometric evaluation of unloaded non-submerged implants in the canine mandible. Journal of Periodontology. 2001;**72**:1372-1383

[137] Buser D, Mericske-Stern R, Dula K, Lang NP. Clinical experience with one-stage, non-submerged dental implants. Advances in Dental Research. 1999;**13**:153-161

[138] Cochran DL. The scientific basis for and clinical experiences with Straumann implants including the ITI dental implant system: A consensus report. Clinical Oral Implants Research. 2000;**11**(Suppl. 1):33-58

[139] Kim S, Jung U-W, Cho K-S, Lee J-S. Retrospective radiographic observational study of 1692 Straumann tissue-level dental implants over 10 years: I. Implant survival and loss pattern. Clinical Implant Dentistry and Related Research. 2018;**20**:860-866

[140] Cosola S, Marconcini S, Boccuzzi M, Menchini Fabris GB, Covani U, Peñarrocha-Diago M, et al. Radiological outcomes of bone-level and tissue-level dental implants: Systematic review. International Journal of Environmental Research and Public Health. 2020;**17**:6920

[141] Atieh MA, Ibrahim HM, Atieh AH. Platform switching for marginal bone preservation around dental implants: A systematic review and meta-analysis. Journal of Periodontology. 2010;**81**:1350-1366

[142] Sasada Y, Cochran D. Implant-abutment connections: A review of biologic consequences and Peri-implantitis implications. The International Journal of Oral & Maxillofacial Implants. 2017;**32**:1296-1307

[143] Elkattan A, Torres-Velázquez N, Blázquez-Hinarejos M, Egido-Moreno S, Ayuso-Montero R, Roselló-Llabrés X, et al. Marginal bone loss around bone-level and tissue-level implants: A systematic review and meta-analysis. Applied Sciences. 2025;**15**:2286

[144] Meloni SM, Jovanovic SA, Lolli FM, Pisano M, Riu GD, Riu ND, et al. Platform switching vs regular platform implants: Nine-month post-loading results from a randomised controlled trial. European Journal of Oral Implantology;**7**:257-265

[145] Chrcanovic BR, Albrektsson T, Wennerberg A. Platform switch and dental implants: A meta-analysis. Journal of Dentistry. 2015;**43**:629-646

[146] Mattheos N, Janda M, Acharya A, Pekarski S, Larsson C. Impact of design elements of the implant supracrestal complex (ISC) on the risk of peri-implant mucositis and peri-implantitis: A critical review. Clinical Oral Implants Research. 2021;**32**:181-202

[147] Paolantoni G, Tatullo M, Miniello A, Sammartino G, Marenzi G. Influence of crestal and sub-crestal implant position on development of peri-implant diseases: A 5-year retrospective analysis. Clinical Oral Investigations. 2023;**28**:16

[148] Wittneben J, Joda T, Weber H, Brägger U. Screw retained vs. cement retained implant-supported fixed dental prosthesis. Periodontology 2000. 2017;**73**:141-151

[149] Wittneben J-G, Millen C, Brägger U. Clinical performance of screw-versus cement-retained fixed implant-supported reconstructions—A systematic review. The International Journal of Oral & Maxillofacial Implants. 2014;**29**:84-98

[150] Linkevicius T, Puisys A, Vindasiute E, Linkeviciene L, Apse P. Does residual cement around implant-supported restorations cause peri-implant disease? A retrospective case analysis. Clinical Oral Implants Research. 2013;**24**:1179-1184

[151] Gehrke P, Bleuel K, Fischer C, Sader R. Influence of margin location and luting material on the amount of undetected cement excess on CAD/CAM implant abutments and cement-retained zirconia crowns: An in-vitro study. BMC Oral Health. 2019;**19**:111

[152] Linkevicius T, Vindasiute E, Puisys A, Linkeviciene L, Maslova N, Puriene A. The influence of the cementation margin position on the amount of undetected cement. A prospective clinical study. Clinical Oral Implants Research. 2013;**24**:71-76

[153] Wilson TG Jr. The positive relationship between excess cement and peri-implant disease: A prospective clinical endoscopic study. Journal of Periodontology. 2009;**80**:1388-1392

[154] Agar JR, Cameron SM, Hughbanks JC, Parker MH. Cement removal from restorations luted to titanium abutments with simulated subgingival margins. The Journal of Prosthetic Dentistry. 1997;**78**:43-47

[155] Lemos CAA, De Souza Batista VE, Almeida DADF, Santiago Júnior JF, Verri FR, Pellizzer EP. Evaluation of cement-retained versus screw-retained implant-supported restorations for marginal bone loss. The Journal of Prosthetic Dentistry. 2016;**115**:419-427

[156] Schuldt Filho G, Dalago HR, Oliveira de Souza JG, Stanley K, Jovanovic S, Bianchini MA. Prevalence of peri-implantitis in patients with implant-supported fixed prostheses. Quintessence International. 2014;**45**:861-868

[157] Katafuchi M, Weinstein BF, Leroux BG, Chen Y, Daubert DM. Restoration contour is a risk indicator for peri-implantitis: A cross-sectional radiographic analysis. Journal of Clinical Periodontology. 2018;**45**:225-232

[158] Yi Y, Koo K, Schwarz F, Ben Amara H, Heo S. Association of prosthetic features and peri-implantitis: A cross-sectional study. Journal of Clinical Periodontology. 2020;**47**:392-403

Chapter 12

Advances in Metabolic Regulation in Periodontal Bone Homeostasis: From Basic Biology to Translational Medicine

Xiaoxiao Wang, Houze Li, Yunyi Xie, Yan Wang, Sun Haipeng and Dan Zhao

Abstract

Periodontal bone homeostasis relies on dynamic interactions between glucose, lipid, and amino acid metabolism in osteoblasts and osteoclasts, regulated by signaling hubs like mammalian target of rapamycin (mTOR), 5′-adenosine monophosphate-activated protein kinase (AMPK), and hypoxia-inducible factor-1α (HIF-1α). Osteoblasts use aerobic glycolysis for early differentiation and fatty acid oxidation for mineralization, while osteoclasts shift from oxidative phosphorylation to glycolysis for resorption. In periodontitis, inflammation impairs osteoblastic glycolysis and mitochondrial function, whereas osteoclasts enhance glycolytic and glutamine metabolism via protein kinase B (AKT)/mTOR/HIF-1α and reactive oxygen species (ROS), driving bone loss. Systemic diseases (e.g., diabetes, hyperlipidemia) exacerbate bone cell metabolic dysfunction, linking metabolism to alveolar destruction. Translational strategies include periodontal treatment to restore metabolic states and "regenerative windows," and drugs like metformin and statins to promote osteogenesis. Metabolic markers (e.g., glucose transporter 1 (GLUT1), lactate) enable personalized regenerative assessment. Future research may focus on mechanistic insights and potential interventions to restore structural and metabolic homeostasis in periodontal tissues.

Keywords: periodontal bone homeostasis, metabolic reprogramming, osteoblasts, osteoclasts, periodontal disease, metabolic-targeted therapy

1. Introduction

Periodontal bone homeostasis is fundamental to maintain the integrity and functionality of periodontal tissues, closely under the regulation of metabolic dynamics of osteogenesis and osteoclastogenesis [1, 2]. Recently, it has been recognized that cell metabolism is not only a "background" for energy supply, but an important mechanism in regulating cell fate, differentiation, and functional execution [3, 4]. Cellular metabolism, including glucose metabolism, lipid metabolism, and amino acid metabolism, exhibits significant dynamic changes during the differentiation of osteogenic precursor cells (such as bone marrow mesenchymal stem cells) and osteoclastic precursor cells (such as monocyte/macrophage lineages). Cells undergo metabolic reprogramming to meet specific demands for energy and biosynthesis, thereby maintaining bone homeostasis [5].

As a special bone tissue in the oral environment, the alveolar bone is long-term exposed to complex microbial stimuli, hypoxic microenvironments, chronic inflammatory responses, and high-frequency mechanical stress (masticatory forces), which may lead to characteristic changes in its metabolic dynamics when compared to systemic bone tissues [6]. Lactate accumulation, persistent activation of HIF-1α, and chronic oxidative stress detected in periodontitis lesions may all interfere with the osteoblast-osteoclast balance and bring about metabolic remodeling [7, 8].

This chapter is an overview of how glucose, lipid and amino acid metabolism regulate osteogenic and osteoclastic differentiation to maintain periodontal bone homeostasis. The synergistic and compensatory effects among metabolic pathways and related signaling pathways (such as mTOR, AMPK, and HIF-1α) will be included in the discussion. Based on these fundamental studies, we will introduce novel metabolic-targeted therapeutic strategies for periodontal bone regeneration, including metabolite-based drug interventions, metabolic pathway-targeted therapies, and metabolomics-guided interventions. This chapter tries to provide readers with theoretical supports and potential directions for future individualized and precise periodontal treatments.

2. The basis of periodontal bone homeostasis

2.1 Key pattern of periodontal bone remodeling

Bone remodeling is a dynamic equilibrium process, relying on the balanced interplay between osteoblast-mediated bone formation and osteoclast-driven bone resorption. This process contributes to maintaining bone mass and structural integrity. Osteoclasts originate from hematopoietic precursor cells and form multinucleated cells with bone-resorbing capacity through fusion; whereas osteoblasts differentiate from mesenchymal stem cells and are responsible for matrix secretion and mineralization. In physiological states, bone formation and bone resorption are in balance, ensuring that the alveolar bone can adapt to daily repair and changes in micro-trauma and mechanical loading [9]. However, in pathological states, particularly in periodontitis, this equilibrium is disrupted, leading to progressive alveolar bone resorption and loss of supportive periodontal tissues.

Although the basic cellular composition and remodeling patterns are similar with long bones, the alveolar bone exhibits a higher turnover rate and is closely associated with teeth and periodontal tissues. The alveolar bone is more susceptible to oral infections and mechanical stimuli, thus the remodeling mechanism is more complicated [2, 10]. (1) The alveolar bone endures cyclic mechanical loading from masticatory forces, which locally induces bone remodeling to meet functional demands. (2) The bone surface can be affected with dental plaque microbiome, thus suffering from continuous influences from microbial communities and their metabolites. (3) Under pathological conditions such as periodontitis, chronic inflammation triggered by bacterial infections can disrupt the balance between bone resorption and formation by locally secreting abundant inflammatory cytokines (e.g., tumor necrosis factor-α (TNF-α) and interleukin-1 beta (IL-1β)), which promote osteoclastogenesis and inhibit osteoblastic function [11]. This imbalance exacerbates alveolar bone resorption and undermines tooth support.

Therefore, compared with systemic bone biology, the dynamics of periodontal bone are more active and vulnerable due to its microbial, inflammatory, and mechanical microenvironments. This unique biological pressure serves as a key pathological basis for periodontal disease progression.

2.2 Metabolic demand of periodontal bone

Processes, such as cell differentiation, migration, matrix synthesis, and bone resorption, are all highly energy-dependent biological activities. The metabolic systems provide energy and metabolic intermediates for the differentiation and functional activities of osteocytes [12]. In mature osteoblasts, aerobic glycolysis accounts for approximately 80% of adenosine triphosphate (ATP) production, which enables a rapid generation of ATP and a stable supply of synthetic precursors such as lactate and metabolic intermediates. Glycolysis also maintains the NAD+/NADH (nicotinamide adenine dinucleotide/nicotinamide adenine dinucleotide + hydrogen) balance to meet the demand for collagen and non-collagen protein synthesis [13]. In the latter phase of differentiation, fatty acid oxidation and mitochondrial genes are upregulated to sustain the continuous energy supply required for the long-term mineralization. Additionally, glutamine metabolism plays a key role in osteogenesis by replenishing tricarboxylic acid (TCA) cycle intermediates through α-ketoglutaric acid and maintaining redox balance via NADPH (nicotinamide adenine dinucleotide phosphate) production, thereby enhancing cellular tolerance to oxidative stress [14].

Osteoclasts exhibit phase-specific metabolic characteristics during differentiation and functioning. In the early phase of differentiation, osteoclasts gradually enhance oxidative phosphorylation to support cell expansion, fusion, and bone surface attachment until the formation of multinucleated, mitochondria-rich mature osteoclasts [15]. Conversely, mature osteoclasts show a significant glycolytic preference during active bone resorption, with upregulated expression of lactate dehydrogenase A (LDHA) and monocarboxylate transporter 4 (MCT4), leading to a significant increase in intra- and extracellular lactate levels [16, 17]. This switch in metabolic patterns is crucial for maintaining osteoclastic functional integrity.

In pathological conditions such as periodontitis, Pg-LPS (*Porphyromonas gingivalis* lipopolysaccharide) triggers ROS production and inflammatory cascades in periodontium, exposing osteocytes to a complex microenvironment characterized by hypoxia, hyper-inflammation, and nutrient restriction [18]. Inflammatory cytokines and ROS disrupt glycolysis and mitochondrial function in osteoblasts, inducing metabolic dysfunction and apoptosis. In contrast, osteoclasts maintain their resorptive function and survival advantage through metabolic reprogramming, enhancing glycolysis and glutamine uptake. This asymmetric change in bone metabolic adaptation serves as a critical basis for the imbalance in periodontal bone remodeling.

3. Metabolic characteristics in bone formation

3.1 Glucose metabolism in osteogenesis

Glucose metabolism exerts a critical regulatory role in the differentiation process of osteoprogenitor cells by providing both energy and biosynthetic precursors.

Studies indicate that osteoblasts significantly enhance aerobic glycolysis during the early differentiation stage, even under aerobic conditions. Approximately 80% of adenosine triphosphate (ATP) is generated via glycolysis, rather than mitochondrial oxidative phosphorylation [13]. This "glycolytic bias" not only provides ATP more rapidly but also supplies essential precursors and reducing equivalents for cell functions such as collagen synthesis [13]. Glucose metabolites, such as pyruvate, enter the tricarboxylic acid (TCA) cycle to generate intermediates (e.g., α-ketoglutarate (α-KG), citric acid), which participate in energy metabolism and the biosynthesis of lipids and amino acids, thereby supporting the functional development of osteoblasts.

Multiple key signaling pathways have been validated to regulate glucose metabolic reprogramming during osteogenic differentiation. The Wnt (wingless-related integration site) signaling pathway upregulates the expression of glucose transporters (e.g., GLUT1) and key glycolytic enzymes (e.g., hexokinase 2 (HK2)) through β-catenin-dependent mechanisms, promoting glucose uptake and glycolytic activity in osteoblasts and enhancing their osteogenic potential [19–21]. Parathyroid hormone (PTH) indirectly stimulates glycolytic flux via the cyclic adenosine 3,5-monophosphate (cAMP)/protein kinase A (PKA) pathway while inducing insulin-like growth factor 1 (IGF-1) expression, further amplifying the activity of the phosphoinositide-3-kinase (PI3K)-protein kinase B (Akt)-mTOR signaling axis to promote osteoblast proliferation and matrix secretion [22]. IGF-1 itself facilitates osteoblast proliferation, glucose metabolism, and differentiation via the Akt pathway, playing a pivotal role in maintaining bone homeostasis [23].

In the periodontal microenvironment, chronic inflammation leads to significant elevations in local hypoxia and oxidative stress, disrupting the normal glycolysis-oxidative phosphorylation balance in osteoblasts [24]. Persistent oxidative stress from chronic inflammation causes mitochondrial dysfunction, inhibiting the metabolic utilization efficiency of glucose in osteoblasts. Meanwhile, tumor necrosis factor-α (TNF-α) suppresses the osteogenic transcription factor such as runt-related transcription factor 2 (Runx2) by upregulating micro RNA 23b (miR-23b) expression, thereby interfering with osteogenic differentiation. Collectively, local metabolic dysfunction combined with downregulated osteogenic signaling ultimately results in impaired periodontal bone formation and exacerbated disruption of bone homeostasis [25].

3.2 Lipid metabolism in osteogenesis

Osteoblasts exhibit a high dependency on lipid metabolism, particularly fatty acid β-oxidation, in differentiation and function [26]. Lipid metabolism enables the energy supply and microenvironmental adaptation needed for bone formation. When differentiation progresses, osteoblasts enhance fatty acid uptake and oxidation to replenish tricarboxylic acid (TCA) cycle and maintain high-level energy supply [27]. Fatty acid β-oxidation not only provides adenosine triphosphate (ATP) for cells, but also regulates nicotinamide adenine dinucleotide (NAD^+) levels through sirtuin 1 (SIRT1) and peroxisome proliferator-activated receptor-γ coactivator 1α (PGC-1α), sustaining mitochondrial function and antioxidant capacity [27]. Studies showed that the Wnt signaling pathway not only participates in osteogenic differentiation, but also activates fatty acid oxidation (including the regulation of carnitine palmitoyltransferase 1A, CPT1A) to meet the metabolic demands of osteocytes to support osteoblastic metabolic activity [21].

Beyond energy metabolism, some lipid molecules directly engage in osteogenic signal regulation [26]. Phospholipids, critical for cell membrane structure and signal transduction, regulate osteoblastic functions such as secretion and polarization [28]. Gangliosides like monosialotetrahexosylganglioside (GM1), by accumulating in lipid raft regions, modulate the membrane localization and activity of osteogenic signaling receptors (e.g., fibroblast growth factor [FGF], bone morphogenetic protein [BMP] receptors), thereby accelerating osteogenic gene expression and differentiation. Upregulation of gangliosides has been confirmed to correlate closely with the activation of osteogenic transcription factors such as Runx2 [21].

Lipid metabolism is perturbed by inflammation when periodontitis occurs. Oxidative stress disrupts fatty acid metabolism and impairs mitochondrial β-oxidation function, thereby weakening the energy supply and antioxidant capacity of osteoblasts [29]. Simultaneously, the accumulation of peroxidized lipid products in inflamed microenvironments damages mitochondrial function in osteoprogenitor cells and induces cell apoptosis. The changes of lipid metabolism in periodontitis suppress differentiation and bone-forming activity, which further destabilizes periodontal bone homeostasis [30].

3.3 Amino acid metabolism in osteogenesis

Amino acid metabolism not only serves as the foundation for protein synthesis but also plays critical roles in maintaining energy metabolism, redox balance, and epigenetic regulation during osteoblast differentiation. Among these amino acids, glutaminolysis stands out as particularly important. Glutamine transporters (e.g., solute carrier family 1 member 5 (SLC1A5)) are highly expressed in osteoblasts and responsible for encoding amino acid transporters to uptake glutamine. In osteogenic differentiation, osteoprogenitor cells upregulate SLC1A5 to support the production of glutamate and α-ketoglutarate, thereby meeting the energy and biosynthetic demands of bone differentiation [31, 32]. Glutaminolysis also generates NADPH via the TCA cycle and its ancillary pathways, bolstering the antioxidant defense system of osteoblasts, maintaining redox balance, and promoting their survival and functional execution [14].

Additionally, certain non-essential amino acids (e.g., aspartate, arginine) play auxiliary roles in osteogenic differentiation. Aspartate acts as a TCA cycle anaplerotic substrate, promoting metabolic flux, whereas arginine activates the expression of osteogenesis-related transcription factors such as Runx2 via the nitric oxide synthase pathway, enhancing osteogenic activity [31, 33].

Chronic inflammation and hypoxia significantly perturb the amino acid metabolic network of osteoblasts. At the local site of periodontitis lesions, sustained high levels of oxidative stress inhibit glutamine transport and catabolism efficiency, suppressing α-ketoglutarate synthesis and TCA cycle activity. This metabolic disorder restricts cellular ATP production and disrupts the balance between bone resorption and formation, exacerbating periodontal tissue destruction [29].

4. Metabolic characteristics in bone resorption

4.1 Glucose metabolism in osteoclastogenesis

Osteoclasts undergo remarkable glucose metabolic remodeling during differentiation. Early osteoclast precursors mainly rely on mitochondrial oxidative phosphorylation (OXPHOS) to provide energy for cell fusion and maturation. However, as differentiation progresses, mature osteoclasts shift to a glycolysis-dominated energy production mode. Glycolysis not only provides rapid cell energy but also enhances the expression of receptor activator of nuclear factor-kappa B (NF-κB) ligand (RANKL) and lactate production [34]. The increased lactate production by osteoclasts contributes to inducing acidification of the surrounding microenvironment, thereby promoting bone resorption [20]. This metabolic switch is governed by the AKT/mTOR/HIF-1α pathway: RANKL activates HIF-1α via the AKT/mTOR pathway and thereby upregulates the expression of glycolytic enzymes (e.g., LDHA, HK2) and GLUT1, significantly enhancing glucose uptake and lactate production [35–37].

Beyond the AKT/mTOR/HIF-1α axis, osteoclastic metabolic reprogramming is synergistically regulated by multiple auxiliary signaling pathways. The RANKL-NFATc1 (Nuclear Factor of Activated T cells 1) pathway also plays a role in osteoclastic metabolic regulation. As a key transcription factor downstream of the RANKL pathway, NFATc1 regulates osteoclast-specific gene expression and promotes the transcriptional activity of metabolic genes [38, 39]. The Myc signaling pathway is activated in early osteoclast precursors, promoting glycolysis and glutamine metabolism to support the high-energy demands of osteoclastogenesis [40]. Additionally, reactive oxygen species (ROS), as byproducts of oxidative stress, function as intracellular signaling molecules in osteoclasts to amplify glycolytic flux, thereby enabling cells to sustain activity under hypoxic and high-inflammatory microenvironments [29].

Within the periodontitis microenvironment, chronic hypoxia and inflammatory stimuli synergistically augment the glycolytic dependence of osteoclasts [3, 20]. Sustained activation of HIF-1α induces the expression of glycolytic enzymes, such as GLUT1, HK2, and LDHA, promoting lactate accumulation. Concomitantly, the generation of ROS and activation of the advanced glycation end products (AGEs)-RAGE (the receptor for advanced glycation end products) pathway increase metabolic load, enabling osteoclasts to maintain efficient bone resorption in inflammatory environments. Collectively, the AKT/mTOR/HIF-1α pathway serves as the regulatory core for glucose metabolic reprogramming in osteoclasts, while its interactive crosstalk with NFATc1, Myc, and ROS signaling pathways collectively orchestrates the metabolic remodeling process. These signaling pathways jointly establish the metabolic basis for enhanced osteoclastic activity and aggravated bone loss in periodontitis lesions [35, 37].

4.2 Lipid metabolism in osteoclastogenesis

Osteoclastic differentiation and its functioning are highly dependent on lipid metabolism. Early in differentiation, osteoclast precursors rely on fatty acid oxidation for energy to facilitate multinuclear fusion and cell maturation [41]. During active bone resorption by osteoclasts, lipid metabolites modulate plasma membrane lipid rafts, vesicle trafficking systems, and osteoclastic secretion. These lipid metabolites facilitate the precise localization of proton-translocating adenosine triphosphatase (H^+-ATPase) and efficient deployment of osteolytic enzymes in osteoclasts [42].

Cholesterol and its oxidized derivatives play unique roles in osteoclastic metabolism. Physiological cholesterol levels facilitate proper lipid structural remodeling during precursor cell fusion, a pivotal step in multinucleated osteoclastogenesis [43]. However, when hyperlipidemia or chronic inflammation occurs, excessive cholesterol and its oxidation products significantly increase osteoclast number and bone resorptive activity, and trigger cholesterol-sensing pathways (liver X receptor (LXR)/cluster of differentiation 36 (CD36), etc.) to induce bone loss [44, 45]. The main cholesterol oxidation product, oxidized low-density lipoprotein (OxLDL), elevates reactive oxygen species (ROS) in osteoclasts and activates inflammation-related pathways such as NF-κB. This process upregulates tartrate-resistant acid phosphatase (TRAP) and osteolytic enzyme expression, thereby enhancing osteoclastic activity [46]. Additionally, excess lipids promote osteoclastic metabolic flux and osteoclastogenetic programs by activating ROS production, thereby augmenting bone resorptive efficiency [41, 44].

Dysregulated lipid metabolism has been identified as a critical bridge connecting metabolic disorders (e.g., hyperlipidemia, diabetes) and periodontal tissue destruction [47]. When periodontitis occurs, osteocytes under hyperlipidemic conditions exhibit heightened sensitivity to lipid stimuli, synergizing with inflammatory factors to promote osteoclast activation—a converging pathway linking metabolic diseases and periodontal bone loss. Local lipid accumulation not only increases osteoclast numbers, but also accelerates alveolar bone resorption by disrupting the osteoblast-osteoclast coupling balance [48].

4.3 Amino acid metabolism in osteoclastogenesis

Osteoclastogenesis is dependent on amino acid metabolism, particularly the regulation of glutamine metabolism, during cell differentiation and functional maturation. Early osteoclast precursors maintain an active TCA cycle by increasing glutamine uptake, meeting the demands of energy and metabolic intermediates for cell fusion, proliferation, and initial functional formation [49, 50]. Elevated GLS (glutaminase) activity not only supports energy supply, but also drives osteoclastic metabolic reprogramming and maturation by regulating mammalian target of rapamycin complex 1 (mTORC1) signaling [50]. As a central amino acid-sensing hub, mTORC1 promotes protein synthesis and cellular proliferation in the early differentiation stage of osteoclasts. Meanwhile, its activity attenuated during osteoclast fusion and maturation to enable multinuclear formation and the establishment of osteolytic functionality [51].

Beyond glutamine, other amino acids such as leucine and serine serve as cofactors in osteoclastic metabolism. Leucine directly activates the mTORC1 pathway to enhance osteoclast precursor proliferation, while serine metabolites are closely associated with nucleic acid synthesis and methylation, exerting positive effects on osteoclast division and metabolic regulation [50, 52, 53].

Osteoclasts exhibit enhanced dependence on amino acid metabolism in periodontitis. Chronic inflammation increases local metabolic stress, with elevated expression of inflammatory cytokines such as granulocyte colony-stimulating factor (G-CSF). Under high metabolic load, G-CSF induces activation of glutamine metabolism to promote TCA cycle-driven energy production. The enhanced energy production supports continuous bone resorption of osteoclasts in the inflamed periodontal microenvironment [54, 55]. Moreover, inflammation-associated molecules (e.g., TNF-α, IL-1β) participate in amino acid metabolism by upregulating mTORC1 and its downstream effectors, thereby amplifying osteoclastic metabolic activity and accelerating alveolar bone loss [56].

5. Metabolic synergy and signal integration in periodontal bone

5.1 Interactions and compensation of metabolic pathways

The cells in bone do not rely on any single metabolic pathway, but maintain physiological functions through the interplay and compensation of three major metabolic systems: glycolysis, fatty acid β-oxidation, and amino acid metabolism [12, 14]. Glucose metabolism supports cellular biosynthesis by providing rapid energy and metabolic intermediates. When glycolysis is constrained, osteoblasts sustain ATP production and metabolic activity by activating fatty acid oxidation pathways (e.g., CPT1A) [27, 57]. Amino acid metabolism replenishes TCA cycle intermediates (e.g., α-ketoglutarate), serving as a bridge in carbon source and energy supply [58]. Glucose, lipids, and amino acids are not metabolically independent but exhibit coordinated compensation. For instance, glycolytic end products (e.g., pyruvate) can enter the TCA cycle or serve as precursors for fatty acid synthesis. Under low-glucose conditions, lipid and amino acid metabolism provide metabolic intermediates to sustain cellular viability.

During different stages of differentiation and functional activity, osteoblasts face diverse energy and biosynthetic demands, which necessitate synergistic regulation and stage-specific transitions of metabolic pathways. During periods of vigorous proliferation and matrix synthesis, aerobic glycolysis is markedly activated, enabling rapid production of matrix proteins and supply of energy and synthetic precursors. Under nutrient-limiting conditions (e.g., glucose deprivation), osteoblasts mobilize fatty acids stored in lipid droplets and generate energy via fatty acid β-oxidation [59]. The osteoblast survival and functional stability are ensured by enhanced glutamine metabolism, replenishing energy and producing NADPH to reinforce the antioxidant system.

In contrast, osteoclasts rely on fatty acid oxidation and the TCA cycle for energy in early differentiation phase, but shift to glycolysis for rapid lactic acid production upon maturation to meet the high metabolic demands of bone resorption [36]. During pathway transitions, osteoclasts maintain dynamic balance of energy and metabolic intermediates by flexibly regulating substrate utilization.

This interaction and stage-specific reprogramming of metabolic pathways in osteoblasts and osteoclasts form a critical metabolic basis for their adaptive response to functional changes and maintenance of bone homeostasis. Inflammation and hypoxia often disrupt certain metabolic pathways during periodontitis, thereby forcing cells in periodontium to rely on metabolic compensation and synergy for survival and function. For example, osteoblasts upregulate fatty acid oxidation to sustain energy supply when glycolysis is impaired, while osteoclasts adapt to hypoxic and pro-inflammatory conditions by replenishing the TCA cycle through glutamine metabolism [60, 61]. Such metabolic synergy and compensation represent essential adaptive strategies of osteoblasts and osteoclasts to extreme microenvironmental stress.

5.2 Integration nodes of signaling pathways in bone metabolism

The dynamic regulation of bone metabolism relies on the integration and precise coordination of multiple signaling pathways. As sensors of nutrient, oxygen, and energy status, the protein mTOR, HIF-1α, and AMPK, respectively, orchestrate autophagy, metabolism, inflammation, and bone turnover in osteoblasts and osteoclasts, serving as core hubs of metabolic control [62, 63]. mTORC1 (mammalian target of rapamycin complex 1) senses amino acid, glucose, and fatty acid availability in osteocytes, and regulates cell growth, protein synthesis, and metabolic reprogramming [64]. During osteoblast differentiation, mTORC1 promotes glycolysis, fatty acid oxidation, and expression of osteogenic genes. In early osteoclast differentiation, mTORC1 is essential for sustaining energy supply and fusion capacity, whereas suppression of mTORC1 in mature osteoclasts enhances bone resorptive function.

HIF-1α (hypoxia-inducible factor-1α), a main regulator of oxygen homeostasis, elevates GLUT1 and VEGF (vascular endothelial growth factor) expression in osteoblasts, enhancing glycolysis and angiogenesis to support osteogenic remodeling [65]. Osteoclasts rely on HIF-1α to upregulate GLUT1 and key glycolytic enzymes under hypoxic conditions. During chronic inflammation, acute HIF-1α activation responds to the energy demands. However, the accumulated HIF-1α exacerbates bone loss and leads to a chronic inflammation-induced bone destruction [66].

AMPK (5′-adenosine monophosphate-activated protein kinase), an energy sensor, inhibits mTORC1 activity during energy deficit to promote fatty acid oxidation and autophagy, maintaining metabolic homeostasis [67]. In osteoblasts, AMPK activation not only initiates autophagy but also suppresses mTORC1-dependent inflammation, supporting mitochondrial function and fatty acid oxidation to ensure survival under inflammatory and nutrient-deprived conditions [62, 63]. Conversely, AMPK activation in osteoclasts suppresses differentiation by attenuating mTORC1 signaling, implying potential antiresorptive effects on bone [68].

ROS (reactive oxygen species), as oxidative stress signals, play dual roles in bone metabolic regulation. Moderate ROS level facilitates RANKL-induced osteoclast differentiation, whereas excessive ROS in inflamed environments like periodontitis disrupts osteoblast metabolism and function [38, 69].

In the periodontal microenvironment, the interplay of these signaling pathways dictates the metabolic choices and functional fates of cells. Under chronic inflammation, excessive HIF-1α activation, persistent mTORC1 signaling, and diminished AMPK activity collectively establish an osteoclast-predominant metabolic milieu, accelerating alveolar bone resorption [7, 70, 71]. Targeted modulation of signaling hubs such as mTORC1, HIF-1α, and AMPK may restore osteogenesis-osteoclastogenesis balance and enable precise reprogramming of bone metabolic pathways, facilitating the development of efficient and personalized clinical paradigms for periodontal therapy.

5.3 Metabolic coordination in cellular function

Upon entering the functional execution phase, the bone cells undergo dynamic metabolic adaptations to meet persistent functional demands [72]. The cell function includes robust matrix secretion and mineralization by osteoblasts, as well as efficient bone resorption by osteoclasts. During this stage, bone metabolism exhibits highly complex coordination and adjustment to sustain high-energy and high-throughput functional requirements.

Osteoblasts maintain sustained aerobic glycolysis during matrix synthesis and mineralization to provide rapid energy and synthetic substrates. Concurrently, enhanced fatty acid oxidation ensures protein synthesis, mitochondrial function, and membrane system stability—critical for prolonged energy supply in osteoblasts [27, 73]. Glutamine metabolism supports redox balance via NADPH production at this stage, reinforcing antioxidant system stability and maintaining an intracellular environment conducive to sustained secretory function [57]. In pathological conditions such as periodontitis, these metabolic pathways are suppressed, weakening osteoblastic matrix synthesis and reducing mineralization efficiency.

Osteoclasts derive energy from glycolysis during bone resorption, rapidly producing lactic acid to maintain an acidic microenvironment for bone resorption [36]. This metabolic profile not only promotes osteolytic enzyme activity and bone matrix degradation, but also stabilizes pH homeostasis for osteoclast function. Mature osteoclasts exhibit persistent demand for substrates like glutamine to sustain the TCA cycle, supporting mitochondrial energy metabolism under inflammatory and metabolic stress [41]. Chronic inflammatory stimuli heighten osteoclasts' sensitivity to signals such as HIF-1α and ROS, thereby amplifying metabolic activity and sustaining prolonged excessive bone resorption.

The metabolic profiles of osteoblasts and osteoclasts during the functional phase reflect profound task-specific adaptations and energy strategy divergence: the former prioritizes anabolic metabolism and mitochondrial homeostasis, while the latter emphasizes rapid energy production and microenvironmental remodeling. Periodontitis disrupts this balance by aberrantly regulating osteocyte secretion of RANKL and sclerostin, thereby promoting bone resorption and inhibiting formation [74]. Elucidating the bone metabolic adaptation mechanisms during functional phases can help clinical decisions on intervention timing, drug window selection, and local microenvironment optimization.

6. Effects of local and systemic diseases on periodontal bone homeostasis

6.1 Periodontal metabolic alterations in local inflammation

In periodontitis lesions, persistent colonization of Gram-negative bacteria and their endotoxins within the gingival crevicular fluid and root surface microenvironment triggers sustained RANKL secretion and other pro-inflammatory mediators [75]. Infiltrating immune cells (neutrophils, macrophages, T cells) release high levels of IL-1β and TNF-α [29, 76], which not only drive immune activation but directly disrupt osteocyte metabolic pathways, mediating metabolic reprogramming and impairing osteoblast-osteoclast balance.

In osteoblasts, TNF-α and IL-1β inhibit metabolic activity and differentiation via NF-κB/MAPK signaling, downregulating the downstream Runx2, alkaline phosphatase (ALP), and GLUT1 expression [29]. This disrupts glycolytic function, mitochondrial membrane potential, and ROS clearance [77]. Concomitant reduction in glutamine metabolism impairs TCA cycle flux and antioxidant defenses, leading to diminished matrix deposition and mineralization efficiency.

Osteoclasts, in contrast, gain a metabolic advantage under inflammatory conditions. Inflammatory cytokines can promote the expression of receptor activator of nuclear factor-kappa B (NF-κB) ligand (RANKL), enhance the expression of its downstream hypoxia-inducible factor-1α (HIF-1α), and elevate the RANKL/osteoprotegerin (OPG) ratio in gingival fibroblasts [78, 79]. This significantly promotes osteoclast differentiation in vitro, further upregulating their glycolytic activity and bone resorption capacity. Lactate, a glycolytic product, not only provides rapid energy but also helps create an acidic environment in the resorption lacunae, enhancing the efficiency of bone dissolution. Meanwhile, inflammation-induced elevation of reactive oxygen species (ROS) forms a positive feedback loop, promoting the continuous increase in metabolic activity and maintaining the high-functional state of osteoclasts under inflammatory conditions. In the local inflammatory environment, this dynamic imbalance of "inhibition of osteogenic metabolism—activation of osteoclastic metabolism" constitutes the core mechanism of continuous alveolar bone destruction.

Studies support the metabolic change in periodontitis: in patients with severe periodontitis, the levels of RANKL and interleukin-1 beta (IL-1β) are significantly elevated, while OPG expression is downregulated, indicating enhanced osteoclastogenesis and suppressed osteogenesis [80]. While periodontal treatment can effectively manage inflammation, it is incapable of fully reinstating the mitochondrial enzyme activity and restoring osteogenic metabolism within periodontal tissues [81]. Therefore, periodontal treatment should not only focus on inflammation control, but also concentrate on reestablishing metabolic equilibrium and restoring the metabolic adaptation and functional potential of the bone cells.

6.2 Periodontal metabolic alterations in systemic diseases

In addition to local inflammatory factors, periodontal disease is associated with a variety of systemic diseases, including diabetes and obesity [82]. Diseases such as diabetes, hyperlipidemia, and osteoporosis influence the energy supply, signal transduction, and functional stability of bone cells through chronic metabolic disorders. This leads to reduced responsiveness to periodontal treatment and compromised regenerative capacity, contributing to insufficient bone filling in refractory periodontal disease.

In the periodontal tissues of patients with diabetes, there is a continuous accumulation of advanced glycation end products (AGEs) and downregulation of sirtuin 3 (SIRT3). This change in diabetes results in mitochondrial dysfunction and decreased osteogenic differentiation ability, indicating oxidative damage related to high blood glucose [83]. Research indicates that under diabetic conditions, the expression of metabolic regulators such as glucose transporter 1 (GLUT1) generally declines, while reactive oxygen species (ROS) continuously accumulate. The low GLUT1 and high ROS together present a dual impairment of insufficient energy supply and oxidative damage in bone cells [84, 85]. Moreover, high glucose, inflammation, and HIF-1α activation induce gene expression change: an increase of RANKL, interleukin-1 beta (IL-1β), interleukin-6 (IL-6), interleukin-8 (IL-8), monocyte chemoattractant protein-1 (MCP-1), interleukin-10 (IL-10), and a decrease of osteoprotegerin (OPG). This bone-related gene expression pattern is an important mechanism for osteoclast activation [86, 87]. Clinically, the common occurrence of incomplete bone filling and poor treatment response in periodontal regenerative therapy for patients with diabetes are attributed to their metabolic dysfunction.

Another common metabolic disorder, hyperlipidemia, affects periodontal bone metabolism mainly through lipotoxicity and cholesterol accumulation [88, 89]. Oxidized low-density lipoprotein (OxLDL) binds to Toll-like receptor 4 (TLR4) to activate the nuclear factor-kappa B (NF-κB) pathway in osteoclasts, thereby triggering the CD36-TLR4-TLR6 (Toll-like receptor 6) inflammatory response. These molecules induce the TLR4 inflammatory response through MyD88 (myeloid differentiation primary response 88)-dependent and/or MyD88-independent pathways, promoting the expression of NF-κB and enhancing osteoclast fusion and resorption functions [90]. Regarding osteoblasts, OxLDL can be internalized by osteoblasts but not degraded. At high concentrations, OxLDL can lead to a decrease in osteoblast viability and lysosomal membrane damage, and even cause cell death [91]. Some animal experiments have found that the alveolar bone loss in mice fed a high-fat diet is significantly higher than that in the low-fat diet group, suggesting that abnormal lipid metabolism significantly reduces the effectiveness of periodontal bone repair [92, 93].

In patients with osteoporosis, due to systemic estrogen decline and reduced energy metabolism capacity, the overall metabolic level of bone cells is weakened [94]. The decreased activities of SIRT1 and AMPK limit mitochondrial biogenesis, rendering osteoblasts less responsive to regenerative signals. Meanwhile, in the absence of hormonal inhibition, the metabolic activity of osteoclasts is relatively enhanced, amplifying the bone resorption [95, 96]. In either elderly women or menopausal women, this metabolic background makes them a high-risk group for periodontal bone regeneration. Thus, combined metabolic assessment and adjuvant therapies are required to enhance the regenerative response.

Currently, an increasing number of researchers advocate for metabolic assessment as a routine pre-evaluation step in periodontal regenerative treatment. Through the detection of metabolic markers and individual nutritional assessment, preoperative classification of metabolic status can be achieved for individualized periodontal treatment. For patients with metabolic abnormalities, a combination of systemic metabolic treatment and periodontal treatment can be considered. This approach restores the osteogenic metabolic basis and improves the efficiency of alveolar bone regeneration.

7. Translational medicine: Metabolic-targeted strategies for periodontal treatment

The therapeutic goal of periodontitis extends beyond inflammation control and prevention of alveolar bone resorption; it aims to reconstruct the structural and functional integrity of periodontal tissues. With deeper insights into the metabolic mechanisms of bone cells, metabolic regulation has emerged as a novel target for periodontal regeneration. Unlike traditional approaches focusing solely on "structural repair, " metabolic interventions emphasize cellular functional states, microenvironmental plasticity, and personalized adaptability. In recent research, growing attention has been paid to the metabolic alterations after non-surgical periodontal therapy [8, 97]. Meanwhile, metabolic-targeted drugs and other metabolism-related interventions have been applied to repair bone defects in periodontitis, establishing a translational pathway that integrates metabolism and regeneration.

7.1 Metabolic regulation of periodontal treatment

Periodontal treatment is used to target the removal of dental plaque and the suppression of inflammation, but recent studies have gradually revealed its profound regulatory effects on bone metabolism. In periodontitis lesions, bone cells often exhibit functional imbalance: osteoblasts show decreased glycolytic capacity, mitochondrial damage, and reactive oxygen species (ROS) accumulation; while osteoclasts display a "metabolic advantage" characterized by increased glycolytic flux and enhanced bone resorption ability. Periodontal treatment helps in the restoration of cellular metabolic states by mechanically eliminating infection sources and reducing the burden of inflammatory cytokines. Both clinical and animal studies supported that the expressions of RANKL and OPG decreased in gingival tissues after periodontal treatment, indicating a reduction in the activity of bone resorption [98]. For patients with diabetes and periodontitis, scaling and root planing (SRP) significantly improves periodontal index and glycated hemoglobin (HbA1c) levels. SRP continuously regulates the expressions of inflammatory and osteoclastic factors within 12 months afterwards [99, 100].

The metabolic significance of periodontal treatment is not only limited to "repair" but also embodies a "prospective" role: it establishes a window of metabolic adaptability for regeneration. Studies indicate that within 4 weeks after non-surgical treatment, levels of IL-1β, IL-8, and matrix metalloproteinase-8 (MMP-8) in gingival crevicular fluid decrease significantly. This suggests a gradual restoration of cellular glycolysis, glutamine metabolism, and matrix synthesis programs in the periodontal microenvironment [101]. This timepoint can be considered as an optimal node for implanting bone substitute materials or initiating other regenerative interventions. Thus, periodontal treatment should be regarded as a "metabolic pre-conditioning" step, as it not only reconstructs the cellular environment but also influences the entire regenerative cascade. It is possible that detecting metabolic markers in gingival crevicular fluid or saliva can serve as an indicator to determine whether periodontal tissues have entered a "regenerative sensitive phase" in the future.

Despite that periodontal treatment can partially alleviate inflammation-induced metabolic inhibition, it is incapable of completely reestablishing bone metabolic homeostasis. Multiple studies have demonstrated that the recovery of inflammatory regulators (matrix metalloproteinase-1 (MMP-1), etc.) and osteogenic proteins (osteopontin (OPN), etc.) before and after SRP remains limited. Osteoblasts continue to exhibit metabolic stress and impaired differentiation [102, 103], particularly in high-risk populations (e.g., patients with diabetes, elderly patients, or patients with severe bone resorption), where periodontal treatment alone cannot satisfy the metabolic requisites for bone regeneration. Consequently, adjuvant strategies like local metabolic regulatory agents (e.g., AMPK activators, α-KG supplements) have emerged as necessary approaches. By optimizing cellular activity and metabolic signaling responsiveness, these strategies can significantly enhance regenerative efficiency and tissue reconstruction quality.

Therefore, periodontal treatment is not only the starting point for inflammation control but also a critical window for metabolic reconstruction. Integrating periodontal treatment into the entire regenerative intervention and collaborating with metabolic strategies represent a fundamental transition from "anti-inflammation" to "homeostatic regeneration."

7.2 Metabolite-targeted drug therapy for periodontal diseases

Metabolic regulatory drugs were initially applied to systemic diseases (e.g., diabetes, osteoporosis), but their potential in treating periodontitis-related bone resorption is being increasingly explored. Signaling pathways such as AMPK, mTOR, HIF-1α, and SIRT1 serve as core metabolic regulatory axes, governing glycolysis, fatty acid oxidation, and antioxidant systems in osteoblasts, while also participating in osteoclast function regulation [104, 105].

Metformin, a classic AMPK activator widely used in patients with diabetic periodontitis, has recently been demonstrated to improve alveolar bone metabolic status through local administration. Researches show that metformin promotes [^{18}F] fluorodeoxyglucose ([^{18}F]FDG) uptake in osteoblasts, enhances GLUT1 expression in a dose-dependent manner, and strengthens bone formation. Concurrently, it inhibits mTOR-NF-κB activity in osteoclasts, alleviating inflammation and bone resorption [106, 107]. Preliminary clinical applications have shown that applying metformin gel to periodontal regeneration sites significantly improves bone filling and attachment levels [108].

Statin drugs such as simvastatin have also demonstrated promising potential for periodontal regeneration. They promote osteogenic differentiation by upregulating the gene expression of BMP-2 (bone morphogenetic protein-2) and OCN (osteocalcin), while mitigating bone resorption in inflamed microenvironments to facilitate bone defect repair [109]. Multiple clinical studies have shown that local application of statins to bone defects or implant sites can increase bone density and improve primary implant stability, with particularly pronounced effects observed in smokers and individuals with metabolic abnormalities [110, 111].

HIF-1α stabilizers enhance bone-vascular co-reconstruction by mimicking hypoxic adaptive responses, inducing osteoblastic glycolysis and VEGF expression within the periodontal hypoxic microenvironment. α-KG promotes osteogenesis by polarizing anti-inflammatory M2 macrophages and upregulating osteogenic-related factors, thereby improving bone regenerative capacity in inflamed conditions [112]. These metabolism-targeted drugs have all exhibited significant osteogenic effects in animal models of periodontitis-induced bone defects, providing a potential therapeutic approach for personalized periodontal regenerative strategies.

7.3 Periodontal treatment based on precision monitoring of metabolic markers

As periodontal regenerative therapy enters the era of precision medicine, metabolic markers are emerging as dynamic indicators that guide precision periodontal regeneration by reflecting bone cell activity, local inflammation and bone remodeling potential [113]. Analysis of metabolites in saliva, gingival crevicular fluid, or tissue fluid can not only assist in determining regenerative windows and selecting surgical methods, but also facilitate early monitoring and feedback regulation in postoperative management.

The metabolic profile of local tissues reflects the homeostatic balance between osteoblasts and osteoclasts, making metabolic changes a valuable tool for monitoring the optimal window for bone regeneration. Elevated glycolytic metabolites (lactate, LDHA, etc.) and decreased osteogenesis-related metabolites (glutamine, α-ketoglutaric acid, etc.) often indicate a periodontal microenvironment dominated by bone resorption with suppressed bone formation [114, 115]. Studies have shown that after inflammation control, the expression of metabolic markers such as GLUT1, Runx2, and PGC-1α gradually recovers, suggesting reactivation of the osteogenic program. Accurate identification of this sensitive window can define the optimal timing for regenerative material implantation and bone reconstruction. Such a critical window is elusive with traditional periodontal examinations and imaging techniques, while metabolic changes offer advanced diagnostic insights.

Metabolic markers also provide critical references for optimizing personalized treatment strategies. Significant interpatient variability exists in metabolic adaptability, inflammatory response, and tissue regenerative potential [114, 116, 117]. For example, pre-evaluations indicating low glutamine metabolism or insufficient TCA cycle flux may warrant the use of energy-supplementary scaffold materials based on pyruvate or α-KG [114]. Conversely, persistent elevation of oxidative stress markers may favor combination therapies with AMPK activators or ROS scavenging biomaterials. This strategy of matching biomaterials and drugs to metabolic profiles represents a pivotal step in shifting regenerative interventions from "standard protocols" to "individualized precision."

In the postoperative stage, metabolic markers exhibit rapid responsiveness and high sensitivity, enabling the detection of abnormalities before the manifestation of osteogenic failure or heightened osteoclast activity [118]. In contrast to traditional assessments like imaging and periodontal probing—which are inherently delayed and reflect historical bacterial insults rather than active disease states—metabolic markers provide timely insights into ongoing pathological processes, thereby overcoming the limitations of conventional methods in identifying early signs of bone reconstruction failure [119]. For example, a decline in keratinocyte growth factor (KGF) levels in gingival crevicular fluid after reaching a peak has been correlated with poor periodontal repair outcomes [120]. Moreover, metabolic bone markers such as ICTP (cross-linked C-telopeptide of type I collagen) exhibit a strong association with disease activation and possess the ability to predict future disease activity level [121]. Dynamic monitoring of metabolic changes not only provides real-time guidance for periodontal treatment adjustments, but also has the potential to serve as an early warning signal for recurrence risk in long-term management.

Emerging technologies such as metabolism-imaging fusion are continuously expanding the boundaries of monitoring methodologies. By integrating metabolic imaging techniques—including positron emission tomography (PET) and magnetic resonance spectroscopy (MRS)—with metabolomics data, researchers can achieve spatial visualization of metabolic states in alveolar bone defect regions [122]. This integration holds broad prospects for two key applications: (1) preoperatively pinpointing "metabolically hyporeactive zones" to guide surgical planning; (2) postoperatively tracking neobone activity development to assess regenerative efficacy. Further integration of machine learning models with clinical data is expected to establish a complete chain of "metabolic decision- surgical modality adaptation-real time feedback", leading periodontal regenerative therapy into a new era of metabolism-driven intelligence.

8. Conclusion

Periodontal bone homeostasis is dynamically regulated by the interplay of glucose, lipid, and amino acid metabolism in osteoblasts and osteoclasts, with signaling pathways such as mTOR, AMPK, and HIF-1α serving as key regulatory hubs. Physiologically, these metabolic processes adapt to energy demands during bone remodeling. However, periodontitis disrupts this balance: osteoblasts exhibit impaired glycolysis and mitochondrial function under inflammatory conditions, while osteoclasts enhance glycolytic and glutamine metabolism to sustain resorptive activity. Systemic conditions like diabetes and hyperlipidemia further exacerbate metabolic dysfunction in bone cells, establishing a link between metabolic disorders and alveolar bone loss.

Metabolic-targeted therapies offer promising translational opportunities. Periodontal treatment not only reduces inflammation but also restores cellular metabolic states, creating a "regenerative window" for bone repair. Drugs such as metformin and statins, along with metabolites like α-KG, have demonstrated efficacy in preclinical models by enhancing osteogenesis and inhibiting osteoclastogenesis. Precision monitoring of metabolic markers (e.g., GLUT1, lactate) enables personalized assessment of regenerative potential and treatment response, overcoming the limitations of traditional imaging techniques.

While significant progress has been made, challenges persist in deciphering the crosstalk between metabolic pathways and translating preclinical findings into clinical practice. Future research should prioritize mechanistic insights and develop safe, scalable metabolic interventions to achieve precise periodontal regenerative therapies that restore both bone structure and metabolic homeostasis.

Acknowledgements

The work described in this paper was substantially supported by grants from the Shenzhen Science and Technology Program (JCYJ20230807152400001) and TaiKang Healthcare Research Fund (Youth Incubation Program) (2024020).

Author details

Xiaoxiao Wang[1,2*†], Houze Li[3,4†], Yunyi Xie[4], Yan Wang[4], Sun Haipeng[2] and Dan Zhao[5*]

1 Oral Medical Center, Shenzhen Qianhai Taikang Hospital, Shenzhen, China

2 Shenzhen Stomatology Hospital, Shenzhen, China

3 West China School of Stomatology, Chengdu, China

4 Guangdong Provincial Key Laboratory of Stomatology, Hospital of Stomatology, Guanghua School of Stomatology, Sun Yat-Sen University, Guangzhou, China

5 Beijing Stomatological Hospital, Capital Medical University, Beijing, China

*Address all correspondence to: wxiaox7@163.com; zhaodanashley@hotmail.com

† These authors contributed equally.

References

[1] Zhou J, Zhu Y, Ai D, Zhou M, Li H, Fu Y, et al. Low-intensity pulsed ultrasound regulates osteoblastosteoclast crosstalk via EphrinB2/EphB4 signaling for orthodontic alveolar bone remodeling. Frontiers in Bioengineering and Biotechnology. 2023;**11**:1192720. DOI: 10.3389/fbioe.2023.1192720

[2] Li Y, Ling J, Jiang Q. Inflammasomes in alveolar bone loss. Frontiers in Immunology. 2021;**12**:691013. DOI: 10.3389/fimmu.2021.691013

[3] Li T, Du Y, Yao H, Zhao B, Wang Z, Chen R, et al. Isobavachin attenuates osteoclastogenesis and periodontitis-induced bone loss by inhibiting cellular iron accumulation and mitochondrial biogenesis. Biochemical Pharmacology. 2024;**224**:116202. DOI: 10.1016/j.bcp.2024.116202

[4] Galli C, Passeri G, Macaluso GM. FoxOs, Wnts and oxidative stress-induced bone loss: New players in the periodontitis arena? Journal of Periodontal Research. 2011;**46**:397-406. DOI: 10.1111/j.1600-0765.2011.01354.x

[5] Ledesma-Colunga MG, Passin V, Lademann F, Hofbauer LC, Rauner M. Novel insights into osteoclast energy metabolism. Current Osteoporosis Reports. 2023;**21**:660-669. DOI: 10.1007/s11914-023-00825-3

[6] Fraser D, Ganesan S. Microbiome, alveolar bone, and metabolites: Connecting the dots. Frontiers in Dental Medicine. 2023;**3**:1074339. DOI: 10.3389/fdmed.2022.1074339

[7] Qi X, Bie M, Jiang R, Kang F. HIF-1α regulates osteoclastogenesis and alveolar bone resorption in periodontitis via ANGPTL4. Archives of Oral Biology. 2023;**153**:105736. DOI: 10.1016/j.archoralbio.2023.105736

[8] Shan C, Xia Y, Wu Z, Zhao J. HIF-1α and periodontitis: Novel insights linking host-environment interplay to periodontal phenotypes. Progress in Biophysics and Molecular Biology. 2023;**184**:50-78. DOI: 10.1016/j.pbiomolbio.2023.09.002

[9] Wang L, You X, Zhang L, Zhang C, Zou W. Mechanical regulation of bone remodeling. Bone Research. 2022;**10**:16. DOI: 10.1038/s41413-022-00190-4

[10] Omi M, Mishina Y. Roles of osteoclasts in alveolar bone remodeling. Genesis New York, N.Y. 2000. 2022;**60**:e23490. DOI: 10.1002/dvg.23490

[11] Epsley S, Tadros S, Farid AR, Kargilis DC, Mehta S, Rajapakse C. The effect of inflammation on bone. Frontiers in Physiology. 2021;**11**:511799. DOI: 10.3389/fphys.2020.511799

[12] Shen L, Hu G, Karner CM. Bioenergetic metabolism In osteoblast differentiation. Current Osteoporosis Reports. 2022;**20**:53-64. DOI: 10.1007/s11914-022-00721-2

[13] Lee W-C, Ji X, Nissim I, Long F. Malic enzyme couples mitochondria with aerobic glycolysis in osteoblasts. Cell Reports. 2020;**32**:108108. DOI: 10.1016/j.celrep.2020.108108

[14] Lungu O, Toscani D, Burroughs-Garcia J, Giuliani N. The metabolic features of osteoblasts: Implications for multiple myeloma (MM) bone disease. International Journal of Molecular Sciences. 2023;**24**:4893. DOI: 10.3390/ijms24054893

[15] Guntur AR, Gerencser AA, Le PT, DeMambro VE, Bornstein SA, Mookerjee SA, et al. Osteoblast-like MC3T3-E1 cells prefer glycolysis for ATP production but adipocyte-like 3T3-L1 cells prefer oxidative phosphorylation. Journal of Bone and Mineral Research: The Official Journal of the American Society for Bone and Mineral Research. 2018;**33**:1052-1065. DOI: 10.1002/jbmr.3390

[16] Nishioku T, Anzai R, Hiramatsu S, Terazono A, Nakao M, Moriyama M. Lactatedehydrogenaseinhibitionprevents RANKL-induced osteoclastogenesis by reducing enhanced glycolysis. Journal of Pharmacological Sciences. 2023;**153**:197-207. DOI: 10.1016/j.jphs.2023.09.005

[17] Taubmann J, Krishnacoumar B, Böhm C, Faas M, Müller DIH, Adam S, et al. Metabolic reprogramming of osteoclasts represents a therapeutic target during the treatment of osteoporosis. Scientific Reports. 2020;**10**:21020. DOI: 10.1038/s41598-020-77892-4

[18] Pham TH, Kim E-N, Trang NM, Jeong G-S. Gallic acid induces osteoblast differentiation and alleviates inflammatory response through GPR35/GSK3β/β-catenin signaling pathway in human periodontal ligament cells. Journal of Periodontal Research. 2024;**59**:204-219. DOI: 10.1111/jre.13208

[19] Zhu S, Chen W, Masson A, Li Y-P. Cell signaling and transcriptional regulation of osteoblast lineage commitment, differentiation, bone formation, and homeostasis. Cell Discovery. 2024;**10**:71. DOI: 10.1038/s41421-024-00689-6

[20] Yu Y, Jiang L, Li J, Lei L, Li H. Hexokinase 2-mediated glycolysis promotes receptor activator of NF-κB ligand expression in *Porphyromonas gingivalis* lipopolysaccharide-treated osteoblasts. Journal of Periodontology. 2022;**93**:1036-1047. DOI: 10.1002/JPER.21-0227

[21] Vlashi R, Zhang X, Wu M, Chen G. Wnt signaling: Essential roles in osteoblast differentiation, bone metabolism and therapeutic implications for bone and skeletal disorders. Genes & Diseases. 2023;**10**:1291-1317. DOI: 10.1016/j.gendis.2022.07.011

[22] DeMambro VE, Tian L, Karthik V, Rosen CJ, Guntur AR. Effects of PTH on osteoblast bioenergetics in response to glucose. Bone Reports. 2023;**19**:101705. DOI: 10.1016/j.bonr.2023.101705

[23] Ruan X, Jin X, Sun F, Pi J, Jinghu Y, Lin X, et al. IGF signaling pathway in bone and cartilage development, homeostasis, and disease. FASEB Journal: official publication of the Federation of American Societies for Experimental Biology. 2024;**38**:e70031. DOI: 10.1096/fj.202401298R

[24] Li Y, Xu C, Mao J, Mao L, Li W, Liu Z, et al. ZIF-8-based nanoparticles for inflammation treatment and oxidative stress reduction in periodontitis. ACS Applied Materials & Interfaces. 2024;**16**:36077-36094. DOI: 10.1021/acsami.4c05722

[25] Sun X, Li M, Ban J, Li Z. miR-23b mediates TNF-α-inhibited osteogenic differentiation of human periodontal ligament stem cells by targeting Runx2. International Journal of Medical Sciences. 2021;**18**:3674-3683. DOI: 10.7150/ijms.64312

[26] Alekos NS, Kushwaha P, Kim SP, Li Z, Abood A, Dirckx N, et al. Mitochondrial β-oxidation of adipose-derived fatty acids by osteoblasts fuels parathyroid hormone-induced bone formation. JCI Insight. 2023;**8**:e165604. DOI: 10.1172/jci.insight.165604

[27] Bai Y, Wu Z, Leary SC, Fang C, Yu M, Genth H, et al. Focal adhesion kinase alleviates simulated microgravity-induced inhibition of osteoblast differentiation by activating transcriptional Wnt/β-catenin-BMP2-COL1 and metabolic SIRT1-PGC-1α-CPT1A pathways. International Journal of Molecular Sciences. 2025;**26**:1669. DOI: 10.3390/ijms26041669

[28] Astudillo AM, Balboa MA, Balsinde J. Compartmentalized regulation of lipid signaling in oxidative stress and inflammation: Plasmalogens, oxidized lipids and ferroptosis as new paradigms of bioactive lipid research. Progress in Lipid Research. 2023;**89**:101207. DOI: 10.1016/j.plipres.2022.101207

[29] Yang K, Yang Y, Long T, Wang X, Chen Y, He C, et al. Hyperhomocysteinaemia aggravates periodontitis by suppressing the Nrf2/HO-1 signalling pathway. Redox Report: Communications in Free Radical Research. 2025;**30**:2475691. DOI: 10.1080/13510002.2025.2475691

[30] Zhang X, Jiang Y, Mao J, Ren X, Ji Y, Mao Y, et al. Hydroxytyrosol prevents periodontitis-induced bone loss by regulating mitochondrial function and mitogen-activated protein kinase signaling of bone cells. Free Radical Biology & Medicine. 2021;**176**:298-311. DOI: 10.1016/j.freeradbiomed.2021.09.027

[31] Sharma D, Yu Y, Shen L, Zhang G-F, Karner CM. SLC1A5 provides glutamine and asparagine necessary for bone development in mice. eLife. 2021;**10**:e71595. DOI: 10.7554/eLife.71595

[32] Shen L, Sharma D, Yu Y, Long F, Karner CM. Biphasic regulation of glutamine consumption by WNT during osteoblast differentiation. Journal of Cell Science. 2021;**134**:jcs251645. DOI: 10.1242/jcs.251645

[33] Qu Z, Zhao S, Zhang Y, Wang X, Yan L. Natural compounds for bone remodeling: Targeting osteoblasts and relevant signaling pathways. Biomedicine & Pharmacotherapy = Biomedecine & Pharmacotherapie. 2024;**180**:117490. DOI: 10.1016/j.biopha.2024.117490

[34] Li B, Lee W-C, Song C, Ye L, Abel E, Long F. Both aerobic glycolysis and mitochondrial respiration are required for osteoclast differentiation. The FASEB Journal. 2020;**34**:11058-11067. DOI: 10.1096/fj.202000771R

[35] Yang S, Song D, Wang Z, Su Y, Chen J, Xian Y, et al. AKT/GSK3β/NFATc1 and ROS signal axes are involved in AZD1390-mediated inhibitory effects on osteoclast and OVX-induced osteoporosis. International Immunopharmacology. 2022;**113**:109370. DOI: 10.1016/j.intimp.2022.109370

[36] Chu W, Peng W, Lu Y, Liu Y, Li Q, Wang H, et al. PRMT6 epigenetically drives metabolic switch from fatty acid oxidation toward glycolysis and promotes osteoclast differentiation during osteoporosis. Advanced Science (Weinheim, Baden-Wurttemberg, Germany). 2024;**11**:e2403177. DOI: 10.1002/advs.202403177

[37] Xiao D, Zhou Q, Gao Y, Cao B, Zhang Q, Zeng G, et al. PDK1 is important lipid kinase for RANKL-induced osteoclast formation and function via the regulation of the Akt-GSK3β-NFATc1 signaling cascade. Journal of Cellular Biochemistry. 2020;**121**:4542-4557. DOI: 10.1002/jcb.29677

[38] AlQranei MS, Aljohani H, Majumdar S, Senbanjo LT, Chellaiah MA. C-phycocyanin attenuates

RANKL-induced osteoclastogenesis and bone resorption in vitro through inhibiting ROS levels, NFATc1 and NF-κB activation. Scientific Reports. 2020;**10**:2513. DOI: 10.1038/s41598-020-59363-y

[39] Nakagawa S, Omori K, Nakayama M, Mandai H, Yamamoto S, Kobayashi H, et al. The fungal metabolite (+)-terrein abrogates osteoclast differentiation via suppression of the RANKL signaling pathway through NFATc1. International Immunopharmacology. 2020;**83**:106429. DOI: 10.1016/j.intimp.2020.106429

[40] Gao Y, Kraus FV, Seebach E, Chakraborty S, Schaack D, Schenz J, et al. Acod1 negatively impacts osteoclastogenesis via GPR91-mediated NFATc1 activation. bioRxiv. 2022;**27**(12):111455. DOI: 10.1101/2022.04.07.487467

[41] Kong X, Tao S, Ji Z, Li J, Li H, Jin J, et al. FATP2 regulates osteoclastogenesis by increasing lipid metabolism and ROS production. Journal of Bone and Mineral Research: The Official Journal of the American Society for Bone and Mineral Research. 2024;**39**:737-752. DOI: 10.1093/jbmr/zjae034

[42] Kim H, Oh B, Park-Min K-H. Regulation of osteoclast differentiation and activity by lipid metabolism. Cells. 2021;**10**:89. DOI: 10.3390/cells10010089

[43] Kitano VJF, Ohyama Y, Hayashida C, Ito J, Okayasu M, Sato T, et al. LDL uptake-dependent phosphatidylethanolamine translocation to the cell surface promotes fusion of osteoclast-like cells. Journal of Cell Science. 2020;**133**:jcs243840. DOI: 10.1242/jcs.243840

[44] Sul O-J, Kim J-E, Ke K, Suh J-H, Choi H-S. Atherogenic diet-induced bone loss is primarily due to increased osteoclastogenesis in mice. The Journal of Nutritional Biochemistry. 2020;**79**:108337. DOI: 10.1016/j.jnutbio.2019.108337

[45] Che Y, Yang J, Tang F, Wei Z, Chao Y, Li N, et al. New function of cholesterol oxidation products involved in osteoporosis pathogenesis. International Journal of Molecular Sciences. 2022;**23**:2020. DOI: 10.3390/ijms23042020

[46] Sul O-J, Li G, Kim J-E, Kim E-S, Choi H-S. 7-ketocholesterol enhances autophagy via the ROS-TFEB signaling pathway in osteoclasts. The Journal of Nutritional Biochemistry. 2021;**96**:108783. DOI: 10.1016/j.jnutbio.2021.108783

[47] Anagnostis P, Florentin M, Livadas S, Lambrinoudaki I, Goulis DG. Bone health in patients with dyslipidemias: An underestimated aspect. International Journal of Molecular Sciences. 2022;**23**:1639. DOI: 10.3390/ijms23031639

[48] Zhang J, Hu W, Zou Z, Li Y, Kang F, Li J, et al. The role of lipid metabolism in osteoporosis: Clinical implication and cellular mechanism. Genes & Diseases. 2024;**11**:101122. DOI: 10.1016/j.gendis.2023.101122

[49] Catheline S, Smith CO, McArthur M, Yu C, Brookes PS, Eliseev RA. Energy metabolism in osteoprogenitors and osteoblasts: Role of the pentose phosphate pathway. The Journal of Biological Chemistry. 2024;**301**:4515-4541. DOI: 10.1016/j.jbc.2024.108016

[50] Peng R, Dong Y, Zheng M, Kang H, Wang P, Zhu M, et al. IL-17 promotes osteoclast-induced bone loss by regulating glutamine-dependent energy metabolism. Cell Death & Disease. 2024;**15**:111. DOI: 10.1038/s41419-024-06475-2

[51] Yuping Q, Yijun L, Limei W. Low concentrations of tumor necrosis factor-alpha promote human periodontal ligament stem cells osteogenic differentiation by activation of autophagy via inhibition of AKT/mTOR pathway. Molecular Biology Reports. 2023;**50**:3329-3339. DOI: 10.1007/s11033-022-08173-8

[52] Bae S, Oh B, Tsai J, Park PSU, Greenblatt MB, Giannopoulou EG, et al. The crosstalk between MYC and mTORC1 during osteoclastogenesis. Frontiers in Cell and Developmental Biology. 2022;**10**:920683. DOI: 10.3389/fcell.2022.920683

[53] Saad M, Rauber S, Schett G, Ramming A. OP0241 il9 modulation of osteoclasts differentiation and impacts on bone metabolism. Annals of the Rheumatic Diseases. 2020;**79**:152. DOI: 10.1136/annrheumdis-2020-eular.1676

[54] Yu H, Zhang T, Lu H, Ma Q, Zhao D, Sun J, et al. Granulocyte colony-stimulating factor (G-CSF) mediates bone resorption in periodontitis. BMC Oral Health. 2021;**21**:299. DOI: 10.1186/s12903-021-01658-1

[55] Udumula MP, Sakr S, Dar S, Morris R, Buekers T, Munkarah A, et al. Epithelial ovarian cancer microenvironment regulates myeloid cell metabolism to confer immunosuppression via glutamine metabolism. The Journal of Immunology. 2021;**206**:101.08. DOI: 10.4049/jimmunol.206. Supp.101.08

[56] ALQ d F, Chaves HV, JMO d F, LHT d S, ATA P, MAS L, et al. Molecular docking study and antireabsorptive activity of a semi-synthetic coumarin derivative from Platymiscium floribundum in the ligature-induced periodontitis in rats: The involvement of heme oxygenase-1. Clinical Oral Investigations. 2022;**26**:1701-1711. DOI: 10.1007/s00784-021-04143-9

[57] Pieles O, Höring M, Adel S, Reichert TE, Liebisch G, Morsczeck C. Energy metabolism and lipidome are highly regulated during osteogenic differentiation of dental follicle cells. Stem Cells International. 2022;**2022**:3674931. DOI: 10.1155/2022/3674931

[58] Guo L, Chen S, Ou L, Li S, Ye Z-N, Liu H-F. Disrupted alpha-ketoglutarate homeostasis: Understanding kidney diseases from the view of metabolism and beyond. Diabetes, Metabolic Syndrome and Obesity: Targets and Therapy. 2022;**15**:1961-1974. DOI: 10.2147/DMSO.S369090

[59] Nandy A, Helderman RCM, Thapa S, Jayapalan S, Richards A, Narayani N, et al. Lipolysis supports bone formation by providing osteoblasts with endogenous fatty acid substrates to maintain bioenergetic status. Bone Research. 2023;**11**:62. DOI: 10.1038/s41413-023-00297-2

[60] Wu X, Sun Y, Cui R, Qiu W, Zhang J, Hu Z, et al. A novel adiponectin receptor agonist (AdipoAI) ameliorates type 2 diabetes-associated periodontitis by enhancing autophagy in osteoclasts. Journal of Periodontal Research. 2022;**57**:381-391. DOI: 10.1111/jre.12969

[61] Nantakeeratipat T, Fujihara C, Nogimori T, Matsumoto M, Yamamoto T, Murakami S. Lysosomal acid lipase regulates bioenergetic process during the cytodifferentiation of human periodontal ligament cells. Biochemical and Biophysical Research Communications. 2023;**662**:84-92. DOI: 10.1016/j.bbrc.2023.04.041

[62] Wang J, Zhang Y, Cao J, Wang Y, Anwar N, Zhang Z, et al. The role

of autophagy in bone metabolism and clinical significance. Autophagy. 2023;**19**:2409-2427. DOI: 10.1080/15548627.2023.2186112

[63] Tong X, Ganta RR, Liu Z. AMP-activated protein kinase (AMPK) regulates autophagy, inflammation and immunity and contributes to osteoclast differentiation and functionabs. Biology of the Cell. 2020;**112**:251-264. DOI: 10.1111/boc.202000008

[64] Zhang S, Lin X, Hou Q, Hu Z, Wang Y, Wang Z. Regulation of mTORC1 by amino acids in mammalian cells: A general picture of recent advances. Animal Nutrition (Zhongguo Xu Mu Shou Yi Xue Hui). 2021;7:1009-1023. DOI: 10.1016/j.aninu.2021.05.003

[65] Kierans S, Taylor C. Regulation of glycolysis by the hypoxia-inducible factor (HIF): Implications for cellular physiology. The Journal of Physiology. 2020;**599**(1):23-37. DOI: 10.1113/JP280572

[66] Knowles HJ. Distinct roles for the hypoxia-inducible transcription factors HIF-1α and HIF-2α in human osteoclast formation and function. Scientific Reports. 2020;**10**:21072. DOI: 10.1038/s41598-020-78003-z

[67] Sharma A, Anand SK, Singh N, Dwivedi UN, Kakkar P. AMP-activated protein kinase: An energy sensor and survival mechanism in the reinstatement of metabolic homeostasis. Experimental Cell Research. 2023;**428**:113614. DOI: 10.1016/j.yexcr.2023.113614

[68] Tanaka M, Inoue H, Takahashi N, Uehara M. AMPK negatively regulates RANKL-induced osteoclast differentiation by controlling oxidative stress. Free Radical Biology & Medicine. 2023;**205**:107-115. DOI: 10.1016/j.freeradbiomed.2023.05.033

[69] Peng C, Wang G, Li J. Ros-responsive and scavenging bifunctional hydrogel enables co-delivery of anti-inflammatory agent and osteogenetic nanoparticle for periodontitis treatment. Materials & Design. 2024;**239**:112777. DOI: 10.1016/j.matdes.2024.112777

[70] Feng C, Liu Y, Zhang B-Y, Zhang H, Shan F-Y, Li T-Q, et al. Rapamycin inhibits osteoclastogenesis and prevents LPS-induced alveolar bone loss by oxidative stress suppression. ACS Omega. 2023;**8**:20739-20754. DOI: 10.1021/acsomega.3c01289

[71] Li H, Zhang P, Lin H, Gao H, Yin J. ETC-1002 attenuates *Porphyromonas gingivalis* lipopolysaccharide-induced inflammation in RAW264.7 cells via the AMPK/NF-κB pathway and exerts ameliorative effects in experimental periodontitis in mice. Disease Markers. 2022;**2022**:8583674. DOI: 10.1155/2022/8583674

[72] Nandy A, Helderman RCM, Thapa S, Peck SH, Richards A, Jayapalan S, et al. Enhanced fatty acid oxidation in osteoprogenitor cells provides protection from high-fat diet induced bone dysfunction. Journal of Bone and Mineral Research: The Official Journal of the American Society for Bone and Mineral Research. 2025;**40**:283-298. DOI: 10.1093/jbmr/zjae195

[73] Kim SP, Li Z, Riddle RC. Evaluation of fatty acid oxidation in cultured bone cells. Journal of Visualized Experiments: JoVE. 2022;**182**:e63638. DOI: 10.3791/63638

[74] Huang X, Xie M, Xie Y, Mei F, Lu X, Li X, et al. The roles of osteocytes in alveolar bone destruction in periodontitis. Journal of Translational Medicine. 2020;**18**:479. DOI: 10.1186/s12967-020-02664-7

[75] AlQranei MS, Chellaiah MA. Osteoclastogenesis in periodontal diseases: Possible mediators and mechanisms. Journal of Oral Biosciences. 2020;**62**:123-130. DOI: 10.1016/j.job.2020.02.002

[76] Kim Y-G, Kim MO, Kim S-H, Kim HJ, Pokhrel NK, Lee JH, et al. 6-Shogaol, an active ingredient of ginger, inhibits osteoclastogenesis and alveolar bone resorption in ligature-induced periodontitis in mice. Journal of Periodontology. 2020;**91**:809-818. DOI: 10.1002/JPER.19-0228

[77] Jiang X, Ding X, Wei J, Lv X, Zhang Y, Yang Y, et al. Dioscin alleviates periodontitis by inhibiting NLRP3 inflammasome activation via regulation of K+ homeostasis and mitochondrial function. International Journal of Biological Sciences. 2024;**20**:1375-1388. DOI: 10.7150/ijbs.85851

[78] Chakraborty S, Handrick B, Yu D, Bode KA, Hafner A, Schenz J, et al. Gαq modulates the energy metabolism of osteoclasts. Frontiers in Cellular and Infection Microbiology. 2022;**12**:1016299. DOI: 10.3389/fcimb.2022.1016299

[79] Yan K, Lin Q, Tang K, Liu S, Du Y, Yu X, et al. Substance P participates in periodontitis by upregulating HIF-1α and RANKL/OPG ratio. BMC Oral Health. 2020;**20**:27. DOI: 10.1186/s12903-020-1017-9

[80] Relvas M, Silvestre R, Gonçalves M, Cabral C, Mendes-Frias A, Monteiro L, et al. Analysis of salivary levels of IL-1β, IL17A, OPG and RANK-L in periodontitis using the 2017 classification of periodontal diseases-An exploratory observational study. Journal of Clinical Medicine. 2023;**12**:1003. DOI: 10.3390/jcm12031003

[81] Parveen S. Impact of fasting intervention on inflammatory markers and mitochondrial enzyme complex activity of periodontal tissue and systemic inflammation. Texila International Journal of Public Health. 2024;**12**:1-12. DOI: 10.21522/TIJPH.2013.12.01.Art004

[82] Aizenbud I, Wilensky A, Almoznino G. Periodontal disease and its association with metabolic syndrome—A comprehensive review. International Journal of Molecular Sciences. 2023;**24**:13011. DOI: 10.3390/ijms241613011

[83] Tang H, Zhou Y, Ma L, et al. SIRT3 alleviates mitochondrial dysfunction and senescence in diabetes-associated periodontitis by deacetylating LRPPRC. Free Radical Biology and Medicine. 2025;**227**:407-419. DOI: 10.1016/j.freeradbiomed.2024.11.033

[84] Zhong S, Huang L, Lin T, Li Y, Deng B, Kong D, et al. The glucagon-like Peptide-1 (GLP-1) receptor agonist liraglutide regulates sirtuin-1-mediated neutrophil extracellular traps to improve diabetes-induced bone metabolism imbalance. Iranian Journal of Pharmaceutical Research: IJPR. 2024;**23**:e148139. DOI: 10.5812/ijpr-148139

[85] Zhang Y, An Y, Sun L-J, Qu H, Li X, He X, et al. NADPH-dependent ROS accumulation contributes to the impaired osteogenic differentiation of periodontal ligament stem cells under high glucose conditions. Frontiers in Endocrinology. 2023;**14**:1152845. DOI: 10.3389/fendo.2023.1152845

[86] Kwon H, Lim W, Kim J, Jeon S, Kim S, Karna S, et al. Effect of 635 nm irradiation on high glucose-boosted inflammatory responses in LPS-induced MC3T3-E1 cells. Lasers in Medical Science. 2013;**28**:717-724. DOI: 10.1007/s10103-012-1122-3

[87] García-Hernández A, Arzate H, Gil-Chavarría I, Rojo R, Moreno-Fierros L. High glucose concentrations alter the biomineralization process in human osteoblastic cells. Bone. 2012;**50**:276-288. DOI: 10.1016/j.bone.2011.10.032

[88] Tran T-T, Lee G, Huh YH, Chung K-H, Lee SY, Park KH, et al. Disruption of cholesterol homeostasis triggers periodontal inflammation and alveolar bone loss. Experimental & Molecular Medicine. 2023;**55**:2553-2563. DOI: 10.1038/s12276-023-01122-w

[89] Tran T-T, Lee G, Huh YH, Chung K-H, Lee SY, Park KH, et al. Acceleration of HDL-mediated cholesterol efflux alleviates periodontitis. Journal of Dental Research. 2024;**103**:1109-1118. DOI: 10.1177/00220345241271075

[90] Rocha DM, Caldas AP, Oliveira LL, Bressan J, Hermsdorff HH. Saturated fatty acids trigger TLR4-mediated inflammatory response. Atherosclerosis. 2016;**244**:211-215. DOI: 10.1016/j.atherosclerosis.2015.11.015

[91] Brodeur MR, Brissette L, Falstrault L, Ouellet P, Moreau R. Influence of oxidized low-density lipoproteins (LDL) on the viability of osteoblastic cells. Free Radical Biology & Medicine. 2008;**44**:506-517. DOI: 10.1016/j.freeradbiomed.2007.08.030

[92] Muluke M, Gold T, Kiefhaber K, Al-Sahli A, Celenti R, Jiang H, et al. Diet-induced obesity and its differential impact on periodontal bone loss. Journal of Dental Research. 2016;**95**:223-229. DOI: 10.1177/0022034515609882

[93] Varela-López A, Bullón P, Ramírez-Tortosa CL, Navarro-Hortal MD, Robles-Almazán M, Bullón B, et al. A diet rich in saturated fat and cholesterol aggravates the effect of bacterial lipopolysaccharide on alveolar bone loss in a rabbit model of periodontal disease. Nutrients. 2020;**12**:1405. DOI: 10.3390/nu12051405

[94] Li J, Karim MA, Che H, Geng Q, Miao D. Deletion of p16 prevents estrogen deficiency-induced osteoporosis by inhibiting oxidative stress and osteocyte senescence. American Journal of Translational Research. 2020;**12**:672-683

[95] Zhou D, Ran Y, Yu R, Liu G, Ran D, Liu Z. SIRT1 regulates osteoblast senescence through SOD2 acetylation and mitochondrial dysfunction in the progression of osteoporosis caused by cadmium exposure. Chemico-Biological Interactions. 2023;**382**:110632. DOI: 10.1016/j.cbi.2023.110632

[96] Huh J-E, Shin JH, Jang ES, Park SJ, Park DR, Ko R, et al. Sirtuin 3 (SIRT3) maintains bone homeostasis by regulating AMPK-PGC-1β axis in mice. Scientific Reports. 2016;**6**:22511. DOI: 10.1038/srep22511

[97] Yan N, Hu B, Xu J, et al. Stem cell Janus patch for periodontal regeneration. Nano Today. 2022;**42**:101336. DOI: 10.1016/j.nantod.2021.101336

[98] Dereka XE, Markopoulou CE, Fanourakis G, Tseleni-Balafouta S, Vrotsos IA. RANKL and OPG mRNA level after non-surgical periodontal treatment. Inflammation. 2010;**33**:200-206. DOI: 10.1007/s10753-009-9174-7

[99] Santos VR, Ribeiro FV, Lima JA, Miranda TS, Feres M, Bastos MF, et al. Partial- and full-mouth scaling and root planing in type 2 diabetic subjects: A 12-mo follow-up of clinical parameters and levels of cytokines and osteoclastogenesis-related factors. Journal of

Periodontal Research. 2012;**47**:45-54. DOI: 10.1111/j.1600-0765.2011.01403.x

[100] Sinha S, Sonoo PR, Siddhartha R, Singh SK, Singh A. Effect of conventional periodontal treatment (scaling and root planing) on Type-2 diabetic patient with moderate generalized chronic periodontitis: A clinical study. Journal of Pharmacy & Bioallied Sciences. 2021;**13**:S706-S710. DOI: 10.4103/jpbs.JPBS_692_20

[101] Konopka L, Pietrzak A, Brzezińska-Błaszczyk E. Effect of scaling and root planing on interleukin-1β, interleukin-8 and MMP-8 levels in gingival crevicular fluid from chronic periodontitis patients. Journal of Periodontal Research. 2012;**47**:681-688. DOI: 10.1111/j.1600-0765.2012.01480.x

[102] Mercia M, Soeroso Y, Lessang R, Bachtiar BM. Expression of osteopontin mRNA during periodontal healing following scaling and root planing. Pesquisa Brasileira em Odontopediatria e Clínica Integrada. 2020;**19**:e4991. DOI: 10.4034/PBOCI.2019.191.101

[103] Patricia M, Lessang R, Tadjoedin FM, Bachtiar BM. The effects of scaling and root planing on mRNA expression of matrix metalloproteinase-1 and clinical parameters. Journal of International Dental and Medical Research. 2019;**12**:612-616

[104] Chen J, Zhang Y, Gao J, Li T, Gan X, Yu H. Sirtuin 3 deficiency exacerbates age-related periodontal disease. Journal of Periodontal Research. 2021;**56**:1163-1173. DOI: 10.1111/jre.12930

[105] Cui D, Kong N, Ding L, Guo Y, Yang W, Yan F. Ultrathin 2D titanium carbide MXene (Ti3 C2 T x) nanoflakes activate WNT/HIF-1 α -mediated metabolism reprogramming for periodontal regeneration. Advanced Healthcare Materials. 2021;**10**:2101215. DOI: 10.1002/adhm.202101215

[106] Han Q, Li J, Deng H, Shi S, Zhou M, Cai X, et al. Tetrahedral framework nucleic acid (tFNA)-loaded metformin (met) modulates cellular pyroptosis and AMPK to ameliorate type II diabetic periodontitis. Small. 2025;**21**(20):e2411740. DOI: 10.1002/smll.202411740

[107] de Araújo AA, CACX d PASBF d M, RFC d BGAC d L, de Araújo LS, PMM G, Hiyari S, et al. Effects of metformin on inflammation, oxidative stress, and bone loss in a rat model of periodontitis. PLoS One. 2017;**12**:e0183506. DOI: 10.1371/journal.pone.0183506

[108] Pradeep AR, Nagpal K, Karvekar S, Patnaik K, Naik SB, Guruprasad CN. Platelet-rich fibrin with 1% metformin for the treatment of intrabony defects in chronic periodontitis: A randomized controlled clinical trial. Journal of Periodontology. 2015;**86**:729-737. DOI: 10.1902/jop.2015.140646

[109] Inbarajan A, Mubeena S, Punnoose AM, Gvv G, Anusha D, David J. Effects of simvastatin on gene expression and alkaline phosphatase activity in the MG-63 cell line treated with hyperglycemia for bone regeneration. Cureus. 2024;**16**:e55482. DOI: 10.7759/cureus.55482

[110] Kumari M, Martande SS, Pradeep AR. Subgingivally delivered 1.2% atorvastatin in the treatment of chronic periodontitis among smokers: A randomized, controlled clinical trial. Journal of Investigative and Clinical Dentistry. 2017;**8**:e12213. DOI: 10.1111/jicd.12213

[111] Cao R, Li Q, Chen Y, Yao M, Wu Q, Zhou H. Efficacy of locally-delivered statins adjunct to non-surgical

periodontal therapy for chronic periodontitis: A Bayesian network analysis. BMC Oral Health. 2019;**19**:105. DOI: 10.1186/s12903-019-0789-2

[112] Li Y, Liu L, Li Y, Song W, Shao B, Li H, et al. Alpha-ketoglutarate promotes alveolar bone regeneration by modulating M2 macrophage polarization. Bone Reports. 2023;**18**:101671. DOI: 10.1016/j.bonr.2023.101671

[113] Fujihara C, Nantakeeratipat T, Murakami S. Energy metabolism in osteogenic differentiation and reprogramming: A possible future strategy for periodontal regeneration. Frontiers in Dental Medicine. 2022;**3**:1-6. DOI: 10.3389/fdmed.2022.815140

[114] Mao C, Yu W, Lin L, Yang R, Hu S, Li G, et al. Alpha-ketoglutarate alleviates systemic lupus erythematosus-associated periodontitis in a novel murine model. Journal of Clinical Periodontology. 2025;**52**:457-470. DOI: 10.1111/jcpe.14080

[115] Lee Y-L, Lin S-K, Hou K-L, Kok S-H, Lai EH-H, Wang H-W, et al. Sirtuin 6 attenuates periapical lesion propagation by modulating hypoxia-induced chemokine (C-C motif) ligand 2 production in osteoblasts. International Endodontic Journal. 2018;**51**(Suppl 2):e74-e86. DOI: 10.1111/iej.12742

[116] Marchetti E, Monaco A, Procaccini L, Mummolo S, Gatto R, Tetè S, et al. Periodontal disease: The influence of metabolic syndrome. Nutrition & Metabolism. 2012;**9**:88. DOI: 10.1186/1743-7075-9-88

[117] Zebrowitz E, Aslanukov A, Kajikawa T, Bedelbaeva K, Bollinger S, Zhang Y, et al. Prolyl-hydroxylase inhibitor-induced regeneration of alveolar bone and soft tissue in a mouse model of periodontitis through metabolic reprogramming. Frontiers in Dental Medicine. 2022;**3**:992722. DOI: 10.3389/fdmed.2022.992722

[118] Salvi GE, Roccuzzo A, Imber J-C, Stähli A, Klinge B, Lang NP. Clinical periodontal diagnosis. Periodontology 2000. 2023;**00**:1-19. DOI: 10.1111/prd.12487

[119] Schulze-Späte U, Turner R, Wang Y, Chao R, Schulze PC, Phipps K, et al. Relationship of bone metabolism biomarkers and periodontal disease: The osteoporotic fractures in men (MrOS) study. The Journal of Clinical Endocrinology and Metabolism. 2015;**100**:2425-2433. DOI: 10.1210/jc.2014-4180

[120] Rakmanee T, Calciolari E, Olsen I, Darbar U, Griffiths GS, Petrie A, et al. Expression of growth mediators in the gingival crevicular fluid of patients with aggressive periodontitis undergoing periodontal surgery. Clinical Oral Investigations. 2019;**23**:3307-3318. DOI: 10.1007/s00784-018-2752-z

[121] Kinney JS, Ramseier CA, Giannobile WV. Oral fluid-based biomarkers of alveolar bone loss in periodontitis. Annals of the New York Academy of Sciences. 2007;**1098**:230-251. DOI: 10.1196/annals.1384.028

[122] Ventura M, Boerman OC, Franssen GM, Bronkhorst E, Jansen JA, Walboomers XF. Monitoring the biological effect of BMP-2 release on bone healing by PET/CT. Journal of Controlled Release: Official Journal of the Controlled Release Society. 2014;**183**:138-144. DOI: 10.1016/j.jconrel.2014.03.044

Section 4

Perspective Chapters

Chapter 13

Perspective Chapter: Customized Membranes for Alveolar Ridge Augmentation

Ziad Albash, Ali Khalil and Nadim Sleman

Abstract

Alveolar ridge augmentation is critical for successful dental implant placement, particularly in cases of bone deficiency caused by trauma, periodontal disease, or tooth extraction. Guided bone regeneration (GBR) has emerged as a reliable technique, utilizing barrier membranes to exclude non-osteogenic tissues and promote osteogenesis. While traditional prefabricated membranes have demonstrated efficacy, their limitations—such as poor fit and intraoperative adjustments—have driven the development of customized membranes tailored to patient-specific defects. This chapter explores the evolution of GBR membranes, focusing on digital workflows (CBCT, CAD/CAM) and advanced materials, including titanium, zirconia, and polyether ether ketone (PEEK). Customized membranes offer superior adaptation, space maintenance, and reduced complication rates compared to standard options. Titanium remains the gold standard for complex defects due to its mechanical strength, though exposure risks persist. Zirconia's biocompatibility and tolerance to oral exposure make it promising for aesthetic zones, while PEEK's radiolucency and flexibility address soft tissue irritation. Emerging materials like biodegradable polymers (PLA, PCL) and magnesium alloys show potential but require further clinical validation. Key challenges include membrane exposure, the need for secondary surgeries (non-absorbable materials), and material-specific limitations (e.g., zirconia's brittleness). Future directions emphasize bioactive coatings, optimized porosity, and long-term clinical studies. Customized membranes represent a paradigm shift in GBR, enhancing precision and outcomes in alveolar ridge augmentation, though material selection must balance biomechanical needs with biological performance.

Keywords: guided bone regeneration, customized membranes, alveolar ridge augmentation, titanium mesh, zirconia, PEEK, digital dentistry

1. Introduction

Dental implant rehabilitation has become a cornerstone of modern dentistry, significantly enhancing patients' quality of life by improving function and aesthetics. However, the prerequisite for successful and long-term stable implant placement is adequate alveolar bone volume and quality at the implant site. Alveolar ridge defects, whether vertical or horizontal, are common and arise from various factors, including periodontal disease, endodontic pathology, trauma, and post-extraction alveolar bone resorption [1, 2]. Among the various bone augmentation techniques, guided bone regeneration (GBR) has emerged as a reliable and predictable method for reconstructing alveolar bone and managing peri-implant bone defects [3, 4].

GBR involves the use of barrier membranes, often in conjunction with bone grafts, to selectively guide bone growth within a defined space [5, 6]. Traditional barrier membranes, available in prefabricated standard sizes and shapes, have played an effective role in many successful GBR procedures [7]. However, these solutions often require intraoperative trimming and adjustment to fit the specific morphology of the bone defect, which can be technically demanding and may lead to complications [8].

The improvement of digital technologies such as cone-beam computed tomography (CBCT), computer-aided design (CAD), computer-aided manufacturing (CAM), and additive manufacturing techniques like 3D printing has revolutionized GBR by enabling the fabrication of customized barrier membranes tailored to the unique anatomical characteristics of a given bone defect. These patient-specific membranes overcome some limitations of prefabricated membranes, improving predictability, efficiency, and complication rates in alveolar ridge augmentation procedures [8, 9].

2. Guided bone regeneration

2.1 Principles of guided bone regeneration

Guided bone regeneration (GBR) is a well-established and widely used surgical technique aimed at regenerating lost or deficient alveolar bone to facilitate dental implant placement or enhance overall functional and aesthetic outcomes [3]. The concept of GBR relies on excluding non-osteogenic cells from the bone defect site while preserving space for the migration and proliferation of osteogenic cells [10–13]. The technique involves placing a barrier membrane over the bone defect to prevent the infiltration of rapidly proliferating connective and epithelial tissues, which would otherwise occupy the defect space and hinder bone formation [3, 10, 11]. This barrier function allows slower-migrating osteogenic cells, originating from the surrounding host bone; periosteum (in some cases); and osteoinductive graft materials to fill the defect and regenerate new bone tissue [10–13].

The success of GBR procedures also depends on several other critical factors, often summarized by the "PASS" principles [14, 15]: 1—primary wound closure (to ensure proper healing and prevent bacterial contamination), 2—angiogenesis (to provide blood supply and nutrients for regenerating tissues), 3—space maintenance (to create and preserve adequate volume for new bone formation), and 4—wound stability (to prevent micromotion that could disrupt healing). The barrier membrane plays a key role in space maintenance by providing structural support to the bone graft and preventing soft tissue collapse into the defect. Additionally, the membrane can contribute to wound stability by serving as a scaffold for tissue integration and preventing graft displacement [14].

2.2 Barrier membranes and space-maintaining devices

2.2.1 Overview

Barrier membranes are essential tools in GBR procedures, acting as physical barriers to prevent unwanted cell infiltration into the bone defect. These membranes are fabricated from various materials and are broadly classified based on their resorbability into absorbable (biodegradable) and non-absorbable (non-biodegradable) types [16, 17]. The choice of membrane material depends on several factors, including the size and shape of the bone defect, the need for space maintenance, the selected graft material, and clinician preference. Ideally, a barrier membrane should exhibit biocompatibility to minimize adverse tissue reactions, provide effective barrier function to exclude non-osteogenic cells, possess sufficient mechanical properties to maintain space and resist soft tissue collapse, and be easy to handle during surgical procedures [16, 17].

2.2.2 Absorbable membranes

Absorbable membranes are made from materials that degrade and are resorbed by the body over time, eliminating the need for a second surgical removal procedure. Common absorbable materials include collagen [18] (derived from bovine, porcine, or equine sources) and synthetic biodegradable polymers such as polyglycolic acid (PGA) [19], polylactic acid (PLA) [20, 21], polycaprolactone (PCL) [22], and their copolymers.

Collagen membranes are widely used in GBR due to their excellent biocompatibility, ability to promote cell adhesion and tissue healing, and positive interaction with soft tissues. They facilitate oxygen exchange, nutrient diffusion, and blood perfusion, which are critical factors for healing [18]. Moreover, collagen membranes can absorb growth factors released from autogenous bone chips, potentially enhancing bone regeneration. Studies have shown that collagen membranes can achieve long-term performance comparable to non-absorbable membranes in certain defects, particularly dehiscence-type defects [18].

However, a significant limitation of some collagen membranes is their rapid degradation rate and low mechanical strength, which may compromise their ability to maintain space, especially in larger defects [18, 23]. To address this, cross-linked collagen membranes have been developed to slow degradation and improve enzymatic resistance. While cross-linking extends the membrane's functional lifespan and better preserves the graft, it has also been associated with higher exposure rates and, in some cases, foreign body reactions during resorption (**Table 1**) [24, 25].

2.2.3 Non-absorbable membranes

Non-absorbable membranes are made from materials not readily resorbed by the body, requiring a second surgical procedure for removal. Common non-absorbable materials used in GBR include expanded polytetrafluoroethylene (ePTFE), dense polytetrafluoroethylene (d-PTFE), titanium mesh, and titanium-reinforced ePTFE membranes (**Table 1**) [26, 27].

Expanded polytetrafluoroethylene (ePTFE) membranes were among the first synthetic polymers used in GBR and are considered biologically inert and stable, resisting degradation and eliciting minimal immune responses [28]. Their unique microporous structure, composed of solid nodes interconnected by fine fibrils, facilitates tissue

Property	Absorbable membranes	Non-absorbable membranes
Materials	Collagen, PGA, PLA, PCL	ePTFE, d-PTFE, titanium mesh
degradation time	Weeks to months (varies by cross-linking)	Non-degradable (requires removal)
Barrier function	Moderate (may lose integrity over time)	High (stable long-term)
Space Maintenance	Poor for large defects	Excellent (rigid structure)
Clinical use	Small defects, minimal soft tissue pressure	Large/vertical defects, high tension areas
Advantages	No secondary surgery, biocompatible	Predictable space maintenance
Disadvantages	Rapid degradation, weak mechanical strength	Exposure risk, secondary surgery needed

Table 1.
Comparison of absorbable vs. non-absorbable membranes.

integration [29, 30]. Despite their effectiveness in promoting bone regeneration, a major drawback of ePTFE membranes is the need for a second surgery and the risk of membrane exposure, which can lead to bacterial contamination and compromised outcomes [31, 32].

d-PTFE membranes are denser than ePTFE membranes and are often used in cases with a higher risk of membrane exposure, as they are believed to be less susceptible to bacterial contamination [33, 34]. Some studies have reported successful use of d-PTFE membranes without primary closure. However, like ePTFE membranes, d-PTFE membranes require surgical removal and may cause soft tissue irritation due to their stiffness [33, 34].

2.2.4 Titanium mesh

Titanium mesh is a non-absorbable space-maintaining device widely used in GBR, particularly for large defects and vertical bone augmentation [35–37]. Titanium exhibits excellent mechanical properties, including high rigidity and a degree of plasticity, allowing it to be adapted to the shape and size of the bone defect [38]. The rigidity of titanium mesh provides superior space maintenance, preventing soft tissue collapse and graft displacement, which is critical for successful GBR, especially in defects where space cannot be maintained with barrier membranes alone. In vertical augmentation procedures, non-absorbable membranes like titanium mesh are often preferred due to their high rigidity and space-maintaining capacity, which may be insufficient with absorbable membranes [38]. Titanium mesh can be used with various graft materials, including autogenous bone grafts [35], allografts [39, 40], xenografts [41], and synthetic substitutes [42].

Despite its advantages, titanium mesh has some drawbacks. The most notable is the need for a second surgical procedure for removal. Additionally, sharp edges resulting from intraoperative trimming may irritate the overlying mucosa and increase the risk of membrane exposure. Exposure of titanium mesh can lead to bacterial colonization, infection, and potential graft failure [38].

Titanium mesh has been used to repair large bone defects and has gained popularity due to its biocompatibility and superior mechanical properties, particularly its rigidity. This rigidity is essential for maintaining the space required for new bone formation, especially in cases of significant bone loss or vertical augmentation, where soft tissue pressure can easily collapse the less rigid membranes. The microporous structure of some titanium meshes also facilitates angiogenesis, which is critical for graft healing and integration [43, 44].

Studies have demonstrated the efficacy of titanium mesh in achieving horizontal and vertical bone augmentation, often in conjunction with various graft materials [36–45]. It has been successfully used to improve bucco-lingual ridge width and prevent crestal resorption. Compared to absorbable membranes, titanium mesh generally provides more effective space maintenance and allows better three-dimensional reconstruction of bone defects [36–45].

2.2.5 Advantages and disadvantages of prefabricated membranes and meshes

Prefabricated barrier membranes and titanium meshes, available in standardized sizes and shapes, offer immediate availability, relatively low cost, and ease of use, making them suitable for many routine GBR procedures where the defect morphology matches available dimensions. Numerous studies have documented the successful use of these prefabricated membranes in a wide range of clinical cases.

However, a major limitation of prefabricated membranes and meshes is their imperfect fit to bone defects, often requiring intraoperative trimming and adaptation. This can be technically demanding and may compromise ideal barrier function or space maintenance. In the case of titanium mesh, trimming can create sharp edges that increase the risk of mucosal irritation and subsequent membrane exposure. Additionally, achieving optimal adaptation and stability of prefabricated meshes in complex three-dimensional defects can be challenging, potentially leading to micromotion and graft instability. Standard shapes may not always provide adequate coverage or support for the entire defect area, which can affect the predictability of bone regeneration, especially in larger or irregularly shaped defects.

3. Customized membranes

3.1 Definition

Customized or patient-specific barrier membranes are three-dimensional devices designed and fabricated using digital technologies to precisely match the shape and size of a patient's bone defect [8, 46]. Unlike prefabricated membranes, which come in standard sizes and shapes, customized membranes are tailored to the unique anatomical characteristics of a specific bone defect, as determined by pre-operative imaging such as cone-beam computed tomography (CBCT) [8, 46, 47]. This personalized approach allows for precise adaptation to the defect margins, improved space maintenance, and potentially enhanced outcomes in GBR procedures. The fabrication of customized membranes typically involves a series of steps, including data acquisition using CBCT, computer-aided design (CAD) of the membrane, and computer-aided manufacturing (CAM) using techniques like additive manufacturing (3D printing) or subtractive manufacturing (milling) [8, 46–48].

3.2 Historical overview

The concept of customizing medical devices to improve reliability and outcomes has evolved alongside advancements in digital imaging and manufacturing technologies. In the context of GBR, the limitations of prefabricated membranes in addressing complex and irregular bone defects spurred the development of customized solutions. Titanium was among the first materials used to fabricate customized membranes and meshes [8, 46]. Early applications involved manually bending titanium plates or meshes to better fit the defect, but the true era of customization began with the integration of digital planning and manufacturing [46–48].

The introduction of rapid prototyping technologies, such as selective laser sintering (SLS) and electron beam melting (EBM), combined with CBCT imaging and CAD/CAM software, enabled the precise fabrication of patient-specific titanium membranes for bone augmentation. These customized titanium meshes offered improved fit and stability compared to their prefabricated counterparts. As technology matured and became more accessible, the focus shifted toward optimizing design principles, material selection, and clinical evaluation of customized membranes in various augmentation applications. More recently, the exploration of other biocompatible materials, such as zirconia, for customized membrane fabrication has gained momentum, driven by their unique properties and the availability of milling machines in dental laboratories [49, 50].

3.3 Digital manufacturing techniques

The fabrication of customized barrier membranes heavily relies on digital manufacturing technologies that bridge the gap between patient-specific anatomical data and the physical realization of the membrane [50–53]. A typical workflow includes:

1. Data acquisition: High-resolution CBCT scanning of the patient's bone defect provides detailed three-dimensional data on the defect's size and morphology.

2. Digital planning and design (CAD): The CBCT data are imported into specialized CAD software. Using this digital model, the desired bone augmentation contours are planned, and a virtual membrane is designed to precisely fit the defect margins and provide the necessary space for new bone formation. The design may include features such as fixation holes, stability extensions, and specific thicknesses.

3. Manufacturing (CAM): The digitally designed membrane is then fabricated using additive or subtractive manufacturing techniques:

   - Additive manufacturing (3D printing): Techniques like selective laser melting (SLM) and electron beam melting (EBM) are used to build the membrane layer by layer from powdered materials (e.g., titanium alloys or certain polymers). SLM uses a laser to selectively melt and fuse powder particles, while EBM operates in a vacuum environment. These techniques allow for the creation of complex geometries and porous structures if desired. However, EBM-produced surfaces may be rough and require additional polishing.

- Subtractive manufacturing (milling): In this approach, a block of material (e.g., titanium or zirconia) is precisely shaped using computer-controlled milling machines based on the digital design. Five-axis milling machines are commonly used in dental laboratories to fabricate precise patient-specific membranes, especially from zirconia due to its cost-effectiveness and availability.

4. Post-processing stage: Depending on the manufacturing technique and material, the membrane may undergo steps such as cleaning, polishing, or sterilization before clinical use.

3.4 Design considerations for customized membranes

Designing a customized barrier membrane is a critical step that directly influences its clinical performance and GBR outcomes. Leveraging detailed information from pre-operative CBCT data, the membrane is designed to achieve several key objectives:

- Precise fit: The primary goal is to create a membrane that perfectly adapts to the defect margins and sits passively on the surrounding healthy bone. This precise fit helps define the bone regeneration space and reduces the risk of graft displacement or soft tissue ingrowth. Some designs may include specific support points along the bone edges to ensure proper stability and adaptation [49, 54].

- Space maintenance: The membrane is designed to maintain a sufficient three-dimensional space above the defect to accommodate the bone graft material. The rigidity and strength of the chosen material, along with the overall membrane design, contribute to its space-maintaining capacity [49, 54].

- Stability and fixation: The design often incorporates features to secure the membrane to the host bone, such as pre-designed holes for fixation screws [8, 9, 48–50, 54]. Fixation prevents membrane displacement or rotation, which could disrupt healing and compromise bone regeneration. Some designs rely solely on precise fit for initial stability, while others include extensions that wrap around adjacent bone to enhance retention [49, 50]. The "tenting effect" can also be achieved with customized membranes, where the membrane is secured away from the defect to maximize space for bone formation.

- Barrier function: The membrane must prevent the infiltration of non-osteogenic cells from surrounding soft tissues into the defect. While most customized membranes are rigid and non-porous (except for fixation holes), the material properties and precise adaptation to bone margins contribute to their barrier function [8, 48].

- Soft tissue management: The edges and extensions of the customized membrane are designed to minimize irritation of surrounding soft tissues and reduce the risk of membrane exposure. Smooth edges and appropriate extensions beyond the defect boundaries are critical for achieving tension-free primary closure. Some designs may include considerations for simultaneous soft tissue grafting [5, 49, 54, 55].

- Thickness: Membrane thickness is a design parameter that affects its rigidity, ease of handling, and barrier function. Typical reported thicknesses in the literature range from 0.5 to 1 mm for titanium and approximately 0.7 mm for zirconia [8, 48, 49].

3.5 Materials used in customized membrane fabrication

A variety of biocompatible materials have been explored for the fabrication of customized barrier membranes, each with its own advantages and limitations. Material selection depends on factors such as the mechanical requirements of the defect, desired biological response, manufacturing capabilities, and cost considerations (**Table 2**).

3.5.1 Titanium

The use of titanium in customized membranes represents a significant advancement in GBR techniques in dentistry [38, 48, 49]. Titanium, a common material in various medical fields, including dentistry, is used in its pure form or as alloys due to its exceptional properties, such as excellent biocompatibility, mechanical strength, durability, low density, and corrosion resistance [6, 38, 47, 56]. Its biologically inert nature enhances its suitability for bone augmentation procedures [6]. While traditional titanium mesh has been used for decades, the development of CAD/CAM technologies has paved the way for customized titanium membranes, offering several potential advantages [48, 49, 57, 58]. Titanium was the first material used to fabricate customized membranes [49]. The choice of titanium alloy (e.g., Grade 4 or 5) also influences the properties of the customized device [6, 57].

3.5.1.1 Properties of titanium

Titanium possesses several key properties that make it an excellent material for barrier membranes in GBR:

Mechanical strength and space maintenance: Titanium exhibits high strength and rigidity, essential for maintaining the space required for new bone formation. This ability to create and preserve space is particularly valuable in large horizontal and vertical bone defects, where soft tissue pressure could otherwise collapse the graft [48–56, 58–61].

Biocompatibility: Titanium is known for its excellent biocompatibility, promoting a positive tissue response. It is biologically inert and capable of osseointegration, forming a direct connection with bone through the extracellular matrix—a concept that revolutionized dental implantology [6, 38, 46, 61].

Durability and corrosion resistance: Titanium's durability and corrosion resistance ensure long-term stability in the oral environment, which is critical for maintaining barrier function throughout the bone regeneration process [6, 38, 46, 61].

Flexibility and adaptability: Despite its rigidity, titanium has a degree of flexibility, allowing it to be bent and shaped to conform to the bone defect. This is crucial for achieving precise adaptation and optimal bone regeneration outcomes [38, 48, 57, 62].

Macroporosity: Commercially available titanium mesh often features large pores (in the millimeter range), believed to be necessary for maintaining blood flow, promoting healing, and allowing nutrient diffusion through the mesh [38, 56].

DOI: http://dx.doi.org/10.5772/intechopen.1011442

Material	Mechanical properties	Biocompatibility	Degradation	Clinical advantages	Clinical limitations	Common uses
Titanium	High rigidity, ductile, elastic modulus ~110 GPa	Excellent	Non-absorbable	Superior space maintenance, osseointegration, corrosion-resistant	Requires secondary surgery; risk of exposure; radiopaque	Large/vertical defects, atrophic ridges
Zirconia	High strength but brittle (~900–1200 MPa)	Superior (low biofilm adhesion)	Non-absorbable	Smooth surface reduces soft tissue irritation; tolerates oral environment exposure	Brittle (no intraoperative adjustments); high cost	Anterior esthetic zones, horizontal defects
PEEK	Moderate (elastic modulus ~3.6 GPa, close to bone)	Excellent	Non-absorbable	Radiolucent; flexible; reduced mucosal irritation	No osseointegration; expensive	Complex 3D defects, cranial reconstructions
Collagen	Low tensile strength, rapid degradation	Excellent	Absorbable (weeks–months)	Promotes cell adhesion/healing; no secondary surgery	Poor space maintenance; cross-linked versions may cause inflammation	Small defects, dehiscence-type defects
Polyesters (PLA/PGA/PCL)	Moderate (tunable degradation)	Good (may provoke inflammation)	Absorbable (months)	Drug-loading capability; electrospinnable for customization	Inflammatory degradation byproducts; weak for large defects	Experimental/resorbable GBR applications
Chitosan	Weak mechanical strength	Excellent	Absorbable	Antimicrobial properties; promotes wound healing	Limited space maintenance; fragile	Adjunct to other membranes
Magnesium Alloys	Elastic modulus ~45 GPa (close to bone)	Good (with coatings)	Absorbable (months)	Self-degrading; stimulates osteogenesis	Rapid corrosion; gas release during degradation	Experimental (animal studies)
Chromium-Cobalt	High hardness/durability	Poor (ion toxicity)	Non-absorbable	Low cost; high mechanical strength	Toxic ion release; no human clinical data	Not recommended for clinical use
Ceramics (HA/β-TCP)	Brittle, osteoconductive	Excellent	Absorbable (slow)	Enhances bone regeneration; integrates with native bone	Fragility complicates fixation; limited to small defects	Combined with other materials

Table 2.
Comprehensive comparison of materials for customized membranes.

3.5.1.2 Clinical applications of customized titanium membranes

Customized titanium mesh has proven effective in various bone augmentation procedures:

Vertical and horizontal augmentation: This technique is effectively used to increase alveolar ridge width (horizontally) and height (vertically) to secure the bone volume needed for dental implants [9, 38, 56]. Its superior space-maintaining capacity and ability to withstand soft tissue pressure make it suitable for both types of defects [56, 61, 63]. Studies have shown promising results for horizontal ridge augmentation performed concurrently with implant placement using titanium mesh [9, 38].

Large three-dimensional defects: These complex cases often pose challenges in bone augmentation, and customized titanium mesh provides a predictable method for bone grafting in such scenarios [46, 64, 65].

Simultaneous implant placement: This technique enables horizontal bone augmentation using titanium mesh concurrently with implant placement [38, 56].

Atrophic site reconstruction: The use of particulate bone grafts with titanium mesh has been shown to be a successful method for reconstructing atrophic alveolar ridges [54].

3.5.1.3 Complications associated with titanium membranes (including customized)

Despite their advantages, titanium membranes, including customized ones, involve some potential complications:

Membrane exposure: Exposure of titanium mesh, whether prefabricated or customized, is one of the most common and serious complications [54, 55, 60, 64–66]. This can lead to graft failure and loss of graft material and often necessitates immediate membrane removal to prevent infection [49]. Reported exposure rates vary widely. Contributing factors include tension during closure, sharp mesh edges, and surgical inexperience [54, 55, 57, 65]. While customized membranes aim to mitigate some of these factors, they remain susceptible to exposure, often due to overestimating the space that can be adequately closed without tension [64, 65, 67].

Infection: Membrane exposure increases the risk of bacterial contamination and infection at the graft site. Although titanium surfaces may be less prone to contamination than the rough surfaces of some absorbable collagen membranes, exposure to the oral environment remains a significant risk [38, 66, 68].

Need for a second surgery: As non-absorbable materials, titanium mesh requires a second surgical procedure for removal, increasing morbidity, treatment duration, and cost [9, 48, 54, 68].

Soft tissue irritation: Sharp edges, especially in manually adjusted traditional mesh, can cause irritation and trauma to the surrounding soft tissues, potentially leading to mucosal dehiscence and membrane exposure [38, 55, 57, 69].

Radiopacity: The radiopacity of titanium mesh can interfere with post-operative radiographic interpretation, potentially affecting the accuracy of imaging and leading to artifacts in the mesh area [38, 46].

Pseudoperiosteum formation: The formation of a fibrous connective tissue layer (pseudoperiosteum) over newly formed bone may occupy unnecessary space and reduce the volume of regenerated bone [9, 38, 48].

3.5.1.4 Future directions

These trends aim to improve outcomes and reduce complications associated with titanium membranes in alveolar ridge augmentation. Areas of interest include:

Surface modifications: Modifying the surface of titanium membranes to enhance cell adhesion, promote bone regeneration, and potentially reduce bacterial adhesion [38, 61, 70].

Incorporation of bioactive agents: Using barrier membranes loaded with growth factors or antibacterial agents [71].

Optimized custom designs: Refining CAD/CAM techniques and mesh designs to improve fit, reduce stress concentrations, and minimize exposure risks [9, 38, 48, 65].

Comparative studies: More clinical research is needed to directly compare the efficacy and complication rates of different membrane types, including customized titanium mesh versus traditional mesh and other materials like PEEK and zirconia [48, 49].

Long-term follow-up studies: Long-term data on the performance of customized titanium membranes and the stability of regenerated bone are essential to confirm their reliability [47, 72].

3.5.2 Zirconia

3.5.2.1 Introduction

Zirconia (zirconium dioxide) is a polycrystalline ceramic material with excellent biocompatibility, increasingly used in dentistry for fixed prostheses, dental implants, and, more recently, customized membrane fabrication [8, 49, 59, 73]. Its desirable properties include exceptional mechanical strength, hardness, high corrosion resistance, and chemical inertness [6, 8]. Additionally, zirconia exhibits high biocompatibility, resulting in reduced inflammatory responses and lower biofilm adhesion compared to titanium. These properties make zirconia an attractive candidate for use in bone regeneration procedures [8, 49, 59, 73].

3.5.2.2 Advantages of customized zirconia membranes

The use of zirconia in customized barrier membranes offers several potential advantages over traditional materials:

Biocompatibility: Multiple sources highlight zirconia's superior biological response compared to titanium. It promotes better fibroblast response, reduces biofilm adhesion, and elicits a milder inflammatory reaction [8, 49, 59, 73]. This enhanced biocompatibility may be crucial for promoting tissue healing and reducing complications, especially in cases of membrane exposure [74, 75].

Manufacturing process: One of the key advantages of customized zirconia membranes is their fabrication process. They can be easily milled using standard five-axis dental laboratory milling machines, making this subtractive manufacturing approach more accessible and cost-effective than additive techniques like selective laser melting or electron beam melting required for customized titanium mesh. Such techniques require expensive equipment, limiting its widespread adoption. Additionally, additively manufactured titanium surfaces may require additional polishing [8, 49, 59, 73, 75].

Tolerance to oral environment exposure: Several case series and studies have reported that even when customized zirconia membranes are exposed early, minimal signs of infection are observed. This is attributed to zirconia's smooth and biocompatible nature, potentially limiting bacterial colonization compared to materials like ePTFE. This property may allow for a longer period before membrane removal becomes necessary [8, 49, 59, 73].

Clinical success: Case series and reports have demonstrated good clinical and histological performance of customized zirconia barriers in bone augmentation procedures, leading to successful bone regeneration and subsequent implant placement without the need for additional augmentation [8].

3.5.2.3 Disadvantages and limitations of customized zirconia membranes

Despite their advantages, customized zirconia membranes also have potential limitations:

Brittleness: Unlike titanium, ceramic materials like zirconia are brittle and cannot be easily bent or adjusted intraoperatively if design or fabrication errors occur. Care must be taken when tightening fixation screws to avoid fracture. Some studies have produced two identical membranes to mitigate the risk of breakage during placement or fixation [49, 59, 73].

Lack of flexibility: While zirconia's rigidity contributes to space maintenance, it lacks the flexibility of titanium mesh, which can be manually contoured to adapt to complex bone defects. This lack of flexibility demands highly accurate planning and fabrication [74–76].

Rigid, non-porous design: Many customized zirconia membranes described in the literature are rigid and non-perforated. While this design aims to ensure complete graft isolation and simplify membrane removal, the impact of porosity on blood supply, osteogenic cell migration, and growth factor delivery from the periosteum remains debated. Some researchers argue that perforations are necessary for these processes [49, 59, 73].

Limited long-term studies: While preliminary results from case series are promising, more comprehensive research including long-term prospective clinical studies with larger sample sizes is needed to confirm the long-term predictability and efficacy of customized zirconia membranes in various clinical scenarios [8].

3.5.2.4 Clinical applications and outcomes

Customized zirconia membranes have been used for horizontal and vertical bone augmentation in both the maxilla and mandible [49, 59, 73–77]. Even in cases of early membrane exposure, significant bone formation has been observed without evidence of infection [59, 73]. Histological analyses have confirmed the formation of new, dense bone beneath zirconia membranes [59].

Customized zirconia membranes have proven effective in treating horizontal defects. The precise fit of the membrane helps contain the graft material and guides bone regeneration to the desired dimensions. Zirconia has also shown excellent biocompatibility and space-maintaining capacity in posterior jaw regions [49, 74].

3.5.2.5 Future directions

Future research on customized zirconia membranes for GBR should focus on:

Surface modifications: Investigating various surface treatments for zirconia to enhance its properties and further improve bone regeneration.

Porosity: Conducting long-term studies to evaluate and compare the efficacy of porous versus non-porous zirconia membrane designs, balancing the need for barrier function with the potential benefits of cell signaling and migration [8].

Long-term clinical trials: Performing prospective studies with larger patient cohorts and extended follow-up periods to assess the long-term success and predictability of customized zirconia membranes in different clinical indications [8].

Comparative studies: Conducting more direct comparisons between customized zirconia membranes and other materials, including titanium and high-performance polymers like PEEK [8].

3.5.3 Polyether ether ketone (PEEK)

3.5.3.1 Introduction

Polyether ether ketone (PEEK) is a high-performance polymer belonging to the polyaryletherketone (PAEK) family. It is semi-crystalline, described as a linear aromatic polyether ketone, characterized by a stable semi-aromatic structure that enhances its superior mechanical properties and chemical resistance as a thermoplastic [46, 47, 58].

In the field of biomaterials, PEEK has emerged as a prominent high-performance polymer, garnering significant attention for its applications in various medical fields, particularly in dentistry and orthopedics. Belonging to the PAEK family, PEEK is distinguished by its unique chemical composition, which imparts excellent physical and chemical properties and high manufacturability, making it a popular research topic in the development of customized barrier membrane scaffolds. Its exceptional combination of strength, stiffness, toughness, and resistance to environmental factors and wear enhances its appeal for medical applications [46, 47, 58, 78].

3.5.3.2 Properties of PEEK

PEEK possesses a range of properties that make it attractive for use in customized GBR membranes:

Biocompatibility: PEEK is a semi-crystalline thermoplastic with high biocompatibility. In vitro studies have shown no mutagenic or cytotoxic effects. It is also approved by the U.S. Food and Drug Administration (FDA) in the Master File for drugs and devices [46].

Mechanical properties: PEEK exhibits excellent mechanical properties, including an elastic modulus of 3.6 GPa, which can be increased to 18 GPa with carbon fiber reinforcement, a value close to that of cortical bone (15 GPa) [41, 46, 78]. It also has sufficient stiffness, with flexural strength ranging between 140 and 170 MPa, allowing it to withstand masticatory forces. These mechanical properties are essential for space maintenance [41, 46, 57, 58]. Compared to titanium, PEEK demonstrates better tensile strength and flexibility, more closely resembling human bone [46].

Radiolucency: Unlike titanium mesh, PEEK membranes are radiolucent and do not interfere with post-operative radiographic imaging [46].

Manufacturability and process ability: PEEK can be manufactured and processed using subtractive (milling) and additive (3D printing) techniques, offering versatility in creating customized designs [46, 47].

3.5.3.3 Clinical applications

Customized PEEK membranes have been successfully used in the augmentation of atrophic ridges, achieving vertical and horizontal bone gain. PEEK has also been used in maxillofacial surgery applications, such as repairing large cranial defects and mandibular reconstruction, often compared to titanium mesh in terms of cost and operative time. While customized PEEK implants may reduce operative time compared to manually bent titanium mesh, they can be more expensive [41, 46, 47, 58, 66, 78].

3.5.3.4 Advantages of customized PEEK membranes

Customized PEEK membranes share some advantages with customized titanium mesh, such as their ability to be precisely designed to fit bone defects. However, PEEK offers unique advantages:

Superior mechanical properties: PEEK exhibits higher tensile strength and flexibility compared to titanium, with an elastic modulus closer to that of human bone. This may reduce mucosal irritation and potentially lower exposure rates [46, 57, 69, 78].

Radiolucency: PEEK's radiolucent nature does not interfere with post-operative radiographic assessments [46].

Potential for reduced membrane exposure: Due to its smoother surface and better tissue compatibility compared to titanium, customized PEEK membranes may result in lower exposure rates [46].

3.5.3.5 Disadvantages and limitations of customized PEEK membranes

Despite their advantages, customized PEEK membranes have certain drawbacks:

Lack of osseointegration: Pure PEEK is biologically inert and lacks osseointegration properties. This limitation means it cannot fully replace titanium mesh, especially in cases where membrane osseointegration itself might be beneficial, such as supraperiosteal implant placements. As a non-absorbable material, a second surgery is required for its removal [5, 46, 78].

Higher clinical cost: The clinical cost of customized PEEK membranes can be higher compared to traditional titanium mesh, potentially limiting their widespread use [58].

Limited clinical data: Despite their promise, clinical data on the long-term performance of customized PEEK membranes in GBR are relatively scarce compared to established materials like titanium [58].

3.5.3.6 Ongoing research and future directions

These modifications aim to endow PEEK with antibacterial and osteoconductive capabilities, potentially improving wound healing, reducing membrane exposure rates, and enhancing bone regeneration when used in GBR. Future developments will need to consider processing complexity, economic cost, and the practical application of these modifications [46, 57, 69, 78].

To overcome PEEK's limitations, significant research efforts are focused on enhancing its bioactivity. Strategies include surface modification and composite blending.

Surface modification: Techniques such as oxygen and ammonia plasma treatment have been used to modify PEEK surfaces, increasing their hydrophilicity and protein adsorption capacity, which may enhance bone regeneration potential [46].

Composite blending: Incorporating materials like silicon nitride powder into PEEK has shown promising results in significantly improving its osteoconductive and antibacterial properties [46].

3.5.4 Chromium and cobalt

While the primary focus in the field of customized barrier membranes for GBR has been on materials like titanium and PEEK (as discussed earlier), chromium-cobalt (Cr-Co) alloys have also been studied for their potential use in this area. These alloys have a history of medical use, particularly in orthopedic surgery and, to a lesser extent, in dentistry, due to their biocompatibility and good mechanical properties [57, 79, 80].

Chromium-cobalt alloys are considered an alternative to titanium alloys because of their superior hardness and durability. They are also less expensive than titanium while maintaining high mechanical strength and the ability to form solid spaces. One study even reported a significant increase in bone density using a cobalt-chromium membrane in a non-critical bone defect in a rabbit tibia, demonstrating space-maintaining ability [6, 57, 79].

Manufacturing techniques involving CAD and 3D printing of prototypes have been described, which were later used to cast chromium-cobalt-molybdenum alloy membranes. While this process does not directly indicate "customization" as in patient-specific digital design, it highlights the potential to create membranes with specific dimensions and shapes that can be adapted to defect morphologies. Sandblasting these membranes with aluminum oxide particles may enhance their properties by creating surface roughness that promotes bone regeneration [57, 79, 80].

However, there are critical considerations regarding the use of chromium-cobalt alloys. A major drawback is the potential release of toxic chromium and cobalt ions into the body due to corrosion processes. While this is considered less likely in dental implants compared to orthopedic implants due to smaller surface areas and less friction, it remains a concern. The potential release of these ions could destabilize bone, leading to bone resorption and inhibition of bone proliferation and mineralization. Thus, despite promising animal studies, sources indicate that there have been no clinical trials using chromium-cobalt membrane implants in humans, primarily due to their inferior biocompatibility compared to titanium [6, 57, 79, 80].

One study using chromium-cobalt-molybdenum membranes in rabbit tibiae demonstrated new bone formation. The study also found that the physical dimensions and design of the membrane influenced new bone formation. While these results are encouraging, the lack of human clinical data, due to biocompatibility concerns, limits the current use of chromium-cobalt alloys in customized barrier membranes for GBR [57, 79, 80].

In summary, chromium-cobalt alloys offer attractive mechanical properties and lower costs compared to titanium, making them an appealing option for barrier membrane applications. Animal studies have shown promising results in space maintenance and bone regeneration. However, concerns about biocompatibility and the potential release of toxic ions have hindered their clinical application in human GBR procedures, including the development of customized membranes from these materials. Further research is needed to address these biocompatibility issues before chromium-cobalt alloys can be considered a practical alternative to materials like titanium and PEEK.

3.5.5 Other materials

3.5.5.1 Biodegradable polymers

While the focus in customized membranes often leans toward non-absorbable materials due to their space-maintaining ability, the concept of biodegradable customized membranes also exists, potentially eliminating the need for a second surgery [46, 68, 69]. Several biodegradable polymers have been investigated for GBR membranes in general and could theoretically be adapted for customized manufacturing [6, 47, 57, 68].

3.5.5.1.1 Polyesters (PLA, PGA, PCL, and their copolymers)

Aliphatic polyesters such as polylactic acid (PLA), polyglycolic acid (PGA), and polycaprolactone (PCL) have been considered as materials for customized barrier membranes due to their ease of handling, processability, adjustable biodegradation, and drug-loading capabilities [47, 57, 63]. Their degradation can be tuned by selecting different polymers or polymer blends. These materials can be processed using techniques like electrospinning and 3D printing, which may enable the creation of customized shapes and structures. However, a major drawback is their potential to elicit a strong inflammatory response during degradation, which could negatively impact bone regeneration. Their lack of rigidity and stability compared to non-absorbable materials may also limit their use in larger bone defects [47, 57, 63].

3.5.5.1.2 Collagen

Collagen membranes, often derived from bovine or porcine sources, are widely used due to their good biocompatibility, which promotes cell adhesion and tissue healing. These membranes are preferred when a second surgical procedure is undesirable. However, they suffer from poor mechanical properties and rapid degradation, which conflict with the requirements for managing vertical bone defects. While customized collagen structures can be fabricated using techniques like 3D printing, their lack of rigidity may necessitate reinforcement with other materials for space maintenance in customized membrane applications [5, 23, 57, 70].

3.5.5.1.3 Chitosan

Chitosan, a natural polysaccharide, exhibits good biocompatibility and biodegradability and can be processed into membranes using techniques like electrospinning. Customized chitosan membranes could provide an absorbable barrier with additional advantages. However, their weak mechanical strength may limit their ability to maintain space in larger bone defects [5, 54, 57, 63, 68, 69].

3.5.5.2 Ceramic materials

While zirconia has been specifically mentioned, other ceramic materials, including hydroxyapatite (HA) and other calcium phosphate compounds, have been investigated. These materials are known for their osteoconductive properties and have been incorporated into biodegradable membranes to enhance bone regeneration [57, 68, 81]. The drawbacks of customized ceramic membranes include the inherent brittleness of these materials, which complicates the fabrication of thin, adaptable membranes capable of withstanding surgical handling without fracture. This brittleness also poses risks during screw fixation [49, 59, 82].

3.5.5.3 Magnesium and magnesium alloys

Magnesium-based materials are biodegradable metals with the unique ability to self-degrade after tissue repair, eliminating the need for a second surgery. The magnesium-rich environment resulting from degradation can stimulate bone regeneration and improve osteoblast adhesion. Magnesium alloys also have an elastic modulus similar to that of human bone, enabling stress shielding avoidance. While these alloys are primarily used in orthopedic surgery and fracture fixation, the potential exists to fabricate customized magnesium membranes, especially with advancements in metal 3D printing. However, their degradation rate and potential for rapid corrosion must be carefully managed. Studies have explored coating magnesium alloys with materials like calcium phosphate to improve biocompatibility and corrosion resistance.

3.5.5.4 Multiphasic membranes

The concept of multiphasic membranes, which combine different materials or layers with varying properties, can be applied to customized membranes. These membranes are designed to meet the diverse needs of periodontal tissues, enhancing wound healing and bone regeneration. For example, a membrane could feature an outer non-absorbable, mechanically durable layer for space maintenance and an inner absorbable layer loaded with growth factors to promote osteogenesis. Customized manufacturing techniques allow for the precise layering and integration of different materials to create multiphasic membranes tailored to specific defects [46, 63].

4. Conclusions

The advancements in customized membranes for alveolar ridge augmentation have significantly enhanced the predictability and efficacy of guided bone regeneration (GBR) procedures. Traditional prefabricated membranes, while effective in many cases, often require intraoperative adjustments and may not perfectly fit complex bone defects, leading to complications such as membrane exposure, graft displacement, and compromised healing. The integration of digital technologies—including cone-beam computed tomography (CBCT), computer-aided design (CAD), and computer-aided manufacturing (CAM)—has revolutionized the field by enabling the fabrication of patient-specific membranes tailored to the unique anatomical characteristics of each defect.

Customized membranes, fabricated from materials such as titanium, zirconia, and polyether ether ketone (PEEK), offer superior fit, stability, and space-maintaining capabilities compared to their prefabricated counterparts. Titanium remains a gold standard due to its biocompatibility, mechanical strength, and adaptability, though concerns about membrane exposure and the need for secondary surgery persist. Zirconia membranes, with their excellent biocompatibility and resistance to bacterial adhesion, present a promising alternative, particularly in cases where exposure risks are high. PEEK membranes, with their radiolucency and mechanical properties resembling bone, provide another viable option, though further research is needed to validate their long-term performance.

Despite these advancements, challenges remain, including the risk of membrane exposure, the need for secondary surgeries in non-absorbable membranes, and the brittleness of ceramic materials like zirconia. Future research should focus on optimizing membrane designs, exploring bioactive surface modifications, and conducting long-term clinical studies to compare the efficacy of different materials. Additionally, the development of biodegradable customized membranes could eliminate the need for secondary surgeries, further improving patient outcomes.

In conclusion, customized membranes represent a significant leap forward in alveolar ridge augmentation, offering improved precision, reduced complications, and enhanced bone regeneration outcomes. As digital manufacturing technologies continue to evolve, the potential for further innovation in this field remains vast, promising even greater advancements in dental implantology and regenerative therapies.

Acknowledgements

The authors would like to acknowledge the contributions of researchers and clinicians whose work has advanced the field of guided bone regeneration and customized membrane technology.

Author contributions

All authors contributed equally to the conceptualization, writing, and revision of this chapter.

Funding

No external funding was received for the preparation of this chapter.

Conflict of interest

The authors declare no conflicts of interest related to the content of this chapter.

Data availability

No original data were generated for this chapter. All referenced studies are publicly available through their respective sources.

Ethical approval

This chapter is a review of existing literature and does not involve any human or animal subjects; thus, ethical approval was not required.

Author details

Ziad Albash[1*], Ali Khalil[2] and Nadim Sleman[1]

1 Oral and Maxillofacial Surgery Department, Faculty of Dentistry, Latakia University, Latakia, Syria

2 Oral and Maxillofacial Surgery Department, Faculty of Dentistry, Manara University, Latakia, Syria

*Address all correspondence to: zeyadalbash@yahoo.com

References

[1] Stumbras A, Kuliesius P, Januzis G, Juodzbalys G. Alveolar ridge preservation after tooth extraction using different bone graft materials and autologous platelet concentrates: A systematic review. Journal of Oral and Maxillofacial Research. 31 Mar 2019;**10**(1):e2. DOI: 10.5037/jomr.2019.10102

[2] Horowitz R, Holtzclaw D, Rosen PS. A review on alveolar ridge preservation following tooth extraction. Journal of Evidence Based Dental Practice. 2012;**12**(3):149-160. DOI: 10.1016/S1532-3382(12)70029-5

[3] Retzepi M, Donos N. Guided bone regeneration: Biological principle and therapeutic applications. Clinical Oral Implants Research. 2010;**21**(6):567-576. DOI: 10.1111/j.1600-0501.2010.01922.x

[4] Liu J, Kerns DG. Mechanisms of guided bone regeneration: A review. The Open Dentistry Journal. 2014;**8**:56-65. DOI: 10.2174/1874210601408010056

[5] Mizraji G, Davidzohn A, Gursoy M, Gursoy UK, Shapira L, Wilensky A. Membrane barriers for guided bone regeneration: An overview of available biomaterials. Periodontology 2000. 2023;**93**(1):56-76. DOI: 10.1111/prd.12502

[6] Chiapasco J-I, Abe GL, Li A, Thongthai P, Tsuboi R, Kohno T, et al. Barrier membranes for tissue regeneration in dentistry. Biomaterial Investigations in Dentistry. 2021;**8**(1):54-63. DOI: 10.1080/26415275.2021.1925556

[7] Caballé-Serrano J, Munar-Frau A, Ortiz-Puigpelat O, Soto-Penaloza D, Peñarrocha M, Hernández-Alfaro F. On the search of the ideal barrier membrane for guided bone regeneration. Journal of Clinical and Experimental Dentistry. 2018;**10**(5):e477-e483. DOI: 10.4317/jced.54767

[8] Albash Z, Khalil A, Kashkash W. Alveolar ridge augmentation using customized zirconia membranes: A systematic review. The Open Dentistry Journal. 9 Dec 2024;**18**(1). DOI: 10.2174/0118742106356292241122070017

[9] Cucchi A, Vignudelli E, Franceschi D, Randellini E, Lizio G, Fiorino A, et al. Vertical and horizontal ridge augmentation using customized CAD/CAM titanium mesh with versus without resorbable membranes. A randomized clinical trial. Clinical Oral Implants Research. 2021;**32**(12):1411-1424. DOI: 10.1111/clr.13841

[10] Won J, Kim WJ, Shim JS, Ryu JJ. Guided bone regeneration with a nitric-oxide releasing polymer inducing angiogenesis and osteogenesis in critical-sized bone defects. Macromolecular Bioscience. 2022;**22**(10):2200162. DOI: 10.1002/mabi.202200162

[11] Dominiak M, Łysiak-Drwal K, Solski L, Żywicka B, Rybak Z, Gedrange T. Evaluation of healing processes of intraosseous defects with and without guided bone regeneration and platelet rich plasma. An animal study. Annals of Anatomy-Anatomischer Anzeiger. 2012;**194**(6):549-555. DOI: 10.1016/j.aanat.2012.07.007

[12] Turri A, Elgali I, Vazirisani F, Johansson A, Emanuelsson L, Dahlin C, et al. Guided bone regeneration is promoted by the molecular events in the membrane compartment. Biomaterials. 2016;**84**:167-183. DOI: 10.1016/j.biomaterials.2016.01.034

[13] Esteves MET, Bianchini RMG, Gonzatti JPP, Scriboni AB. Guided bone regeneration in implant dentistry: A systematic review. MedNEXT Journal of Medical and Health Sciences. 2023;**4**(S2). DOI: 10.54448/mdnt23S221

[14] Wang H-L, Boyapati L. "Pass" principles for predictable bone regeneration. Implant Dentistry. 2006;**15**(1):8-17. DOI: 10.1097/01.id.0000204762.39826.0f

[15] Kim Y-K, Ku J-K. Guided bone regeneration. Journal of the Korean Association of Oral and Maxillofacial Surgeons. 2020;**46**(5):361-366. DOI: 10.5125/jkaoms.2020.46.5.361

[16] Omar O, Elgali I, Dahlin C, Thomsen P. Barrier membranes: More than the barrier effect? Journal of Clinical Periodontology. 2019;**46**(S21):103-123. DOI: 10.1111/jcpe.13068

[17] Ren Y, Fan L, Alkildani S, Liu L, Emmert S, Najman S, et al. Barrier membranes for guided bone regeneration (Gbr): A focus on recent advances in collagen membranes. International Journal of Molecular Sciences. 2022;**23**(23):14987. DOI: 10.3390/ijms232314987

[18] Bubalo M, Lazic Z, Tatic Z, Milovic R, Magic M. The use of collagen membranes in guided tissue regeneration. Vojnosanitetski Pregled. 2017;**74**(8):767-772. DOI: 10.2298/VSP160117116B

[19] Sehdev B, Bhongade M, Ganji K. Evaluation of effectiveness of hyaluronic acid in combination with bioresorbable membrane (poly lactic acid-poly glycolic acid) for the treatment of infrabony defects in humans: A clinical and radiographic study. Journal of Indian Society of Periodontology. 2016;**20**(1):50. DOI: 10.4103/0972-124X.170809

[20] Li X, Jin Q, Xu H, Zhang S, Wang W, Zhao B. Effect of polylactic acid membrane on guided bone regeneration in anterior maxillary implantation. Medical Science Monitor. International Medical Journal of Experimental and Clinical Research. 18 Mar 2023;**29**:e938566-1. DOI: 10.12659/MSM.938566

[21] Mau LP, Cheng C-W, Hsieh P-Y, Jones AA. Biological complication in guided bone regeneration with a polylactic acid membrane: A case report. Implant Dentistry. 2012;**21**(3):171-174. DOI: 10.1097/ID.0b013e31824eece1

[22] Shim J-H, Won J-Y, Park J-H, Bae J-H, Ahn G, Kim C-H, et al. Effects of 3d-printed polycaprolactone/β-tricalcium phosphate membranes on guided bone regeneration. International Journal of Molecular Sciences. 2017;**18**(5):899. DOI: 10.3390/ijms18050899

[23] Sbricoli L, Guazzo R, Annunziata M, Gobbato L, Bressan E, Nastri L. Selection of collagen membranes for bone regeneration: A literature review. Materials. 2020;**13**(3):786. DOI: 10.3390/ma13030786

[24] Jiménez Garcia J, Berghezan S, Caramês JMM, Dard MM, Marques DNS. Effect of cross-linked vs non-cross-linked collagen membranes on bone: A systematic review. Journal of Periodontal Research. 2017;**52**(6):955-964. DOI: 10.1111/jre.12470

[25] Becker J, Al-Nawas B, Klein MO, Schliephake H, Terheyden H, Schwarz F. Use of a new cross-linked collagen membrane for the treatment of dehiscence-type defects at titanium implants: A prospective, randomized-controlled double-blinded clinical multicenter study. Clinical Oral Implants Research. 2009;**20**(7):742-749. DOI: 10.1111/j.1600-0501.2008.01689.x

[26] Papi P, Di Murro B, Tromba M, Passarelli PC, D'Addona A, Pompa G. The use of a non-absorbable membrane as an occlusive barrier for alveolar ridge preservation: A one year follow-up prospective cohort study. Antibiotics. 2020;**9**(3):110. DOI: 10.3390/antibiotics9030110

[27] Solomon S-M, Sufaru I-G, Teslaru S, Ghiciuc CM, Stafie CS. Finding the perfect membrane: Current knowledge on barrier membranes in regenerative procedures: A descriptive review. Applied Sciences. 2022;**12**(3):1042. DOI: 10.3390/app12031042

[28] Bottino MC, Thomas V, Schmidt G, Vohra YK, Chu T-MG, Kowolik MJ, et al. Recent advances in the development of GTR/GBR membranes for periodontal regeneration—A materials perspective. Dental Materials. 2012;**28**(7):703-721. DOI: 10.1016/j.dental.2012.04.022

[29] Wang G, Feng Y, Gao C, Zhang X, Wang Q, Zhang J, et al. Biaxial stretching of polytetrafluoroethylene in industrial scale to fabricate medical ePTFE membrane with node-fibril microstructure. Regenerative Biomaterials. 2023;**10**:rbad056. DOI: 10.1093/rb/rbad056

[30] Miura H, Nishibe T, Yasuda K, Shimada T, Hazama K, Katoh H, et al. The influence of node-fibril morphology on healing of high-porosity expanded polytetrafluoroethylene grafts. European Surgical Research. 2002;**34**(3):224-231. DOI: 10.1159/000063393

[31] Scott TA, Towle HJ, Assad DA, Nicoll BK. Comparison of bioabsorbable laminar bone membrane and non-resorbable eptfe membrane in mandibular furcations. Journal of Periodontology. 1997;**68**(7):679-686. DOI: 10.1902/jop.1997.68.7.679

[32] Roina Y, Auber F, Hocquet D, Herlem G. ePTFE-based biomedical devices: An overview of surgical efficiency. Journal of Biomedical Materials Research Part B: Applied Biomaterials. 2022;**110**(2):302-320. DOI: 10.1002/jbm.b.34928

[33] Kashkash W, Albash Z. Bone block protection using dense polytetrafluoroethylene membranes in vertical bone augmentation procedures for atrophic maxilla: A case report. The Open Dentistry Journal. 27 Dec 2024;**18**(1). DOI: 10.2174/0118742106356353241211112225

[34] Barber HD, Lignelli J, Smith BM, Bartee BK. Using a dense PTFE membrane without primary closure to achieve bone and tissue regeneration. Journal of Oral and Maxillofacial Surgery. 2007;**65**(4):748-752. DOI: 10.1016/j.joms.2006.10.042

[35] Roccuzzo M, Ramieri G, Spada MC, Bianchi SD, Berrone S. Vertical alveolar ridge augmentation by means of a titanium mesh and autogenous bone grafts. Clinical Oral Implants Research. 2004;**15**(1):73-81. DOI: 10.1111/j.1600-0501.2004.00998.x

[36] Roccuzzo M, Ramieri G, Bunino M, Berrone S. Autogenous bone graft alone or associated with titanium mesh for vertical alveolar ridge augmentation: A controlled clinical trial. Clinical Oral Implants Research. 2007;**18**(3):286-294. DOI: 10.1111/j.1600-0501.2006.01301.x

[37] Poli PP, Beretta M, Cicciù M, Maiorana C. Alveolar ridge augmentation with titanium mesh. A retrospective clinical study. The Open Dentistry Journal. 2014;**8**(1):148-158. DOI: 10.2174/1874210601408010148

[38] Xie Y, Li S, Zhang T, Wang C, Cai X. Titanium mesh for bone augmentation in

oral implantology: Current application and progress. International Journal of Oral Science. 2020;**12**(1):1-12. DOI: 10.1038/s41368-020-00107-z

[39] Chan H-L, Benavides E, Tsai C-Y, Wang H-L. A titanium mesh and particulate allograft for vertical ridge augmentation in the posterior mandible: A pilot study. The International Journal of Periodontics & Restorative Dentistry. 2015;**35**(4):515-522. DOI: 10.11607/prd.1980

[40] Deshpande S, Deshmukh J, Deshpande S, Khatri R, Deshpande S. Vertical and horizontal ridge augmentation in anterior maxilla using autograft, xenograft and titanium mesh with simultaneous placement of endosseous implants. Journal of Indian Society of Periodontology. 2014;**18**(5):661. DOI: 10.4103/0972-124X.142469

[41] Mounir M, Mounir S, Abou-Elfetouh A, Shaker MA. Assessment of vertical ridge augmentation in anterior aesthetic zone using onlay xenografts with titanium mesh versus the inlay bone grafting technique: A randomized clinical trial. International Journal of Oral and Maxillofacial Surgery. 2017;**46**(11):1458-1465. DOI: 10.1016/j.ijom.2017.04.021

[42] Huh J-B, Jung D-H, Kim J-S, Shin S-W. Effects of different sizes of hydroxyapatite/β-tricalcium phosphate particles on vertical bone augmentation. The Journal of Korean Academy of Prosthodontics. 2010;**48**(4):259. DOI: 10.4047/jkap.2010.48.4.259

[43] Senoo M, Hasuike A, Yamamoto T, Ozawa Y, Watanabe N, Furuhata M, et al. Comparison of macro-and micro-porosity of a titanium mesh for guided bone regeneration: An in vivo experimental study. In Vivo. 2022;**36**(1):76-85. DOI: 10.21873/invivo.12678

[44] Briguglio F, Falcomatà D, Marconcini S, Fiorillo L, Briguglio R, Farronato D. The use of titanium mesh in guided bone regeneration: A systematic review. International Journal of Dentistry. 2019;**2019**:1-8. DOI: 10.1155/2019/9065423

[45] Atef M, Tarek A, Shaheen M, Alarawi RM, Askar N. Horizontal ridge augmentation using native collagen membrane vs titanium mesh in atrophic maxillary ridges: Randomized clinical trial. Clinical Implant Dentistry and Related Research. 2020;**22**(2):156-166. DOI: 10.1111/cid.12892

[46] Shi Y, Liu J, Du M, Zhang S, Liu Y, Yang H, et al. Customized barrier membrane (titanium alloy, poly ether-ether ketone and unsintered hydroxyapatite/poly-l-lactide) for guided bone regeneration. Frontiers in Bioengineering and Biotechnology. 2022;**10**:916967. DOI: 10.3389/fbioe.2022.916967

[47] Alauddin MS, Abdul Hayei NA, Sabarudin MA, Mat Baharin NH. Barrier membrane in regenerative therapy: A narrative review. Membranes. 2022;**12**(5):444. DOI: 10.3390/membranes12050444

[48] De Angelis N, Kassim ZH, Mohd Yusof E, Yumang C, Menini M. Bone augmentation techniques with customized titanium meshes: A systematic review of randomized clinical trials. The Open Dentistry Journal. 28 Feb 2023;**17**(1). DOI: 10.2174/18742106-v17-230228-2022-172

[49] Albash Z, Abdallah Y, Moawad S, Khalil A, Assad M, Noureddin H. Horizontal augmentation using customized zirconia membrane: A case

report. The Open Dentistry Journal. 28 Aug 2024;**18**(1). DOI: 10.2174/0118742106332436240820100241

[50] Connors C, Liacouras P, Grant G. Custom titanium ridge augmentation matrix (Ctram): A case report. The International Journal of Periodontics & Restorative Dentistry. 1 Sep 2016;**36**(5). DOI: 10.11607/prd.2620

[51] Di Spirito F, Giordano F, Di Palo MP, Ferraro C, Cecere L, Frucci E, et al. Customized 3d-printed mesh, membrane, bone substitute, and dental implant applied to guided bone regeneration in oral implantology: A narrative review. Dentistry Journal. 2024;**12**(10):303. DOI: 10.3390/dj12100303

[52] Liu Y, Li Y, Dong Z, Wang Y, Han C, Liao Z, et al. Additive manufacturing of personalized, semipermeable and biodegradable polymer/metal composite membrane for guided bone regeneration. Materials Today. 2025;**83**:181-197. DOI: 10.1016/j.mattod.2025.01.001

[53] Felice P, Lizio G, Barausse C, Roccoli L, Bonifazi L, Pistilli R, et al. Reverse guided bone regeneration (R-gbr) digital workflow for atrophic jaws rehabilitation. Applied Sciences. 2022;**12**(19):9947. DOI: 10.3390/app12199947

[54] Chiapasco M, Casentini P, Tommasato G, Dellavia C, Del Fabbro M. Customized CAD/CAM titanium meshes for the guided bone regeneration of severe alveolar ridge defects: Preliminary results of a retrospective clinical study in humans. Clinical Oral Implants Research. 2021;**32**(4):498-510. DOI: 10.1111/clr.13720

[55] Sumida T, Otawa N, Kamata Y, Kamakura S, Mtsushita T, Kitagaki H, et al. Custom-made titanium devices as membranes for bone augmentation in implant treatment: Clinical application and the comparison with conventional titanium mesh. Journal of Cranio-Maxillofacial Surgery. 2015;**43**(10):2183-2188. DOI: 10.1016/j.jcms.2015.10.020

[56] Al Shaikh MS, Gamal AY, Amr AEH. "Customized titanium mesh versus titanium reinforced membrane in localized alveolar ridge augmentation with simultaneously delayed implant placement" A randomized clinical study. Egyptian Dental Journal. 2020;**66**(4-October (Oral Medicine, X-Ray, Oral Biology&Oral Pathology)):2289-2301. DOI: 10.21608/edj.2020.36620.1181

[57] Elgali I, Omar O, Dahlin C, Thomsen P. Guided bone regeneration: Materials and biological mechanisms revisited. European Journal of Oral Sciences. 2017;**125**(5):315-337. DOI: 10.1111/eos.12364

[58] Hao X, Wang W, Wang C, Han J, Zhang Y. Polyetherketoneketone mesh for alveolar bone augmentation: Geometric parameter design and finite element analysis. Journal of Healthcare Engineering. 2023;**2023**(1):8487380. DOI: 10.1155/2023/8487380

[59] Mandelli F, Traini T, Ghensi P. Customized-3D zirconia barriers for guided bone regeneration (Gbr): Clinical and histological findings from a proof-of-concept case series. Journal of Dentistry. 2021;**114**:103780. DOI: 10.1016/j.jdent.2021.103780

[60] Kumar G, Parthasarathy H, Ponnaiyan D. Localized ridge augmentation with simultaneous implant placement followed by soft tissue augmentation in the maxillary anterior region: A case report. World Academy of Sciences Journal. 2022;**4**(5):31. DOI: 10.3892/wasj.2022.166

[61] Seiler M, Kämmerer PW, Peetz M, Hartmann AG. Customized titanium lattice structure in three-dimensional alveolar defect: An initial case letter. Journal of Oral Implantology. 2018;**44**(3):219-224. DOI: 10.1563/aaid-joi-D-17-00084

[62] Rodriguez IA, Selders GS, Fetz AE, Gehrmann CJ, Stein SH, Evensky JA, et al. Barrier membranes for dental applications: A review and sweet advancement in membrane developments. Mouth and Teeth. 2018;**2**(1). DOI: 10.15761/MTJ.1000108

[63] Yang Z, Wu C, Shi H, Luo X, Sun H, Wang Q, et al. Advances in barrier membranes for guided bone regeneration techniques. Frontiers in Bioengineering and Biotechnology. 2022;**10**:921576. DOI: 10.3389/fbioe.2022.921576

[64] Hartmann A, Hildebrandt H, Schmohl JU, Kämmerer PW. Evaluation of risk parameters in bone regeneration using a customized titanium mesh: Results of a clinical study. Implant Dentistry. 1 Dec 2019;**28**(6):543-550. DOI: 10.1097/ID.0000000000000933

[65] Hartmann A, Hildebrandt H, Younan Z, Al-Nawas B, Kämmerer PW. Long-term results in three-dimensional, complex bone augmentation procedures with customized titanium meshes. Clinical Oral Implants Research. 2022;**33**(11):1171-1181. DOI: 10.1111/clr.14000

[66] Mounir M, Shalash M, Mounir S, Nassar Y, El Khatib O. Assessment of three dimensional bone augmentation of severely atrophied maxillary alveolar ridges using prebent titanium mesh vs customized poly-ether-ether-ketone (Peek) mesh: A randomized clinical trial. Clinical Implant Dentistry and Related Research. 2019;**21**(5):960-967. DOI: 10.1111/cid.12748

[67] Hartmann A, Seiler M. Minimizing risk of customized titanium mesh exposures – A retrospective analysis. BMC Oral Health. 2020;**20**(1):36. DOI: 10.1186/s12903-020-1023-y

[68] Gentile P, Chiono V, Tonda-Turo C, Ferreira AM, Ciardelli G. Polymeric membranes for guided bone regeneration. Biotechnology Journal. 2011;**6**(10):1187-1197. DOI: 10.1002/biot.201100294

[69] Patil S, Bhandi S, Bakri MMH, Albar DH, Alzahrani KJ, Al-Ghamdi MS, et al. Evaluation of efficacy of non-resorbable membranes compared to resorbable membranes in patients undergoing guided bone regeneration. Heliyon. 2023;**9**(3):e13488. DOI: 10.1016/j.heliyon.2023.e13488

[70] Kim J-Y, Park J-B. Various coated barrier membranes for better guided bone regeneration: A review. Coatings. 2022;**12**(8):1059. DOI: 10.3390/coatings12081059

[71] Pikos MA, Miron RJ. Bone Augmentation in Implant Dentistry: A Step-by-Step Guide to Predictable Alveolar Ridge and Sinus Grafting. Chicago: Quintessence; 2019

[72] Ciocca L, Lizio G, Baldissara P, Sambuco A, Scotti R, Corinaldesi G. Prosthetically CAD-CAM–guided bone augmentation of atrophic jaws using customized titanium mesh: Preliminary results of an open prospective study. Journal of Oral Implantology. 2018;**44**(2):131-137. DOI: 10.1563/aaid-joi-D-17-00125

[73] Souidan AAE, Ayad SS, Sweedan AO. Augmentation of the anterior maxillary bony defects using custom-made zirconia membranes(a case series). Alexandria Dental Journal. 2023;**48**(1):35-43. DOI: 10.21608/adjalexu.2022.106732.1232

[74] Heikal M, Shuman M, Khalil M. Evaluation of bone regeneration for augmentation of alveolar bone using 3D computer guided ceramic sheets. Al-Azhar Journal of Dental Science. 2020;**23**(4):393-399. DOI: 10.21608/ajdsm.2020.26561.1044

[75] Hofferber CE, Beck C, Liacouras PC. Custom zirconia ridge augmentation matrix (CZRAM) for implant site development: A report of two cases. Journal of Implant and Advanced Clinical Dentistry. 2018;**10**:6-15

[76] Malmström J, Anderud J, Abrahamsson P, Wälivaara D-Å, Isaksson SG, Adolfsson E. Guided bone regeneration using individualized ceramic sheets. International Journal of Oral and Maxillofacial Surgery. 2016;**45**(10):1246-1252. DOI: 10.1016/j.ijom.2016.06.005

[77] Retrum JK, McLaughlin SD, Stancoven BW, Inouye KA, Lincicum AR, Johnson TM. Application of a custom two-piece zirconia device for multidimensional ridge augmentation in a trauma patient: A case report. South Asian Research Journal of Oral and Dental Sciences. 2024;**6**(2):25-33. DOI: 10.36346/sarjods.2024.v06i02.002

[78] El Morsy OA, Barakat A, Mekhemer S, Mounir M. Assessment of 3-dimensional bone augmentation of severely atrophied maxillary alveolar ridges using patient-specific poly ether-ether ketone (Peek) sheets. Clinical Implant Dentistry and Related Research. 2020;**22**(2):148-155. DOI: 10.1111/cid.12890

[79] Decco O, Beltrán V, Zuchuat J, Cura A, Lezcano M, Engelke W. Bone augmentation in rabbit tibia using microfixed cobalt-chromium membranes with whole blood and platelet-rich plasma. Materials. 2015;**8**(8):4843-4856. DOI: 10.3390/ma8084843

[80] Zuchuat J, Berli M, Maldonado Y, Decco O. Influence of chromium-cobalt-molybdenum alloy (Astm f75) on bone ingrowth in an experimental animal model. Journal of Functional Biomaterials. 2017;**9**(1):2. DOI: 10.3390/jfb9010002

[81] Vaquette C, Mitchell J, Ivanovski S. Recent advances in vertical alveolar bone augmentation using additive manufacturing technologies. Frontiers in Bioengineering and Biotechnology. 2022;**9**:798393. DOI: 10.3389/fbioe.2021.798393

[82] Anderud J, Abrahamsson P, Jimbo R, Isaksson SG, Adolfsson E, Malmström J, et al. Guided bone augmentation using ceramic space-maintaining devices: The impact of chemistry. Clinical, Cosmetic and Investigational Dentistry. 12 Mar 2015;**45**:53. DOI: 10.2147/CCIDE.S78589

Chapter 14

Perspective Chapter: Stimulation of Periodontal and Peri-Implant Healing with Bioactive Materials and Devices

Robert A. Horowitz, Gregori M. Kurtzman and Hari S. Prasad

Abstract

Periodontal and peri-implant diseases remain among the most challenging conditions in dentistry, often presenting at advanced stages with significant soft and hard tissue loss. Earlier intervention has consistently been shown to improve predictability and long-term outcomes, yet patients are frequently referred late in the disease process, complicating both surgical and regenerative strategies. Advances in biologically active materials and adjunctive technologies now provide clinicians with an expanded armamentarium to address these complex cases. Growth factor–based therapies, including GEM 21S® and platelet-rich fibrin (PRF), have demonstrated the ability to stimulate both hard and soft tissue regeneration, improving osseointegration and stability around natural dentition and implants. Autogenous dentin grafts offer an osteoinductive scaffold derived from the patient's own tissues, while amnion-chorion–derived barriers, such as BioXclude®, enhance healing through anti-infective and angiogenic properties. Complementary modalities—including laser therapy, photobiomodulation (PBM), and low magnitude high-frequency vibration (LMHFV)—further accelerate healing, reduce microbial load, and optimize regenerative responses. Clinical cases supported by histologic and radiographic evidence highlight the synergistic benefits of combining biologically driven grafting materials with novel devices designed to enhance surgical outcomes. Collectively, these approaches improve bone-to-implant contact, reduce peri-implant bone loss, and contribute to greater long-term predictability. The integration of these regenerative strategies underscores the importance of biologically based, patient-specific therapies in preserving natural dentition, salvaging compromised implants, and reducing the systemic risks associated with chronic oral inflammation.

Keywords: periodontal regeneration, peri-implantitis, growth factors, photobiomodulation (PBM), bone grafting, low magnitude high frequency vibration (LMHFV)

1. Introduction

Patients are often referred to a periodontist or to the clinician managing their periodontal or peri-implant disease at varying stages of soft tissue and/or bone loss.

When patients are evaluated earlier in the disease process, outcomes are generally more predictable. Early intervention increases the likelihood of eliminating the underlying inflammation and may allow for the reversal of gingival and/or alveolar bone loss. Unfortunately, timely referrals or interventions by the treating dentist are not always made.

In cases where deep periodontal or peri-implant pockets are already present, the associated biofilm can contribute not only to localized tissue destruction but also to systemic complications [1, 2]. As bone loss progresses, surgical procedures for reconstruction and, ideally, regeneration become increasingly complex. These cases are often further complicated by systemic conditions such as smoking or diabetes, which may impair healing.

The aim of this chapter is to present clinical cases supported by literature and, where possible, histological evidence that showcase various growth-enhancing devices and bioactive materials designed to improve surgical outcomes. By preserving natural dentition whenever possible, we can delay or even prevent the need for implants and reduce the risk of future bone loss around them.

Multiple studies have shown that sites with previously failed implants are associated with higher failure rates upon retreatment [3–6]. Various bioactive materials and treatment modalities for treatment of periodontal disease with associated bone loss and peri-implantitis will be addressed. Additionally, the utilization of devices to augment and enhance bioactive treatment approaches are discussed. By increasing the amount of vital bone and ideally converting allograft to vital bone, the percentage of bone to implant contact should increase, improving osseointegration, implant stability, implant longevity and decreasing the risk for peri-implant bone loss.

2. Platelet-rich fibrin (PRF)

Platelet-rich fibrin (PRF) is a second-generation platelet concentrate that has gained significant attention in regenerative dentistry due to its ability to promote tissue healing and regeneration. Advantages of PRF over PRP include natural fibrin matrices, a higher concentration of platelets, a longer-term release of growth factors, which are crucial for healing and no need to incorporate additional materials like thrombin [7]. PRF is widely used in periodontal and implant treatment to enhance bone regeneration, improve soft tissue healing, and support the integration of dental implants.

PRF is inexpensive and derived from the patient's own blood. It is a highly biocompatible and safe option for regenerative procedures. Its enhanced healing and regenerative properties promote faster and more efficient healing, reducing postoperative pain, swelling, and inflammation. The variety of procedures in which it is used includes socket preservation, bone grafting, periodontal regeneration, and implant therapy, PRF contains a high concentration of platelets, leukocytes, and growth factors such as platelet-derived growth factor (PDGF), transforming growth factor-beta (TGF-β), and vascular endothelial growth factor (VEGF), all of which play a vital role in tissue healing and regeneration [8]. Different centrifuges which operate at variable speeds and angles may affect the physical and biological properties of the clot formed. Low speed centrifugation, horizontal forces may permit longer release of growth factors improving the clinical and histologic results in regenerated tissues [9, 10].

The mechanism by which PRF works is mainly attributed to PDGF, collagen matrix formation, angiogenesis and its anti-inflammatory effects [11]. Platelet-derived growth factors in the PRF stimulate the recruitment, migration and proliferation of osteoblasts, fibroblasts, and endothelial cells, which are necessary for bone and soft tissue regeneration. Growth factors in PRF encourage the formation of new blood vessels, enhancing oxygen and nutrient supply to the healing tissue, which is especially crucial for both soft and hard tissue regeneration around dental implants and periodontal tissues. Additionally, the anti-inflammatory effects PRF provides have been demonstrated to reduce inflammation in the treated area, accelerating healing and reducing complications after grafting procedures [12, 13]. Clinical evidence and studies on PRF in periodontal and implant treatment support PRF's ability to enhance treatment and clinical outcomes.

In addition to its' biological properties, PRF will clinically enable the surgeon to fabricate "sticky bone" or a "block" of bone out of particulate graft materials [14–17]. In this manner, extra-alveolar defects can be filled to ideal contour to perform ridge augmentation and the graft material can hold its' shape.

2.1 PRF in periodontal and implant-related treatment

Periodontal diseases lead to the destruction of the supporting structures of teeth (bone and periodontal ligament). PRF has proven to be effective in enhancing the healing process and promoting tissue regeneration in these cases [18]. Growth factors in PRF stimulate osteoblast activity, promoting bone formation. PRF additionally supports the regeneration of the periodontal ligament, critical for tooth stability and function. In conjunction with bone grafting, The slow release of growth factors in PRF [19] stimulates the proliferation of periodontal ligament cells, leading to the formation of new attachments between the tooth and alveolar bone, decreasing tooth mobility by increasing its stability.

A meta-analysis study demonstrated that the combination of PRF and bone grafts resulted in improved clinical outcomes in periodontal defect treatment, with enhanced bone fill and attachment gain compared to the use of bone grafts alone [20]. Similar results were reported that PRF significantly enhanced periodontal regeneration, leading to better clinical attachment levels and radiographic bone fill [21].

2.2 PRF in implantology

PRF's use in implantology has become increasingly popular due to its ability to enhance bone regeneration and accelerate the healing process. Following tooth extraction, the alveolar ridge undergoes resorption when socket preservation is not performed. This can complicate subsequent implant placement when a delayed approach is utilized [22–24]. When PRF is combined with bone graft materials, it enhances the integration of the graft material, leading to improved bone volume for later implant placement. This also has benefits when immediate implant placement at time of extraction is planned, aiding in accelerating integration of the implant and promoting faster healing of the surrounding soft tissue [25].

PRF improves bone regeneration in the maxillary sinus, enabling successful implant placement whether placed at time of grafting or in a delayed approach [26]. The incorporation of PRF into the implant surgical site aids in accelerating osseointegration [27]. PRF's growth factors stimulate osteoblast activity, promoting faster and more robust bone healing around the implant leading to quicker functional implant procedures. Its ability to enhance bone regeneration, improve soft tissue healing and support osseointegration makes it an invaluable adjunct to various grafting techniques. As clinical studies continue to demonstrate its efficacy, PRF is increasingly being integrated into dental practices as a cost-effective, safe, and highly beneficial solution to enhance hard and soft tissue regeneration. Throughout this chapter, PRF will be shown in multiple cases of bone grafting, loading and reducing the risk of implant failure [28, 29]. Other uses include placing PRF plugs around healing abutments to thicken the biotype [30] and to enhance root coverage [31].

3. Autogenous dentin grafting

The concept of using dentin as a graft material capitalizes on its biological properties, which include the presence of osteoinductive factors (growth factors and proteins) that promote bone formation and tissue healing. This has led to its increasing application in periodontal and implant treatment.

Physical and chemical similarities between dentin and bone have been reported [31]. Dentin is a viscoelastic material, making it a very effective in bone replacement. These properties include: osteoinductive potential, osteoconductive, biocompatibility and release of bioactive molecules [32]. Dentin's osteoinductive potential comes from multiple growth factors, including bone morphogenetic proteins (BMPs), transforming growth factors (TGF-β), and fibroblast growth factors (FGFs). These are involved in the regulation of osteoblast differentiation and bone formation, stimulating the differentiation of mesenchymal stem cells into osteoblasts and promoting new bone formation in the grafted site [33, 34]. The osteoconductive, mineralized matrix of dentin allows for the attachment, migration, and differentiation of osteoblasts and other cells necessary for bone regeneration [35]. The processed dentin matrix releases bioactive molecules, growth factors that enhance and promote osseous healing and soft tissue regeneration [36]. Autogenous dentin has been proven to be a highly biocompatible and safe material for grafting procedures [37].

3.1 Autogenous dentin graft in periodontal treatment

Autogenous dentin grafts have demonstrated promise in achieving restoration of lost hard and soft tissue through regeneration. They may also be more beneficial in elderly, immunocompromised patients and in large and/or challenging defects - infrabony, furcation defects, and other periodontal lesions that require osseous grafting. The osteoinductive properties of dentin, combined with its osteoconductive scaffold, enhance the healing process, promoting regeneration of missing bone and the periodontal ligament [38]. Clinical studies have indicated that the use of dentin grafts in periodontal defects results in increased bone fill, improved attachment levels, and greater clinical stability compared to non-regenerative procedures [39].

3.2 Case example: Extraction, socket grafting and periodontal furcation repair

A 67-year-old male presented for evaluation of the upper right molars. Continued periodontal breakdown not related to any medical history nor medications taken, was noted on the 1st and 2nd molars in the upper right. A radiograph was taken to evaluate the advanced periodontal condition (**Figure 1**). Both molars were noted to have significant bone loss with advanced furcation involvement (**Figure 2**). While both had hopeless prognoses, the patient expressed a desire to maintain the 1st molar for as long as possible. Treatment was discussed with the patient to extract the 2nd molar, utilize

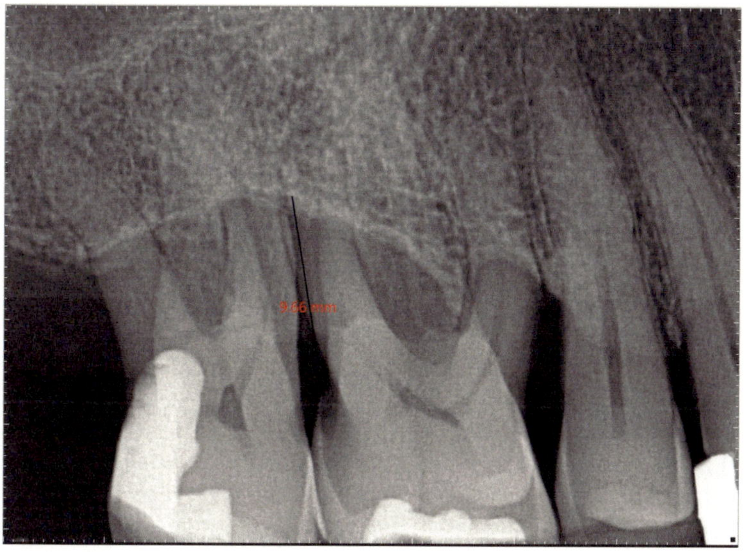

Figure 1.
Initial radiographic presentation of periodontally involved with advanced bone loss and Class 2–4 involved furcations.

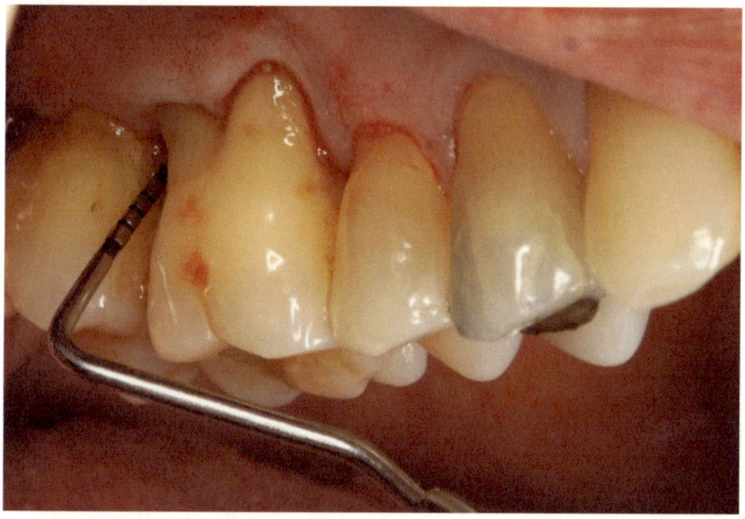

Figure 2.
Initial pocketing of 9 mm in the distal furcation of tooth # 3.

that as graft material for the 2nd molar socket and periodontally around the 1st molar to attempt to improve the periodontal condition of that tooth.

Local anesthetic was administered, and blood was drawn from the patient to fabricate PRF. After the restoration was removed, the 2nd molar was atraumatically extracted. The tooth was debrided of hard and soft accretions, sectioned into pieces and placed into the Smart Dentin Grinder (KometaBio, Ft. Lee, NJ) (**Figure 2**). Following processing (grinding) the resulting particulate was sterilized (cleansed) and partially demineralized according to the manufacturer's directions. It was then mixed with corticocancellous allograft (Maxxeus, Solvita, Dayton, OH) in a 1:1 ratio. PRF from the patient's blood was prepared and added to the graft to create a "block" of bone and set aside. Flaps were elevated to the mesial of the 2nd premolar then the socket and periodontal defects were debrided. The roots were planed and treated with EDTA (Kometabio). The PRF-Allograft-ADG (autologous dentin graft) block was placed into the extraction socket and periodontal defects around the 1st molar. Due to the physical properties of the "block", it was able to be placed and remain stable in a supra-alveolar location. The graft was then covered with an Amnion-Chorion membrane (BioXclude, Solvita, Dayton, Ohio) and L-PRF barriers. As both the membrane and barrier have no memory when they are wet, it takes minimal time to place them over any defect. The flaps were coronally repositioned, sutured and a radiograph was taken.

The patient was seen on 3-month periodontal recare schedule and reevaluated 3 years post grafting. Periodontal probing on the distal of 1st molar was 2-3 mm where pretreatment that probing was 8–9 mm. A periapical radiograph demonstrated bone stability at the extraction socket, above the previous height of the alveolar crests and in the furcations (**Figure 3**). The furcations were closed clinically and radiographically. There appeared to be 6.6 mm of vertical bone gain under the distal CEJ of tooth # 3 which was verified clinically (**Figure 4**). Tooth # 3 which originally had a hopeless prognosis now has a good prognosis.

Diagnosis of the patient, mouth and site are critical in prognosis of the teeth and patient [40]. Many other periodontal non-surgical and surgical procedures which have shown varying degrees of success rates in the treatment of infrabony pockets [41, 42]. This combination of bioactive materials and partially demineralized dentin mixed with a specific allograft (Maxxeus) fabricated into a PRF block and covered by a specific amnion-chorion (BioXclude) barrier has repeatedly shown excellent results in filling infrabony defects and gaining suprabony healing along smooth roots and into

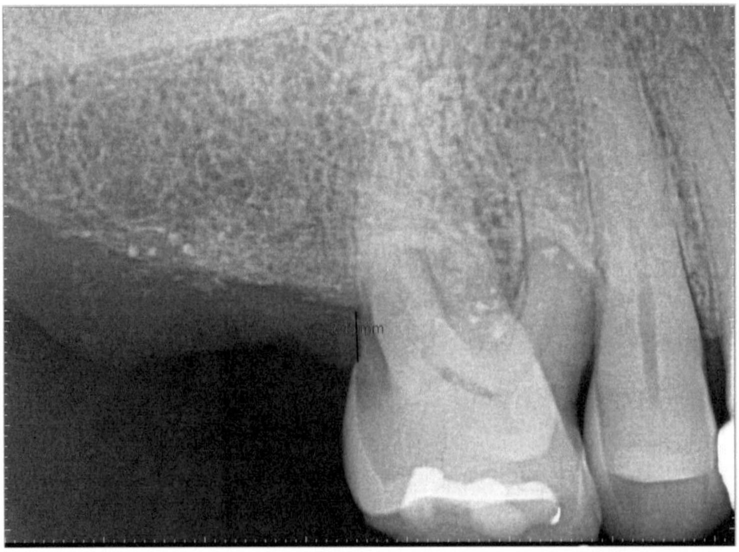

Figure 3.
Three year postop radiograph showing excellent periodontal fill and graft remodeling in socket defect.

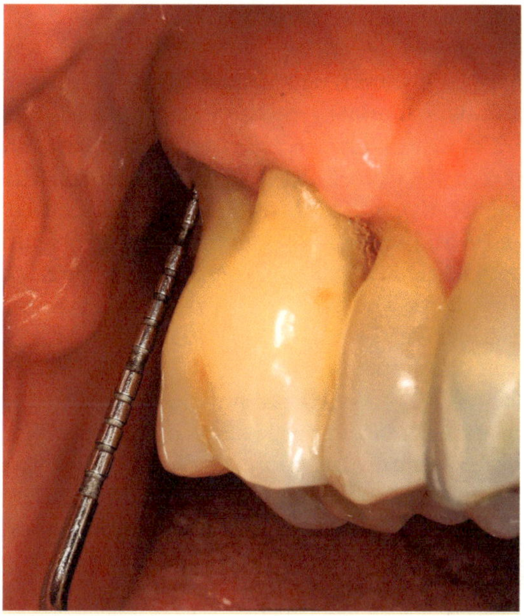

Figure 4.
Three year probing DB of tooth # 3 showing 2 mm pocket, no bleeding, 5 mm CAL gain in the distal furcation.

furcations as shown here. There are very few if any reports in the periodontal literature of other materials performing well in suprabony defects to treat these severely advanced periodontal lesions. Research has reported that autogenous dentin grafting results in better, more vital bone compared to allograft materials currently used when histologically analyzed [43].

3.3 Autogenous dentin graft in implant treatment

After tooth extraction, the alveolar ridge typically undergoes resorption, which can reduce the available bone for implant placement [23]. Socket preservation techniques using autogenous dentin grafts aim to prevent this resorption by promoting the regeneration of bone in the extraction site [24, 25]. Dentin grafts are cost effective to place in the socket. They provide structural support and bioactive molecules, helping to maintain the ridge volume and improve conditions for future implant placement.

The growth factors and bioactive molecules released from the dentin stimulate the conversion of M1 to M2 macrophages [44, 45]. This assists in removal of "debris" from the initial surgery and then formation of bone in the same sites. The released growth factors also stimulate osteoblasts to enhance bone formation around the graft and implant site, leading to a faster and more effective osseointegration. This can yield a higher implant success rate, especially in patients with compromised bone quality.

In periodontal and peri-implant treatments, autogenous dentin grafting significantly improves bone fill in the defect being treated while increasing attachment levels to the affected sites [46, 47]. For patients or dentists who are concerned about infected teeth, a study has been done showing that the manufacturer's cleansing process renders the graft fully sterile without altering levels of growth factors contained [48].

4. BioXclude in periodontal and implant treatment

BioXclude is a tissue-engineered, dehydrated human amnion-chorion membrane (dHACM) which contains numerous growth factors and has been used to enhance wound healing [49]. The material is derived from the amnion and chorion layers of the placenta, rich sources of extracellular matrix proteins, growth factors, and cytokines, which have regenerative and anti-inflammatory properties [50]. Clinically, BioXclude in periodontal and implant treatment has gained significant attention due to its ability to promote tissue healing, enhance bone regeneration, and support the integration of dental implants. The growth factors include vascular endothelial growth factor (VEGF), platelet-derived growth factor (PDGF), and fibroblast growth factors (FGF), critical for promoting tissue regeneration [51, 52]. BioXclude modulates the immune response locally. This is beneficial in periodontal and implant procedures where inflammation can delay healing or lead to complications like infection [53].

BioXclude contributes to faster and more predictable outcomes for implant therapy due to the promotion of osteoblastic activity and enhanced osseointegration. This is particularly useful in cases when peri-implant mucositis or peri-implantitis is noted and requires treatment. Studies and clinical trials have supported the effectiveness of BioXclude in periodontal and implant treatments, demonstrating its role in improving tissue healing, promoting bone regeneration, and enhancing implant integration [54, 55]. BioXclude is highly biocompatible, reducing the risk of rejection or allergic reactions compared to bovine or other non-human membrane products. BioXclude represents a significant advancement in regenerative dentistry, offering numerous benefits in both periodontal and implant treatment.

5. Laser therapy in periodontal and implant treatment

Laser therapy in dentistry has gained significant popularity due to its ability to provide effective, non-invasive, and precise treatment for a variety of dental conditions. In periodontal therapy and implant dentistry, lasers offer significant advantages in promoting tissue healing, reducing pain, and improving clinical outcomes. Lasers have shown an ability to enhance the regenerative capacity of hard and soft tissues, reduce bacterial load in the area being treated, and provide minimally invasive treatment options, making them valuable tools in both periodontal and implant treatment.

A laser's mechanism of action results from emitting focused light energy at specific wavelengths, which are absorbed by tissues depending on their properties. In dental treatment, lasers are typically classified according to the tissue they affect and the wavelength they emit. The most commonly used laser types in periodontal and implant therapy are diodes, Er:YAG and Nd:YAG lasers. Diode lasers typically are utilized for soft tissue procedures, such as gingival contouring, soft tissue surgery, and the treatment of periodontal pockets. These lasers work by emitting light that is absorbed by melanin in the soft tissue, leading to tissue cutting with coagulation and with minimal damage to surrounding structures.

Er:YAG and Nd:YAG lasers are generally used for hard tissue and soft tissue treatments respectively. The Er:YAG laser is particularly effective for hard tissue ablation, such as removing calculus deposits on teeth and implants and minor bone recontouring. Whereas the Nd:YAG laser is most often used for soft tissue applications, such as periodontal debridement, gingival recontouring and the treatment of peri-implantitis.

5.1 Laser therapy in periodontal treatment

Periodontal disease is an inflammatory response in the surrounding tissues of the patient [56, 57]. Long-term, this results in the destruction of alveolar bone, periodontal ligament, and gingiva. The goals of periodontal therapy include to arrest disease progression, regenerate lost tissues, and improve the overall health of the periodontium. Laser therapy has been shown to enhance various aspects of periodontal treatment including targeting specific tissues which cannot be done with most other therapeutic modalities.

Laser-assisted periodontal treatment, such as laser-assisted new attachment procedure (LANAP), incorporates Nd:YAG lasers to treat periodontal disease. The laser targets infected tissue within the periodontal pocket and removes or vaporizes associated specific pathogenic species of bacteria creating a disinfected area [58]. This laser removes inflamed, diseased tissue while promoting healing [59]. The laser also stimulates the regeneration of the periodontal ligament and alveolar bone by encouraging fibroblast and osteoblast activity [60]. As is accepted, untreated gingivitis can progress to periodontitis, involving the bone around teeth and implants leading to moderate periodontal disease. Advanced periodontal disease can then lead to tooth or implant loss. Identifying and treating periodontal, peri-implant issues at an early stage can avoid those potential complications.

Laser periodontal treatment has multiple benefits. A key benefit of laser therapy in periodontal disease is its ability to reduce the bacterial load in the periodontal pocket [61]. The bactericidal effect of specific lasers and specific laser protocols contributes to faster and more effective healing, reducing the risk of infection after periodontal therapy. Lasers are highly effective at killing or neutralizing harmful bacteria, including periodontal pathogens such as *Porphyromonas gingivalis* and *Aggregatibacter actinomycetemcomitans*. Laser therapy, when targeting the pathogenic pigmented bacteria, provides a minimally invasive treatment with less tissue damage than conventional surgical methods. As a result, patients experience less post-treatment discomfort, swelling, and bleeding.

Laser therapy has been utilized for its role in periodontal regeneration. Studies suggest that low-level laser therapy (LLLT) can stimulate the production of growth factors and collagen, which are essential for tissue regeneration [61, 62]. Additionally, laser therapy has been shown to promote osteoblast activity, contributing to the regeneration of alveolar bone in cases of bone loss [63]. Laser usage in treatment of periodontal disease can also help prevent systemic spread of these pathogens [1, 61–63].

5.2 Laser therapy in implant treatment

Laser therapy plays an essential role in various stages of implant treatment, from the initial placement of the implant to the management of peri-implantitis.

Peri-implantitis, an inflammatory condition, is one of the leading causes of implant failure. Laser therapy assists in decontaminating the surface of the implant, removing biofilm, infected tissue, and targeting the pathogenic, pigmented bacteria. It also promotes healing by stimulating tissue regeneration and reducing inflammation, which can help improve the long-term success of implants [64].

5.3 Case example: LANAP and LAPIP treatment

A 75 year-old female patient was referred for evaluation and treatment of full mouth periodontal and peri-implant issues with significant bone loss in the lower left posterior sextant. Review of the medical history noted significant medical history including cancer, heart disease and taking Mounjaro, but no contradictions to surgical or non-surgical therapy. Evaluation of the radiographs sent by the referring dentist noted generalized moderate to advanced pocketing, moderate to advanced bone loss, specifically at the implant at the left mandibular 1st molar (**Figure 5**). Periodontal charting was performed noting generalized significant pocketing and bone loss with exudate evident at the 1st molar (**Figure 6**). Clinical findings were discussed with the patient, recommending full mouth laser treatment of the natural teeth (LANAP) and of the affected implants (LAPIP), which the patient accepted.

The patient presented premedicated with Amoxicillin. Local anesthetic was administered. The LANAP//LAPIP protocol was followed including specific laser applications and scaling was performed with Piezoscaler to remove subgingival calculus and attempt to break up the biofilm. Utilizing an Nd:YAG laser (Periolase® MVP-7™, Millennium Dental Technologies, Cerritos, CA) the fiber tip was introduced into the sulcus and maneuvered around the teeth and implants in the quadrants according to the specific protocols. Upon removal of the tip from the sulcus on the buccal of the implant at the 1st molar necrotic, inflamed gingival tissue was adhered to the tip. A 4 X 8 mm piece of BioXclude membrane (**Figure 7**) was placed into the mesial and distal sulcus prior to hemostasis and two sutures were placed. The patient was given an Oralight (Harrisonburg, PA) LED device and instructed to utilize it once daily for 5 minutes and appointed for treatment of the right quadrants.

The patient was seen at 9 months post-treatment to evaluate healing. An absence of gingival inflammation was noted with no bleeding on probing (**Figure 8**). A radiograph was taken to document the bone crestally related to the implant. Periodontal charting demonstrated improved probing depths on the implants and teeth with an absence of gingival bleeding in the majority of the mouth. She was instructed to continue daily use of the Accelite device and continued on 3-month recall. At the 14 month post treatment recall appointment a radiograph was taken the cupping defects on the mesial and distal of the 1st molar implant were not present, having

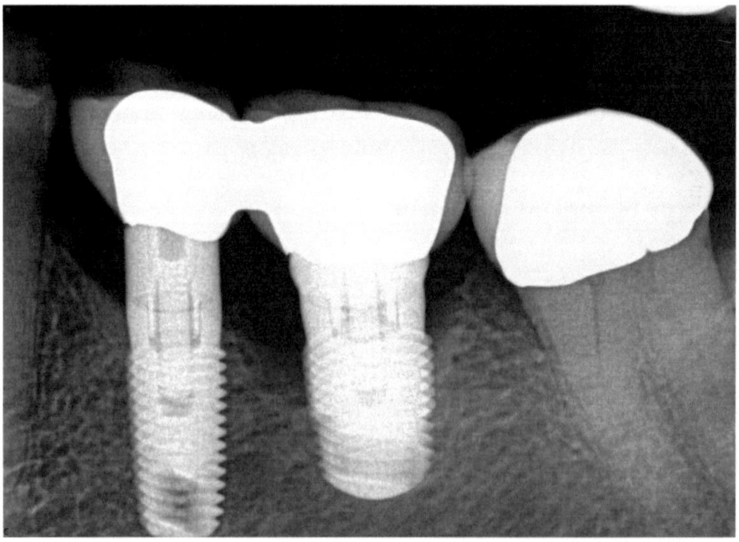

Figure 5.
Initial radiograph demonstrating significant bone loss on the implant at the 1st molar and slight bone loss on the implant at the 2nd premolar.

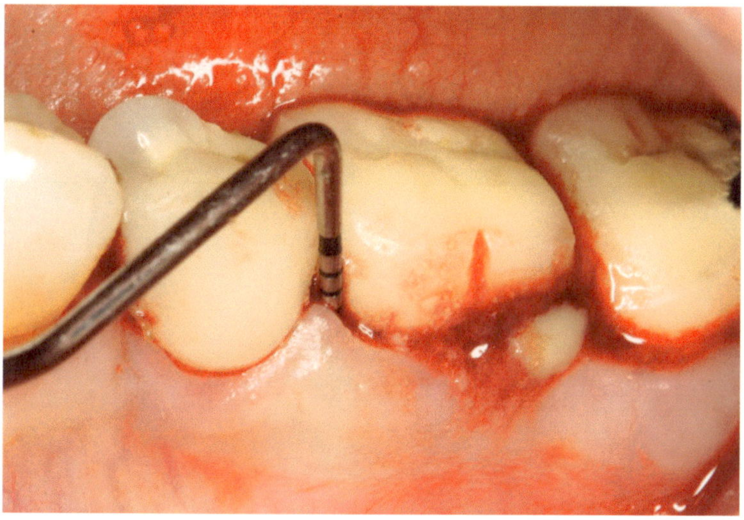

Figure 6.
Periodontal probing on the 1st molar noted exudate in the sulcus.

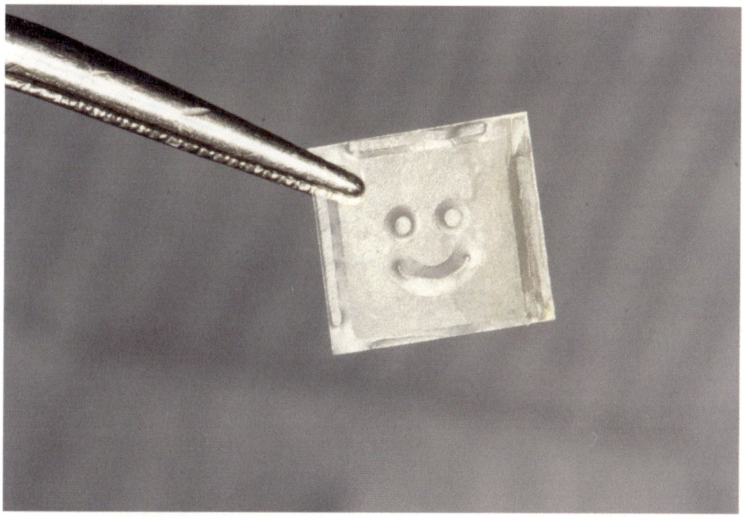

Figure 7.
BioXclude membrane prior to placement in the treated pocket area.

filled above the top thread with bone. A radiograph was taken at the 18-month demonstrated continued bone stability and position relative to the implants (**Figure 9**). Periodontal charting confirmed the quadrant and the rest of the mouth remained stable with no changes in probing depths or bleeding. The patient continued to use the Oralight daily as part of the homecare routine.

5.4 Clinical evidence supporting laser therapy in periodontal and implant treatment

Several clinical studies have demonstrated the effectiveness of laser therapy in periodontal and implant treatments. One study reported that LANAP led to significant

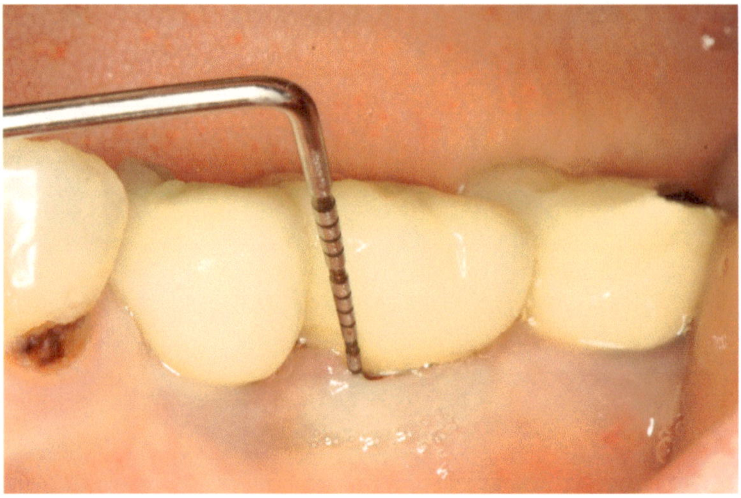

Figure 8.
Periodontal probing 9 months after laser treatment demonstrating improved probing depth and an absence of gingival inflammation.

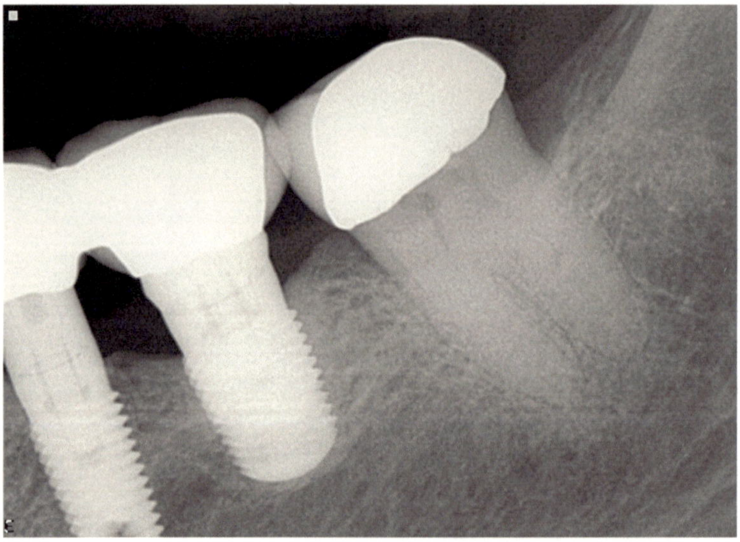

Figure 9.
Radiograph taken 14 months after treatment demonstrating maintenance of bone gain around the implants.

clinical improvements in pocket depth reduction, clinical attachment level gain, and reduced bleeding on probing, compared to traditional surgical methods [65]. Laser therapy (Er:YAG or Nd:YAG) in the treatment of peri-implantitis found that laser decontamination of implant surfaces resulted in significant reductions in probing depth, inflammation, and bleeding, leading to improved clinical outcomes [66]. Additionally, LLLT accelerated soft tissue healing after periodontal surgery, reducing inflammation and postoperative pain while enhancing collagen formation and tissue regeneration [67].

5.5 Advantages of laser therapy

Laser therapy offers a minimally invasive, precise approach for treating periodontal disease and performing implant-related procedures, reducing the need for incisions, flaps and sutures. Patients report less pain, swelling, and bleeding following laser therapy. Laser therapy reduces the bacterial load, decreasing the risk of infection and improving healing outcomes [68–71].

6. Platelet derived growth factor

Gem 21S® (Geistlich North America, Franklin, TN) is a regenerative bioactive material that is used widely in periodontal and implant dentistry. This material contains recombinant human platelet-derived growth factor (rhPDGF-BB). It has shown significant promise in enhancing healing in dentoalveolar, periodontal and peri-implant tissue regeneration [72]. This growth factor works through promotion of cellular recruitment, proliferation, and differentiation, particularly of osteoblasts, periodontal ligament cells, and gingival fibroblasts. rhPDGF-BB is a potent mitogen, specifically stimulates the proliferation of these critical cell types and facilitating the regeneration of periodontal tissues, enhancing bone formation in the areas being treated. This is highly beneficial in the treatment of extraction sockets, ridge augmentation, and periodontal defects.

A graft mixture may be hydrated with GEM 21S® and placed in the socket following tooth extraction to stimulate the regeneration of bone and soft tissues. Numerous studies have demonstrated the use of GEM 21S® resulting in enhanced bone formation and better preservation of the ridge architecture [73–75]. A recent study demonstrated that patients who underwent ridge augmentation with GEM 21S® had higher success rates for implant integration and fewer complications post-surgery [76].

Periodontitis often results in significant hard and soft tissue loss around teeth, many times with tooth loss. Studies have demonstrated that when GEM 21S® is applied in periodontal defects, there is an increase in both osseous fill and periodontal ligament attachment to the tooth being treated [77]. In a clinical trial, rhPDGF-BB was utilized for the treatment of infrabony defects in patients with periodontitis [78]. That study demonstrated that rhPDGF-BB significantly improved clinical attachment levels and radiographic bone fill compared to traditional surgical treatments.

Studies have demonstrated the clinical efficacy of GEM 21S® in ridge augmentation [79] and periodontal regeneration procedures [80]. As reported in a randomized controlled trial, GEM 21S® was evaluated for socket preservation following tooth extraction [81]. The test sites had significantly increased bone density in the extraction socket compared to controls which can lead to improved outcomes for subsequent implant placement [82, 83]. Several studies reported in the treatment of periodontal defect regeneration, GEM 21S® was used in periodontal regeneration for the treatment of Class II furcation defects [84, 85]. The results reported that significant improvements in both clinical attachment and bone levels, with patients experiencing long-term benefits from the treatment. GEM 21S® also has applications in treatment of the missing alveolar structure in peri-implantitis [86].

6.1 Case example: Socket grafting, ridge augmentation and periodontal treatment

A 72-year-old patient presented on referral with a failing lower left mandibular 2nd molar. A radiograph was taken to assist in the clinical analysis. The tooth was tipped mesially and the 1st molar was missing. Probing and mobility confirmed that the tooth was severely periodontally involved, caused the loss of significant periodontal attachment on the mesial of the adjacent 3rd molar and alveolar bone. Extraction of the 2nd molar was recommended. Review of the medical history noted high blood pressure, a thyroid issue and high cholesterol. The patient was on antibiotics, prescribed by her general dentist. The treatment plan was reviewed with the patient who accepted the recommendations.

The consent form was reviewed and signed by the patient. Local anesthetic was administered. Blood was drawn from the patent to create PRF. The mandibular 2nd molar was extracted atraumatically (**Figure 10**). A crestal incision was made at the in the edentulous area and a full thickness flap elevated to expose the area being treated. The socket was curetted to debride it as well as the mesial and buccal aspects of the 3rd molar that had bone loss related to the periodontal issues from the 2nd molar. A graft of Bio-Oss (Geistlich, Princeton, NJ) and Mineralized Cortical Allograft was hydrated with GEM 21S and mixed with DFDBA fibers (Vallos F, Geistlich). This was hydrated and mixed with L- PRF (IntraSpin, BioHorizons, Birmingham, AL) to create a "block" of bone. The graft mixture was placed to fill the extraction socket, fill the defect on the mesial and buccal furcation of the 3rd molar and augment the ridge at the missing 1st molar site. The grafts were covered with BioXclude in all sites with an additional barrier of Ossix Plus (Dentsply Sirona, Charlotte, North Carolina) over the ridge augmentation site in the first molar area. All sites were then covered with L-PRF barriers. The flap margins were reapproximated to get primary closure and secured with PTFE (Osteogenics, Lubbock, TX) sutures. A radiograph was taken to document fill of the socket and defects with the graft material. The patient was dismissed and appointed for a follow-up appointment.

At 11-months post extraction and socket grafting the patient was ready to proceed with implant placement at the 1st and 2nd molar sites. A CBCT was taken to evaluate the grafted area and demonstrated a homogenous appearance of the graft with the surrounding host bone. The consent form was reviewed with the patient and signed. Local

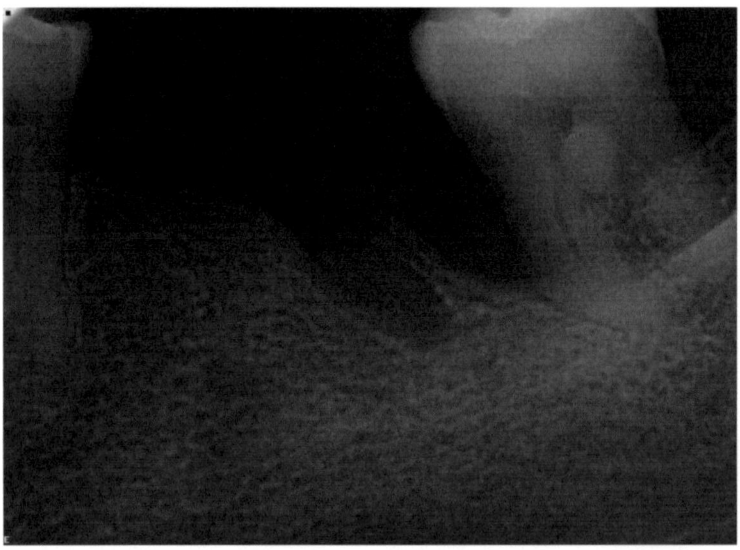

Figure 10.
Radiograph taken following extraction of tooth # 18 showing the size and location of the alveolar and periodontal defects.

anesthetic was administered, and the site was flapped following placement of a crestal incision. The crest presented with fill of the site and blending of the graft material with the host's bone. A core sample was taken at the 2nd molar site utilizing a 3.0 mm trephine drill to be sent for histological analysis. Appropriate length and width dental implants were placed. The flaps were reapproximated to get primary closure following placement of cover screws in the implants and the flaps were secured with sutures. The patient was dismissed, and the core sample was sent for histological analysis.

The core was received at the Hard Tissue Laboratory of the University of Minnesota Dental School. It was mounted, then sectioned and stained with Stevenel's blue and Van Gieson's picric fuchsin dyes. Gross evaluation revealed 81% bone, 100% vital and 18% marrow or fibrous tissue. When analyzed at medium power (40x magnification) very dense trabeculae with a good amount of vital cancellous bone (VB) was noted (**Figure 11**). New bone formation (NB) as well as bone remodeling and delicate marrow space (MS) was noted. This image shows different staining qualities reflect the varying maturity levels of the different areas of the bone, with darker red-staining bone being less mature than the lighter staining bone The different staining qualities reflect the varying maturity levels of the different areas of the bone; darker red-staining bone is less mature than the lighter staining bone. The most interesting finding was that all of the allograft and xenograft had been resorbed and replaced by vital bone, making this site ideal for lacement of dental implants.

The patient presented at 8-months post implant placement to expose the implants and initiate the restorative phase of treatment. Local anesthetic was administered, an incision made, flaps elevated and the implants were exposed. The cover screws were removed and healing abutments placed. Due to the moderate Osstell measurement of 58 on the shorter distal implant, a Magdent (Magdent MED, Bnei Brak, Israel) healing abutment was inserted (**Figure 12**). The healing abutment is activated in a device giving it a magnetic charge. This will last for a month, improving bone density in the site and increasing osseointegration and implant stability. The soft tissue was reapproximated and secured with sutures.

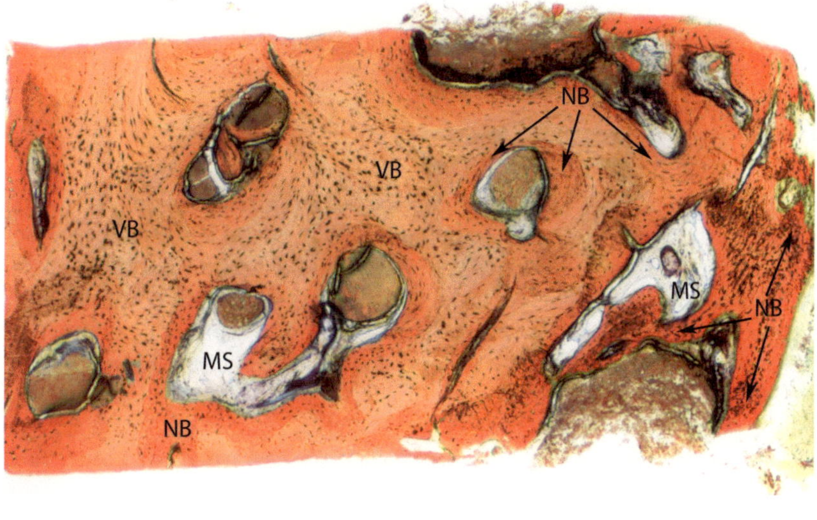

Figure 11.
Histological analysis of the core sample at 40x magnification.

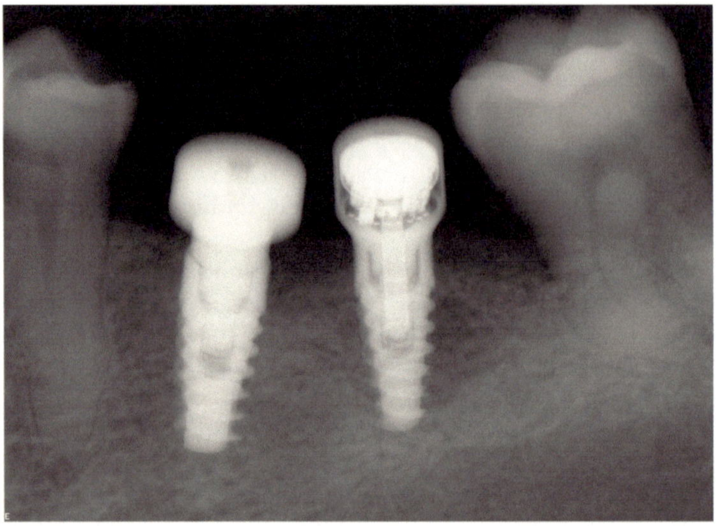

Figure 12.
Periapical radiograph following placement of healing abutments following implant exposure including the magnetic healing abutment (Magdent) to continue to improve osseointegration.

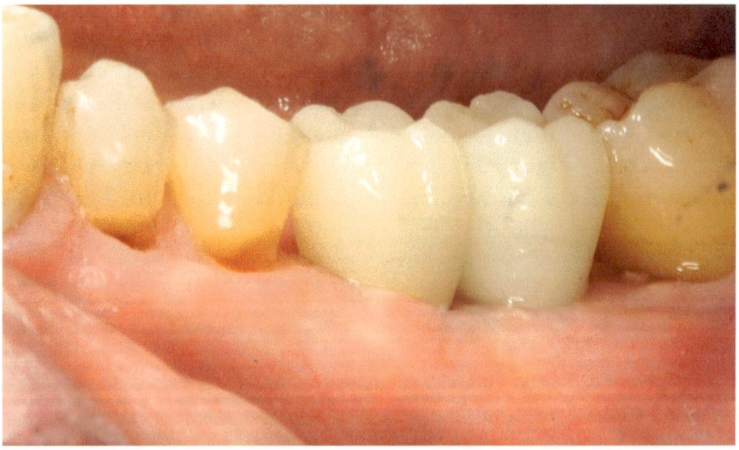

Figure 13.
Clinical view of restored implants.

The patient returned 4 weeks later for impressions for restoration of the implants. The stability of the distal implant had increased to 77 due to the effects of the MagDent healing abutment. As has been reported in the literature, magnetic fields can improve bone healing [18]. This took the implant from one with questionable osseointegration to one the surgeon, restorative dentist and patient can rely upon. The restorations were returned from the lab and inserted intraorally (**Figure 13**).

7. Photobiomodulation (PBM) in periodontal and implant treatment

Photobiomodulation (PBM), also known as low-level laser therapy (LLLT), is an innovative non-invasive therapeutic modality that utilizes light energy to promote tissue healing and regeneration. PBM has gained considerable attention in periodontal therapy and implant dentistry due to its ability to enhance wound healing, reduce inflammation, alleviate pain, improving overall treatment outcomes. PBM operates by applying specific wavelengths of light to targeted tissues, resulting in cellular responses that stimulate tissue repair, regeneration, while modulating the immune response.

The mechanisms of PBM work by delivering low-intensity light, in the red or near-infrared spectrum (600 to 1000 nm), to the tissue. The primary mechanism of PBM is the absorption of light energy by cellular chromophores, mainly cytochrome c oxidase in mitochondria [87]. This leads to several biochemical and physiological effects, eliminate the including and end the prior line with a period. The next paragraphs describe in detail the physiological and biochemical effects.

PBM stimulates the mitochondria, resulting in an increase in adenosine triphosphate (ATP) production and the downstream release of growth factors. Increased ATP production results from absorption of light by cytochrome c oxidase stimulating mitochondrial activity. ATP is the primary energy source for cells, and increased ATP availability promotes cell proliferation, migration, and tissue repair [88]. The binding of growth factors to cell surface receptors induces signaling pathways that transmit to the nucleus for the transcription of genes for increased cellular proliferation, viability, with migration of numerous cell types, including stem cells and fibroblasts [89]. PBM research demonstrated that osteoblasts showed increased mitochondrial ATP production, increased osteoblast activity and proliferation, increased and pro-osteoblast expression in the presence of red and NIR (near infrared) radiation [90]. NIR irradiation further elevated the expression of bone matrix-related genes fostering enhanced deposition and maturation of fibrillar collagen. This study demonstrates that PBM has the potential to enhance osteogenic functionality within a translational organotypic bone culture system [91].

Additionally, PBM has been shown to stimulate fibroblast activity and collagen synthesis, which is crucial for wound healing and tissue regeneration. The density of collagen expression was significantly higher in an in vivo study in the PBM treatment group [92]. PBM has also reported positive photobiostimulatory effects on bone regeneration, accelerating its process regardless of the biomaterials utilized [93]. The anti-inflammatory effects with the use of PBM has reported a reduction in the production of pro-inflammatory mediators, such as cytokines (TNF-α, IL-6) and prostaglandins. Thus, modulating the immune response by decreasing inflammation and promoting tissue homeostasis, is essential for faster and more efficient healing [94]. This enables management of the hyper-inflammatory response characteristic of periodontitis and also following surgical intervention when treatment is being performed [95]. Increased circulation and angiogenesis are also benefits of PBM treatment. As it promotes vasodilation and enhances blood circulation in the treated area, resulting in improved blood flow which increases oxygen, nutrients, and growth factors to the tissue, accelerating healing. Additionally, PBM promotes angiogenesis, which is vital for tissue regeneration and repair [96, 97]. Additionally, PBM has an analgesic effect by stimulating the release of endorphins reducing the transmission of pain signals. This is particularly beneficial in the post-operative period for patients undergoing periodontal or implant treatment [98].

PBM has demonstrated benefits in accelerating tissue regeneration, reducing inflammation, and improving the outcomes of various periodontal procedures. This leads to quicker patient post-operative recovery, a reduced risk of infection, and improved tissue regeneration [99]. PBM is frequently used in GTR procedures to promote the regeneration of the periodontal ligament and alveolar bone, by enhancing osteoblast activity and stimulating collagen production. Thus, supporting regeneration of lost tissues improving the clinical outcomes of GTR. Utilization has proven effective regarding bone repair, when associated with bone regeneration techniques [100]. PBM therapy has shown to improve dentoalveolar-derived mesenchymal stem cells (ddMSCs), with no deleterious effects and a tendency to improve ddMSCs' viability and proliferation [101].

Regarding the treatment of periodontal inflammation, PBM aids in reducing inflammation by modulating the immune response and decreasing the levels of inflammatory cytokines. This leads to reduced swelling and faster resolution of periodontal or peri-implant infections [59]. A reduction of bleeding related to PBM therapy relates to its ability to stimulate vasodilation and enhance blood circulation which can lead to reduced bleeding during and after periodontal surgeries. This improves visibility in the surgical field and enhances the healing process by delivering more oxygen and nutrients to the treated area [102].

PBM can be used as an adjunct to traditional mechanical therapies like scaling and root planing (SRP). It accelerates the healing of gingival tissues, enhancing the reattachment of periodontal ligament fibers (reducing tooth mobility), and reduces post-operative inflammation, contributing to improved clinical outcomes and overall patient comfort [103–106]. PBM provides significant pain relief without the need for medication [107]. The author has noted anecdotally that with over 98% of the surgical and LANAP/LAPIP patients treated, only OTC analgesics are used for control of discomfort. In about 70%, none are taken after the first night.

PBM has been shown to enhance osseointegration by increasing ATP production and promoting the activity of osteoblasts, thereby improving bone formation around the implant [108]. PBM therapy improved new trabecular bone formation and their connectivity which increased the bone surface, indicating the positive effect on alveolar socket repair [109, 110]. In patients that require sinus augmentation (crestal or lateral approach) for implant placement in the maxilla, PBM has demonstrated enhanced healing of the sinus membrane while promoting bone regeneration. By stimulating cell proliferation and collagen synthesis, PBM accelerates bone healing in the sinus cavity, improving the success rate of implant placement there [111].

PBM helps eliminate inflammation and stimulates tissue regeneration, contributing to better outcomes in peri-implantitis therapy [112, 113]. By enhancing collagen production and reducing inflammation, PBM contributes to the formation of healthy and aesthetic peri-implant mucosa [114, 115]. PBM provides significant analgesic effects by stimulating the release of endorphins and reducing the release of inflammatory mediators, offering faster recovery and a more comfortable postoperative experiences [116].

PBM's antimicrobial effects assist in reducing bacterial load, lowering the risk of infection after periodontal and implant surgeries [117, 118]. PBM is non-invasive treatment, making it a comfortable treatment option for patients. Intraoral units allow the patient to use PBM at home, throughout their mouth, on a daily basis to maximize periodontal and implant treatment results and prevent potential issues long-term.

7.1 Case example: Extraction, socket grafting, implant placement with PBM augmentation

A 49-year-old male patient was referred for evaluation and treatment of the lower left molars which presented with loss of the majority of the coronal tooth structure and decay on both teeth (**Figures 14** and **15**). Both teeth were deemed "non-restorable".

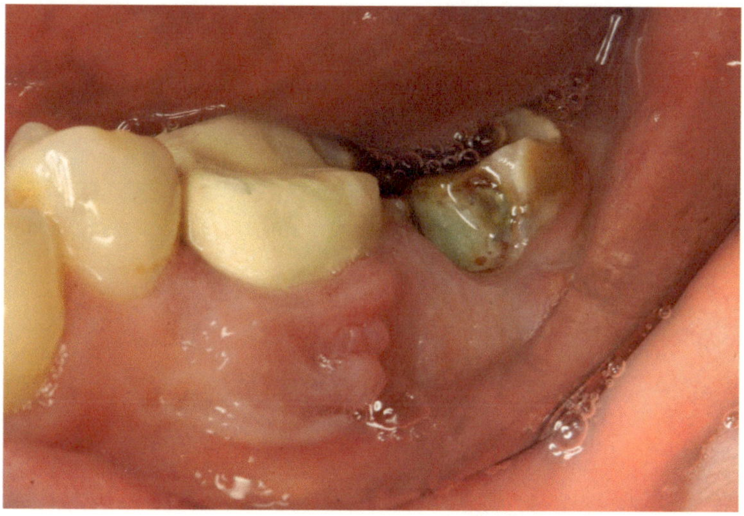

Figure 14.
Clinical appearance of the left mandibular 1st and 2nd molars.

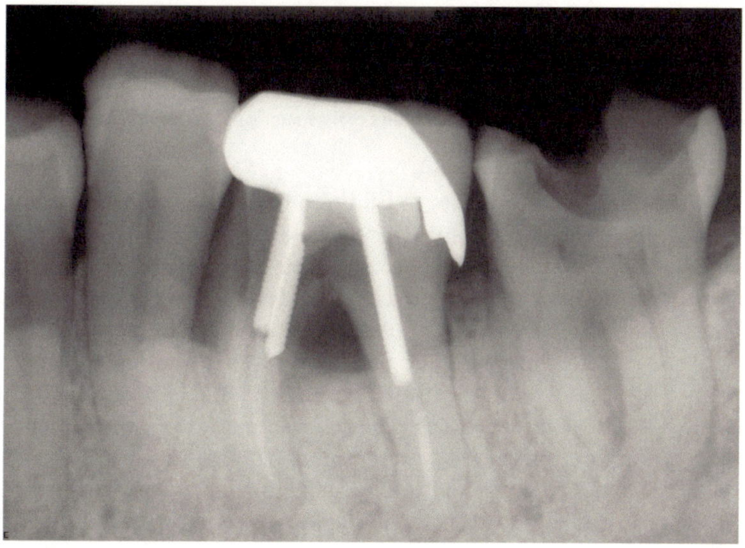

Figure 15.
Periapical radiograph of the mandibular left 1st and 2nd molars demonstrating significant coronal breakdown on the 2nd molar and recurrent caries on the 1st molar with bone loss in the furcation.

Treatment was discussed with the patient and extraction was recommended for both teeth with socket grafting and later implant placement. The patient agreed to the suggested treatment.

The patient presented for treatment and the consent form was reviewed and signed by the patient. Local anesthetic was administered and blood drawn for fabrication of L-PRF. The 1st and 2nd molars were atraumatically extracted and the sockets cleaned and debrided (**Figure 16**). The distal of the 2nd premolar root was planned and treated with citric acid. The L-PRF created from the drawn blood of the patient was mixed with cortico-cancellous bone (Maxxeus) to fabricate a bone "block". This

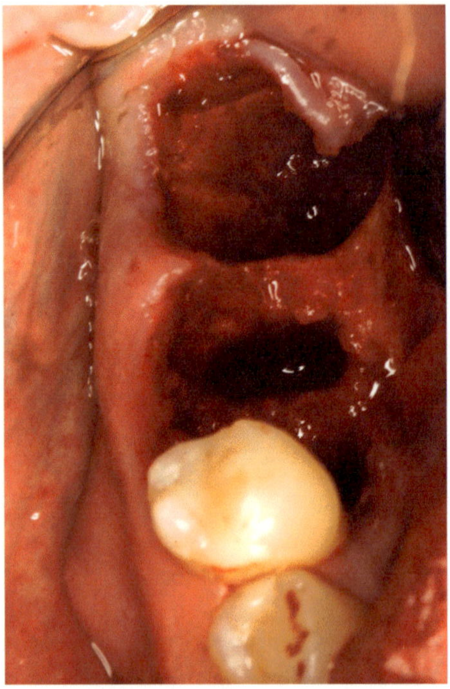

Figure 16.
Extraction sockets following extraction of the 1st and 2nd molars showing significant buccal bone loss.

was placed into the extraction sockets to fill them to the ideal level crestally, which was about 5 mm above the current furcation. The distal surface of tooth # 20 was also grafted supra-alveolarly to ideal height. An amnion-chorion barrier membrane (BioXclude) was placed over the graft material and tucked under the flap margins (**Figure 17**). The site was closed with PGA sutures and postoperative instructions reviewed with the patient. An Oralight PBM device was dispensed and the patient instructed to use it twice daily for 5-minutes each session.

Five months after periodontal treatment and socket grafting the patient presented in preparation for implant placement, indicating he had continued to use the Accelite PBM device as directed. Examination noted the gingival tissue over the healed extraction sites was keratinized and non-inflamed. A periapical radiograph and CBCT were taken and showed the sockets were filled with dense bone similar to adjacent host bone. The surgical consent form was reviewed and signed by the patient. Local anesthetic was administered, and a full thickness flap was elevated. A core was taken at both planned implant sites utilizing a 3 mm outer diameter trephine drill to send a retrieved sample for histological analysis. The alveolar bone was at a significantly elevated height above the initial furcation location in the areas of the extracted teeth, ideal buccal contour was reestablished, and the bone level is now above the initial periodontal defect on the distal of tooth # 20.

Osteotomies were created at both sites and a 5 x 12 mm implant (Kontact, Biotech Dental, Englewood, NJ) was placed into each site (**Figure 18**) achieving good initial stability with an ISQ reading of 75 using the Ostell device. Healing abutments were inserted and the flaps sutured. A periapical radiograph was taken to document the implant placement.

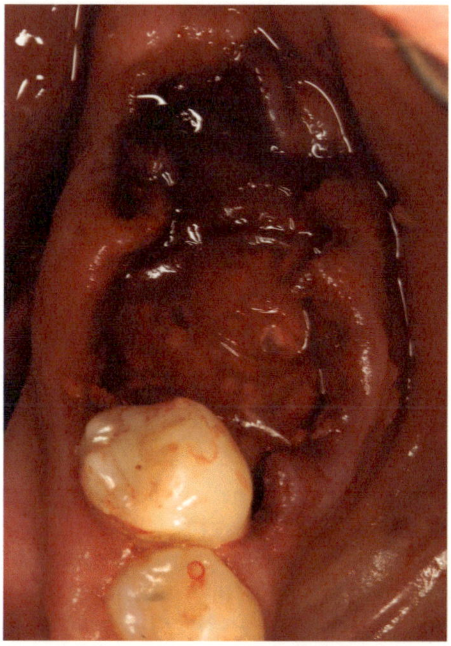

Figure 17.
A BioXclude membrane was placed over the grafted sockets, prior to being covered with PRF and sutures.

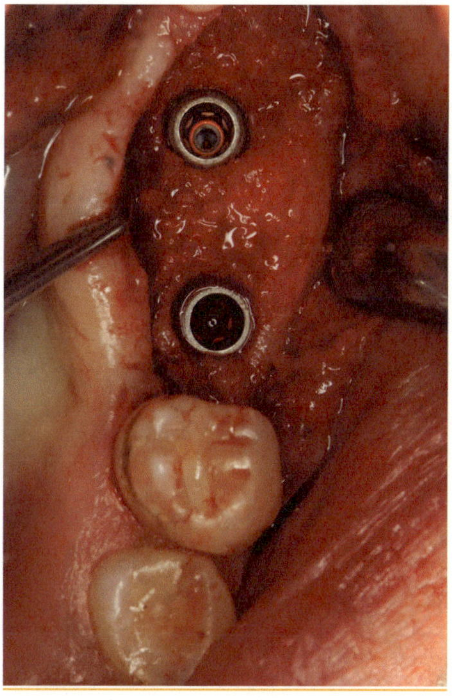

Figure 18.
Implants placed into the previously grafted sites in wide, healthy bone with no visible graft particles.

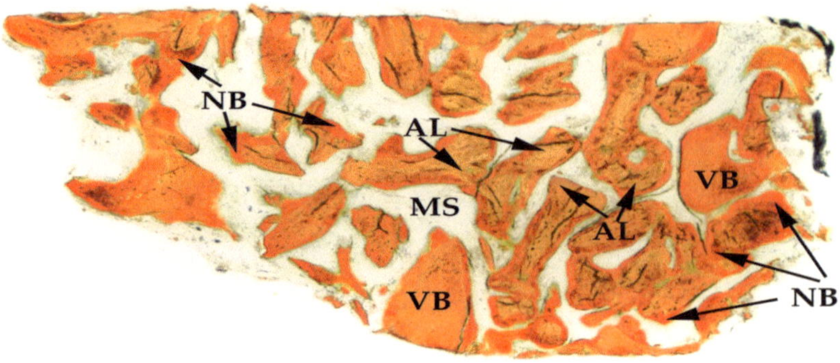

Figure 19.
Histological analysis of site #19 showing allograft converted to vital bone and significant amounts of new and vital bone.

Core samples were processed and stained with Stevenel's blue and Van Gieson's picro fuchsin and analyzed histologically by the lab. Site #19 was analyzed at 20x demonstrating solid, new bone (NB) (**Figure 19**). The majority of the bone is immature, vital bone. The trabeculae are quite thick and numerous and concentrated lacunae filled with osteocyte cells (OC) in the newly formed bone are present. This core shows 67% bone, 92% of which is vital (VB), 8% of which is residual mineralized allograft and 33% marrow. This low-power photomicrograph shows a fairly solid core with good new bone (NB) formation around the few remaining allograft particle. The cancellous network is well formed with good, thick trabeculae bridging among the allograft particle (AL) with good connectivity. The vast majority of the allograft has been replaced by a combination of osteoclastic resorption and vital cell ingrowth into the osteocytic lacunae of the previously non-vital graft particles.

Twelve months after implant placement, the patient presented to begin restoration of the implants. The gingival tissues presented with an absence of inflammation.

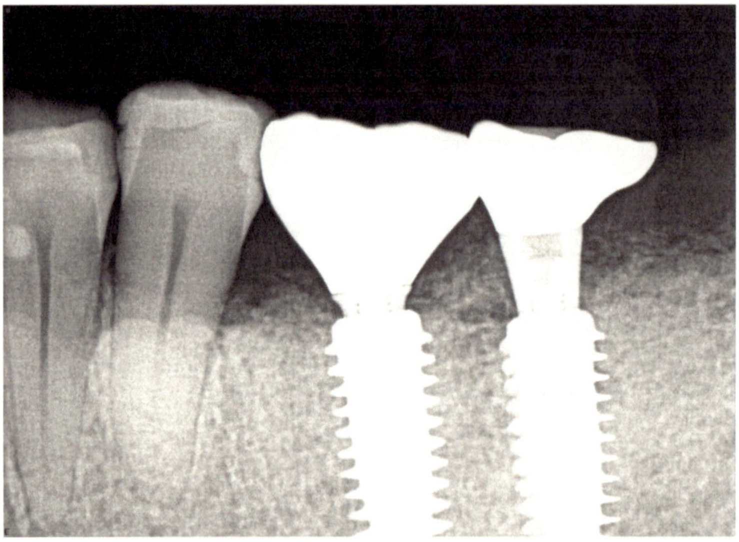

Figure 20.
Periapical radiograph of the implants demonstrating stability of the bone above the initial alveolar crest in all areas 18 months after loading.

Digital impressions were taken to send to the lab. The screw-retained restorations were inserted 2 weeks later. A periapical radiograph was taken to verify mating of the prosthetics with the implant at the connector and document the stability of the bone in relation to the crestal aspect of the implant. The clinical result achieved natural aesthetics. Eighteen months later, the supra-crestal bone is evident between, around the implants and on the distal of tooth # 20 approximately 5 mm higher than at the initiation of therapy (**Figure 20**).

8. Low magnitude high-frequency vibration (LMHFV) in periodontal and implant treatment

Low Magnitude High-Frequency Vibration (LMHFV) therapy is a non-invasive treatment modality utilizing mechanical vibrations of low amplitude and high frequency to stimulate tissue healing and regeneration. It has gained attention in both periodontal and implant dentistry due to its ability to enhance bone regeneration, accelerate healing, improve implant stability, and reduce the risk of complications. LMHFV therapy involves the application of mechanical vibrations that are delivered at low magnitudes at high frequencies (typically in the range of 20 to 50 Hz) to targeted tissues. These vibrations interact with the tissue at a cellular and molecular level, producing beneficial effects [117, 118].

The key mechanisms by which LMHFV works include stimulation of osteoblasts and osteoclasts, expression of bone growth factors, enhance microcirculation, increased collagen synthesis and a reduction in inflammation. This creates a balance between bone formation and resorption, promoting bone remodeling and enhancing bone healing in periodontal tissues (hard and soft tissue) and around dental implants [119]. Osteocytes are sensitive to vibration stimuli and are able to sense LMHFV by producing soluble factors that inhibit osteoclast formation [120]. LMHFV also exhibits a protective effect on osteoblasts by regulating their proliferation, migration and differentiation [121]. The vibrations assist by increasing the expression of bone growth factors such as transforming growth factor-beta (TGF-β), bone morphogenetic proteins (BMPs), and vascular endothelial growth factor (VEGF). Those factors are crucial for stimulating bone formation and angiogenesis, leading to improved osseointegration and bone regeneration [122, 123]. Research in orthopedics has supported these findings that LMHFV enhances bone remodeling and stimulates cells that improve osseous conditions [124–126]. Additionally, LMHFV promotes microcirculation by increasing blood flow to the treated area, which improves oxygen, nutrients, and growth factors. This enhanced circulation accelerates tissue healing, including periodontal tissues and the bone surrounding dental implants [127, 128]. Increased collagen synthesis results from the mechanical vibrations stimulating fibroblast activity. Collagen is essential for wound healing, tissue regeneration, and the stabilization of periodontal and peri-implant tissues [129]. LMHFV has been shown to reduce inflammation in the affected tissues by modulating the inflammatory response. Reduction in the levels of pro-inflammatory cytokines promotes healing of soft and hard tissues [123].

Studies have shown that implants subjected to LMHFV therapy exhibit enhanced stability and improved long-term success rates [130]. When used as an adjunct in the treatment of peri-implantitis by stimulating graft replacement, bone regeneration and reducing inflammation, the therapy enhances healing of all tissues and promotes bone remodeling, which can help save implants affected by peri-implantitis [118, 119].

LMHFV therapy is non-invasive and can be incorporated into the patient's homecare schedule, only requiring one or two 5-minute sessions daily. As the time necessary is minimal, patient compliance is improved. The HF Alveo5 LMHFV device (Houston, TX) device is cordless and compact, placed intraorally and occluded on lightly so that vibration can be felt in the jaws.

8.1 Case example: LMHFV to enhance socket grafting

A 76-year-old male patient presented for extraction of the non-restorable teeth in the right maxillary quadrant. Examination noted a fixed bridge from the right maxillary 1st molar to the right central incisor. There was significant decay in the prosthetic abutments. Site collapse was noted in the edentulous areas and the bridge exhibited Class 2 mobility. The clinical presentation and findings were discussed with the patient, as well as treatment options. The patient indicated he wished a fixed restoration so a treatment plan involving extraction of teeth, socket grafting and delayed placement of implants.

A consent form was reviewed with the patient and signed. Blood was drawn to create PRF (BioPRF, Jupiter, FL). Local anesthetic was administered. The bridge was sectioned and removed (**Figure 21 left**). The 1st molar, residual root at the 2nd premolar, canine and central incisor were atraumatically extracted. The patient did not wish the roots of the 2nd molar extracted. The extraction sockets were cleaned and debrided (**Figure 21 right**). A "block" was fabricated from the PRF mixed with cortico-cancellous bone (Maxxeus). Large defects were noted in the areas of teeth #s 3–4 and 6–7. The extraction sockets were filled with the graft, edentulous areas were grafted to restore ideal volume (**Figure 22 left**). Amnion-chorion barrier membranes

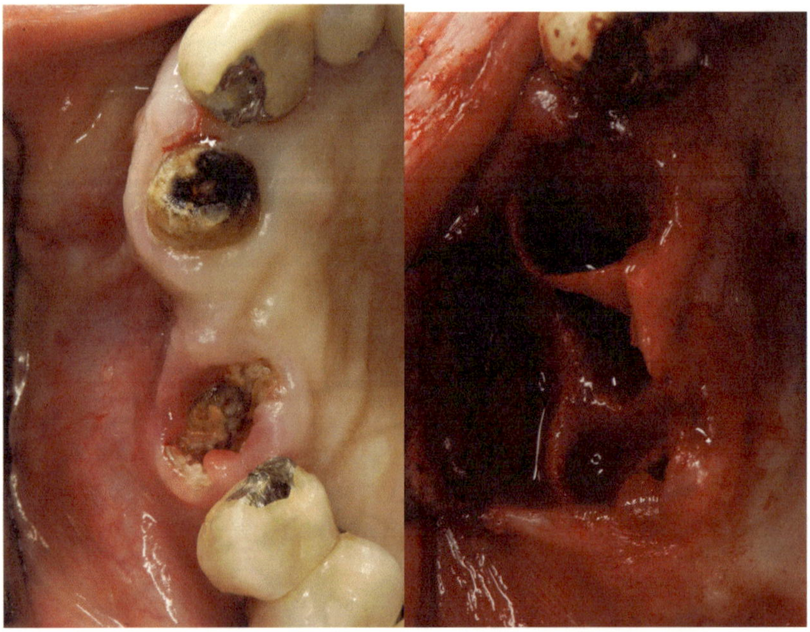

Figure 21.
Initial presentation then the sockets following extraction of the canine and central incisor showing extremely thin buccal plate # 8, missing buccal plate on # 6 and full site collapse at # 7.

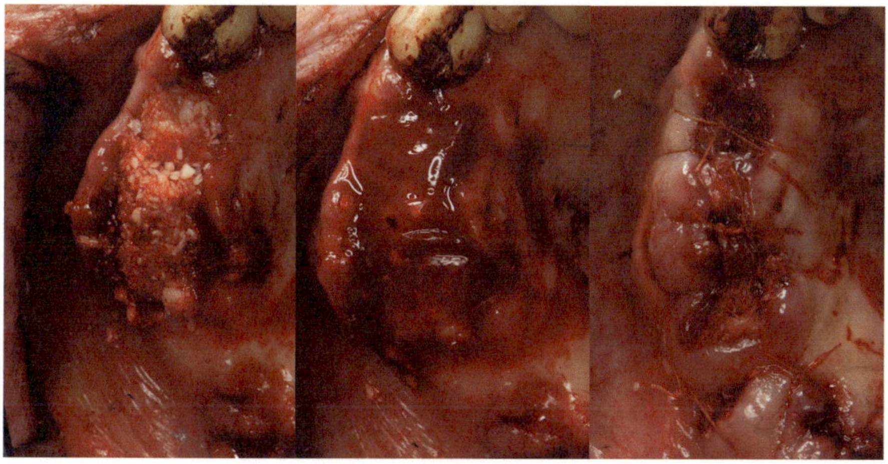

Figure 22.
The extraction sockets were filled with the PRF graft block (left), covered with a BioXclude (middle), PRF and then sutured (right).

(BioXclude) were placed over graft material and tucked under the flap margins (**Figure 22 middle**). The site was covered with a BioPRF barrier, flaps closed with no attempt at primary closure. PGA sutures were placed (**Figure 22 right**) and postoperative instructions reviewed with the patient. The patient was dispensed an Alveo 5 LMHFV device (**Figure 23**) and instructed to use it twice daily for the recommended 5-minutes each session and continue until returning for the post-operative appointment.

At the 6-month post socket grafting appointment the patient presented to initiate implant placement into the grafted ridge. He indicated that since the extraction and socket grafting appointment he had continued to use the Ptech LMHFV device twice daily. Soft tissue overlaying the posterior right quadrant demonstrated healthy

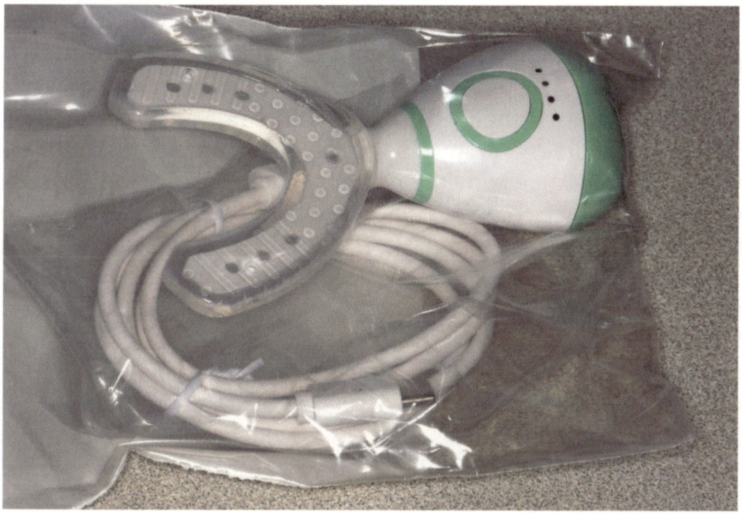

Figure 23.
Alveo5 device with charging cable.

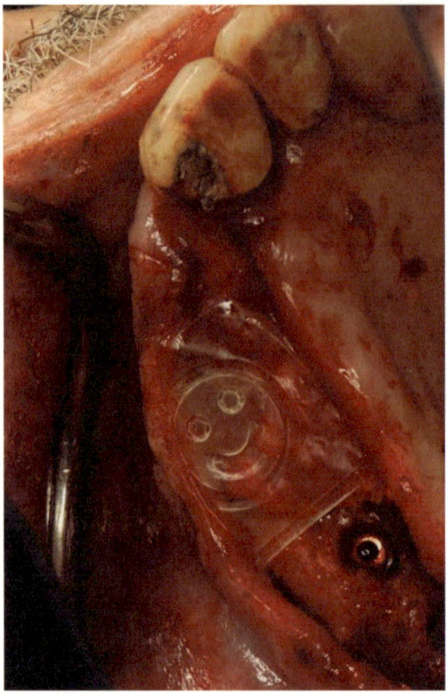

Figure 24.
A BioXclude membrane was placed over the secondary, contour graft, prior to covering with PRF and suturing.

keratinized non-inflamed tissue. Radiographs were taken that demonstrated dense bone in the socket that were grafted blending well with the surrounding host bone (**Figure 24**). The consent form for implant placement was reviewed and signed by the patient. Local anesthetic was administered, and a full thickness flap was elevated.

Evaluation of the CBCT showed excellent bone volume and density in the locations required for implant placement. The crest of the ridge presented with dense bone fill except a slight defect at the 2nd premolar area. Cores were taken from the 2nd premolar, canine and central incisor sites using a 3.0 mm trephine drill for histological analysis. Osteotomies were completed and 4 x 12 mm implants (Kontact, Biotech Dental) were placed at the 2nd premolar, 1st premolar, canine and central incisor sites. Cover screws were placed on the implants. Blood was drawn to create BioPRF to mix with cortico-cancellous bone (Maxxeus) to fill any minor defects and for contour grafting to improve the emergence profile of the soft tissues. A BioXclude membrane was placed over the graft material (**Figure 23**). A BioPRF membrane was placed over the implants and the flap margins reapproximated and sutured. The patient was instructed to continue twice daily use of the Alveo5 LMHFV device.

Core samples were processed and stained with Stevenel's blue and Van Gieson's picro fuchsin and analyzed histologically by the lab. Analysis of the core sample at site #8 noted 77% bone, 100% of which is vital 0% of which is residual mineralized allograft and 23% of marrow. The medium power photomicrograph (40x) shows the dense bone that could be cortical bone or could be very dense trabeculae of cancellous

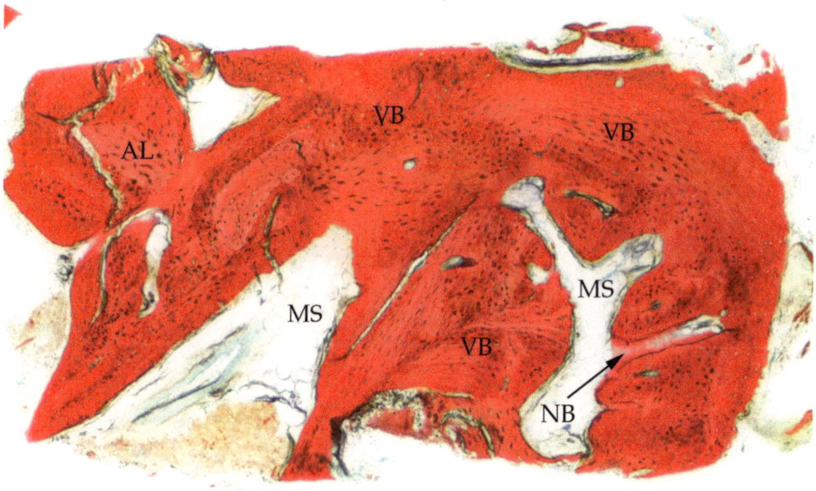

Figure 25.
Histological analysis of site #8 at 40x.

bone (**Figure 24**). Microscopic view emphasizes the immature nature of the bone and shows the thick trabeculae with active new bone formation at the edge of the trabeculae. Most of the bone seems to be vital bone (VB) and new bone (NB) surrounding what is most likely revitalized mineralized allograft (AL) (**Figure 25**). The image shows very delicate, non-inflamed marrow (MS). Conversion of mineralized allograft to vital bone in the absence of growth factors has not previously been reported in the literature. Having complete vital bone around a tooth or implant should greatly improve the longevity of either.

The patient presented at 6-months post implant placement for implant uncovery to initiate the restorative phase of treatment. Local anesthetic was administered, and a full thickness flap was elevated. It was noted that bone was either completely or partially covering the implants. Bone was removed to expose the cover screws. They were removed and healing abutments placed. Implant stability (ISQ) was taken with the Osstell unit – all implants registered 75+. Bond Apatite (Augma Biomaterials, Spotswood, NJ) was mixed and placed filling the area between the healing abutments and covering the crestal aspect of the ridge. The flaps were then sutured. Bond Apatite sets hard and acts as barrier so narrow areas that are not covered do not require a membrane and the soft tissue will migrate over it during healing. The material also converts to bone over time. Periapical radiographs were taken to confirm seating of the healing abutments, graft placement and document the crestal bone level in relation to the implants.

The patient returned at 4 weeks to uncover the implants and gingiva that had covered the graft material. After healing, he was sent for restoration Radiographs of the final bridge demonstrating stable bone around the implants and no pathology around the remaining 2nd molar. The final prosthesis provided an aesthetic result (**Figure 26**). The patient was instructed to continue use of the Alveo5 LMHFV device daily to aid in maintaining the bone in contact with the implants.

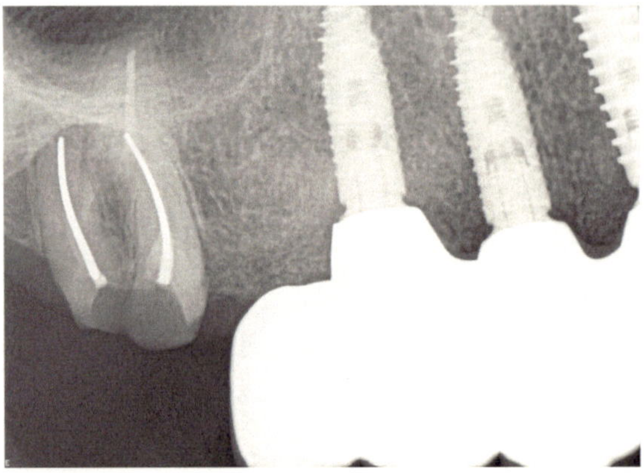

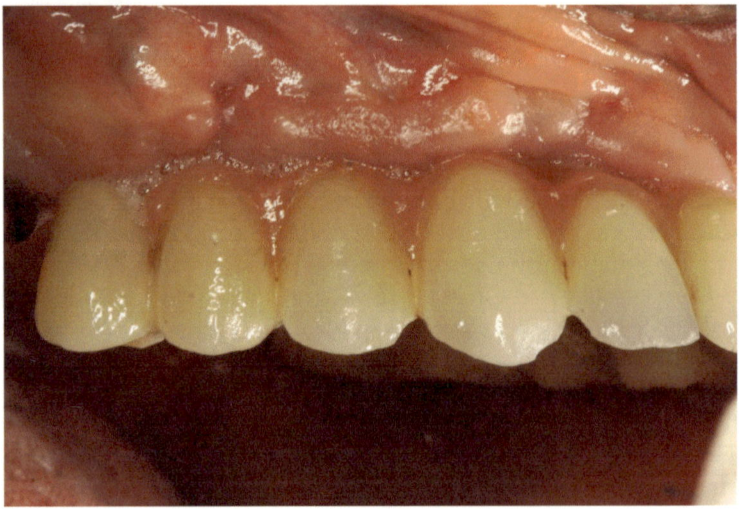

Figure 26.
Radiographic, clinical appearances following placement of the final restoration.

9. Conclusion

The integration of biologically active materials and innovative therapeutic modalities has revolutionized periodontal and peri-implant regeneration, offering clinicians powerful tools to enhance healing and clinical outcomes. The use of growth factors, such as those found in GEM 21S®, Platelet-Rich Fibrin (PRF), BioXclude and autogenous dentin grafts, represents a shift toward biologically driven strategies that optimize tissue regeneration. GEM 21S®, with its regenerative potential through rhPDGF-BB, has proven particularly effective in managing complex cases, such as ridge augmentation, socket preservation, and periodontal defect repair of teeth and implants, leads to more predictable and stable outcomes. When combined with early diagnosis and timely intervention, these growth factors facilitate improved implant prognosis, long-term tissue preservation, and reduced complications associated with advanced tissue breakdown.

PRF and autogenous dentin grafting elevate regenerative strategies by utilizing the body's own healing capabilities. PRF, with its rich concentration of platelets and growth factors, enhances both soft and hard tissue regeneration, accelerating healing and improving surgical predictability. Similarly, autogenous dentin grafts harness the regenerative potential of the patient's own extracted teeth, providing an osteoinductive matrix that supports robust bone and periodontal regeneration. These techniques, while offering numerous benefits, also require clinician expertise and careful case selection to overcome challenges such as technique sensitivity and volume limitations.

BioXclude and laser therapy have elevated clinical results in periodontal and implant dentistry. BioXclude, derived from the human placenta, serves as a natural barrier promoting soft and hard tissue regeneration while reducing inflammation. Unlike other barriers it has been shown to be bioactive and anti-infective, especially important for aging and immunocompromised patients. Specific protocols in laser therapy, with precision and a minimally invasive approach, accelerate healing, reduce pathogenic bacterial loads, and stimulate tissue regeneration, making them invaluable tools in modern regenerative dentistry.

Photobiomodulation (PBM) and Low Magnitude High-Frequency Vibration (LMHFV) each offer significant benefits in regenerative dentistry, enhancing healing and tissue regeneration in unique and non-invasive ways. PBM stimulates cellular metabolism, reduces inflammation, and accelerates recovery by promoting collagen production, angiogenesis, and tissue repair. It is particularly effective in improving soft and hard tissue regeneration and enhancing patient comfort post-surgery. LMHFV, through mechanical activation, stimulates bone and soft tissue regeneration, enhances osseointegration, and accelerates healing. It supports tissue remodeling, bone density, and overall tissue stability, especially in implantology and periodontal treatments. When used separately, both therapies improve clinical outcomes, reduce inflammation, and promote faster healing. Together, PBM and LMHFV offer a comprehensive, non-invasive approach to enhance regeneration, optimize recovery, and improve the long-term success of dental treatments. Histological results of these therapies have been shown here to be ideal for socket regeneration and future osseointegration of dental implants.

When patients present with many issues, dentally and medically, the dental surgeon needs to be able to choose from a variety of biomaterials, techniques and devices to assist them in obtaining optimal health.

The combination of photobiomodulation (PBM) and Low Magnitude High-Frequency Vibration (LMHFV) has introduced a synergistic effect that optimizes healing and reduces discomfort. Together, these therapies enhance osseointegration, stabilize soft and hard tissues, and promote faster postoperative recovery. The integration of PBM and LMHFV into routine dental practices can offer an efficient, predictable, and patient-friendly approach, improving both short-term and long-term clinical outcomes.

As research and technology continue to evolve, these biologically advanced materials and therapeutic modalities are set to become foundational elements in periodontal and implant therapy. Their ability to enhance tissue regeneration, improve clinical predictability, and support long-term success positions them as essential tools in modern dental care, offering effective, comfortable, and biologically sound solutions for patients. This will enable them to preserve teeth and implants for longer periods of time and, maybe more importantly, to have a chance to improve their overall health.

Author details

Robert A. Horowitz[1,2,3*], Gregori M. Kurtzman[4] and Hari S. Prasad[5]

1 Periodontology and Implant Dentistry, Oral Surgery, New York, USA

2 University College of Dentistry, New York, USA

3 Private Practice Scarsdale, New York, USA

4 Private Practice Silver Spring, Maryland, USA

5 Hard Tissue Research Laboratory, Division of Oral and Maxillofacial Pathology, University of Minnesota School of Dentistry Minneapolis, MN, USA

*Address all correspondence to: rahdds@gmail.com

References

[1] Kurtzman GM, Horowitz RA, Johnson R, Pedro Z. Oral biofilm and its connection to Alzheimer's disease. Cureus. 2024;**16**(11):e72841. DOI: 10.7759/cureus.72841

[2] Kurtzman GM, Horowitz RA, Johnson R, Prestiano RA, Klein BI. The systemic oral health connection: Biofilms. Medicine (Baltimore). 2022; **101**(46):e30517. DOI: 10.1097/MD.0000000000030517

[3] Park YS, Lee BA, Choi SH, Kim YT. Evaluation of failed implants and reimplantation at sites of previous dental implant failure: Survival rates and risk factors. Journal of Periodontal & Implant Science. 2022;**52**(3):230-241. DOI: 10.5051/jpis.2105020251

[4] Chatzopoulos GS, Wolff LF. Survival rate of implants performed at sites of previously failed implants and factors associated with failure: A retrospective investigation. Journal of Dental Sciences. 2024;**19**(3):1741-1747. DOI: 10.1016/j.jds.2023.10.012. Epub 2023 Oct 22

[5] Gareb B, Vissink A, Terheyden H, Meijer HJA, Raghoebar GM. Outcomes of implants placed in sites of previously failed implants: A systematic review and meta-analysis. International Journal of Oral and Maxillofacial Surgery. 2025; **54**(3):268-280. DOI: 10.1016/j.ijom.2024.10.006. Epub 2024 Oct 26

[6] Oh SL, Shiau HJ, Reynolds MA. Survival of dental implants at sites after implant failure: A systematic review. The Journal of Prosthetic Dentistry. 2020; **123**(1):54-60. DOI: 10.1016/j.prosdent.2018.11.007. Epub 2019 Apr 23

[7] Pavlovic V, Ciric M, Jovanovic V, Trandafilovic M, Stojanovic P. Platelet-rich fibrin: Basics of biological actions and protocol modifications. Open Medicine (Warsaw, Poland). 2021;**16**(1): 446-454. DOI: 10.1515/med-2021-0259

[8] Goswami P, Chaudhary V, Arya A, Verma R, Vijayakumar G, Bhavani M. Platelet-rich fibrin (PRF) and its application in dentistry: A literature review. Journal of Pharmacy & Bioallied Sciences. 2024;**16**(Suppl. 1):S5-S7. DOI: 10.4103/jpbs.jpbs_435_23. Epub 2024 Feb 29

[9] Dohan DM, Ehrenfest NR, Pinto AP, Jiménez P, Del Corso M, Kang B-S, et al. The impact of the centrifuge characteristics and centrifugation protocols on the cells, growth factors, and fibrin architecture of a leukocyte- and platelet-rich fibrin (L-PRF) clot and membrane. Platelets. 2018;**29**(2): 171-184. DOI: 10.1080/09537104.2017.1293812

[10] Miron RJ, Xu H, Chai J, Wang J, Zheng S, Feng M, et al. Comparison of platelet-rich fibrin (PRF) produced using 3 commercially available centrifuges at both high (~700 g) and low (~200 g) relative centrifugation forces. Clinical Oral Investigations. 2020;**24**(3):1171-1182. DOI: 10.1007/s00784-019-02981-2. Epub 2019 Jul 19. Erratum in: Clin Oral Investig. 2024 Sep 24;28(10):546. doi:10.1007/s00784-024-05949-z

[11] Borie E, Oliví DG, Orsi IA, Garlet K, Weber B, Beltrán V, et al. Platelet-rich fibrin application in dentistry: A literature review. International Journal of Clinical and Experimental Medicine. 2015;**8**(5):7922-7929

[12] Jadali Z, Doroodgar F. Platelet-rich fibrin: Its role in curbing the inflammation and improvement of the wound-healing process. Taiwan Journal

of Ophthalmology. 2024;**15**(1):149-150. DOI: 10.4103/tjo.TJO-D-23-00139

[13] Tanan Karaca G, Duygu G, Er N, Ozgun E. Comparative investigation of anti-inflammatory effect of platelet-rich fibrin after mandibular wisdom tooth surgery: A randomized controlled study. Journal of Clinical Medicine. 2023; **12**(13):4250. DOI: 10.3390/jcm12134250

[14] Kargarpour Z, Panahipour L, Miron RJ, Gruber R. Fibrinogen concentrations in liquid PRF using various centrifugation protocols. Molecules. 2022;**27**(7):2043. DOI: 10.3390/molecules27072043

[15] Feng M, Wang Y, Wei Y, Zhang X, Xiao L, Gong Z, et al. Preparation, characterization and biological properties of a novel bone block composed of platelet rich fibrin and a deproteinized bovine bone mineral. Fundamental Research. 2021;**2**(2): 321-328. DOI: 10.1016/j. fmre.2021.08.003

[16] Dragonas P, Katsaros T, Avila-Ortiz G, Chambrone L, Schiavo JH, Palaiologou A. Effects of leukocyte-platelet-rich fibrin (L-PRF) in different intraoral bone grafting procedures: A systematic review. International Journal of Oral and Maxillofacial Surgery. 2019; **48**(2):250-262. DOI: 10.1016/j. ijom.2018.06.003. Epub 2018 Jul 7

[17] Cortellini S, Castro AB, Temmerman A, Van Dessel J, Pinto N, Jacobs R, et al. Leucocyte- and platelet-rich fibrin block for bone augmentation procedure: A proof-of-concept study. Journal of Clinical Periodontology. 2018; **45**(5):624-634. DOI: 10.1111/jcpe.12877. Epub 2018 Apr 10

[18] Jamjoom AG. From healing to regeneration: A comprehensive review of the efficacy of platelet-rich fibrin in periodontal plastic surgery procedures. Cureus. 2024;**16**(9):e69287. DOI: 10.7759/cureus.69287

[19] Dohan DM, Choukroun J, Diss A, Dohan SL, Dohan AJ, Mouhyi J, et al. Platelet-rich fibrin (PRF): A second-generation platelet concentrate. Part II: Platelet-related biologic features. Oral Surgery, Oral Medicine, Oral Pathology, Oral Radiology, and Endodontics. 2006; **101**(3):e45-e50. DOI: 10.1016/j. tripleo.2005.07.009. Epub 2006 Jan 10

[20] Miron RJ, Moraschini V, Fujioka-Kobayashi M, Zhang Y, Kawase T, Cosgarea R, et al. Use of platelet-rich fibrin for the treatment of periodontal intrabony defects: A systematic review and meta-analysis. Clinical Oral Investigations. 2021;**25**(5):2461-2478. DOI: 10.1007/s00784-021-03825-8. Epub 2021 Feb 20

[21] Miron RJ, Moraschini V, Estrin N, Shibli JA, Cosgarea R, Jepsen K, et al. Autogenous platelet concentrates for treatment of intrabony defects-a systematic review with meta-analysis. Periodontology 2000. 2025;**97**(1): 153-190. DOI: 10.1111/prd.12598. Epub 2024 Oct 19

[22] Horowitz RA, Mazor Z, Miller RJ, Krauser J, Prasad HS, Rohrer MD. Clinical evaluation alveolar ridge preservation with a beta-tricalcium phosphate socket graft. The Compendium of Continuing Education in Dentistry. 2009;**30**(9):588-590, 592, 594 passim; quiz 604, 606

[23] Horowitz R, Holtzclaw D, Rosen PS. A review on alveolar ridge preservation following tooth extraction. The Journal of Evidence-Based Dental Practice. 2012; **12**(3 Suppl.):149-160. DOI: 10.1016/ S1532-3382(12)70029-5

[24] Horowitz RA. Extraction environment enhancement: Critical

evaluation of early socket healing in long-term barrier-protected extraction sockets. The Compendium of Continuing Education in Dentistry. 2005;**26**(10):703-713; quiz 714, 735. Erratum in: Compend Contin Educ Dent. 2005 Nov;26(11):765

[25] Öncü E, Bayram B, Kantarci A, Gülsever S, Alaaddinoğlu EE. Positive effect of platelet rich fibrin on osseointegration. Medicina Oral, Patología Oral y Cirugía Bucal. 2016; **21**(5):e601-e607. DOI: 10.4317/medoral.21026

[26] Petrescu BN, Mirica IC, Miron R, Campian RS, Lucaciu O. Platelet rich fibrin as a gingival tissue regeneration enhancer. Journal of Dental Sciences. 2021;**16**(1):536-539. DOI: 10.1016/j.jds.2020.08.014. Epub 2020 Sep 8

[27] Shiezadeh F, Taher M, Shooshtari Z, Arab H, Shafieian R. Using platelet-rich fibrin in combination with allograft bone particles can induce bone formation in maxillary sinus augmentation. Journal of Oral and Maxillofacial Surgery. 2023; **81**(7):904-912. DOI: 10.1016/j.joms.2023.03.015. Epub 2023 Mar 30

[28] Shetye AG, Rathee M, Jain P, Agarkar V, Kaushik S, Alam M. Effect of advanced platelet-rich fibrin and concentrated growth factor on tissues around implants in maxillary anterior region. Journal of Indian Prosthodontic Society. 2022;**22**(2):169-178. DOI: 10.4103/jips.jips_301_21

[29] Öncü E, Alaaddinoğlu EE. The effect of platelet-rich fibrin on implant stability. The International Journal of Oral & Maxillofacial Implants. 2015; **30**(3):578-582. DOI: 10.11607/jomi.3897

[30] Żurek J, Niemczyk W, Dominiak M, Niemczyk S, Wiench R, Skaba D. Gingival augmentation using injectable platelet-rich fibrin (i-PRF)-A systematic review of randomized controlled trials. Journal of Clinical Medicine. 2024; **13**(18):5591. DOI: 10.3390/jcm13185591

[31] Horowitz RA. Optimizing root coverage with L-PRF. Inside Dentistry. 1 Nov 2011;**7**(10):2-6

[32] Dixit DS, Mundada BP, Bhola N, Agarwal A. Dentin grafts: Navigating the paradigm shift in regenerative dentistry. Cureus. 2024;**16**(10):e70760. DOI: 10.7759/cureus.70760

[33] Kuperschlag A, Keršytė G, Kurtzman GM, Horowitz RA. Autogenous dentin grafting of osseous defects distal to mandibular second molars after extraction of impacted third molars. The Compendium of Continuing Education in Dentistry. 2020;**41**(2): 76-82; quiz 83

[34] Cervera-Maillo JM, Morales-Schwarz D, Morales-Melendez H, Mahesh L, Calvo-Guirado JL. Autologous tooth dentin graft: A retrospective study in humans. Medicina (Kaunas, Lithuania). 2021;**58**(1):56. DOI: 10.3390/medicina58010056

[35] Um IW, Lee JK, Kim JY, Kim YM, Bakhshalian N, Jeong YK, et al. Allogeneic dentin graft: A review on its osteoinductivity and antigenicity. Materials (Basel). 2021;**14**(7):1713. DOI: 10.3390/ma14071713

[36] Olchowy A, Olchowy C, Zawiślak I, Matys J, Dobrzyński M. Revolutionizing bone regeneration with grinder-based dentin biomaterial: A systematic review. International Journal of Molecular Sciences. 2024;**25**(17):9583. DOI: 10.3390/ijms25179583

[37] Sun H, Yin X, Yang C, Kuang H, Luo W. Advances in autogenous dentin matrix graft as a promising biomaterial

for guided bone regeneration in maxillofacial region: A review. Medicine (Baltimore). 2024;**103**(34):e39422. DOI: 10.1097/MD.0000000000039422

[38] Wysłouch E, Sipika A, Grabowska-Jasik N, Tyrakowski M, Kaczmarzyk T, Szuta M. Use of autologous dentin matrix in bone defects augmentation - A literature review. Folia Medica Cracoviensia. 2024;**64**(2):87-91

[39] Yüceer-Çetiner E, Özkan N, Önger ME. Effect of autogenous dentin graft on new bone formation. The Journal of Craniofacial Surgery. 2021; **32**(4):1354-1360. DOI: 10.1097/SCS.0000000000007403

[40] Elsherbini FS, FS, Abdulrahman, M and Mostafa El-Shennawi, M. Evaluation of autogenous tooth graft in regeneration of periodontal vertical alveolar defects: Clinical, radiographic, and experimental study. Journal of Stomatology. 2023; **76**(2):84-93. DOI: 10.5114/jos.2023.128774

[41] Levine RA, Saleh MHA, Dias DR, Ganeles J, Araújo MG, Renouard F, et al. Periodontal regeneration risk assessment in the treatment of intrabony defects. Clinical Advances in Periodontics. 2024; **14**(3):201-210. DOI: 10.1002/cap.10254. Epub 2023 Jul 4

[42] Stavropoulos A, Bertl K, Sculean A, Kantarci A. Regenerative periodontal therapy in intrabony defects and long-term tooth prognosis. Dental Clinics of North America. 2022;**66**(1):103-109. DOI: 10.1016/j.cden.2021.09.002

[43] Kao RT, Nares S, Reynolds MA. Periodontal regeneration - Intrabony defects: A systematic review from the AAP regeneration workshop. Journal of Periodontology. 2015;**86**(2 Suppl.):S77-S104. DOI: 10.1902/jop.2015.130685. Epub 2014 Sep 12

[44] Mazor Z, Horowitz RA, Prasad H, Kotsakis GA. Healing dynamics following alveolar ridge preservation with autologous tooth structure. The International Journal of Periodontics & Restorative Dentistry. 2019;**39**(5): 697-702. DOI: 10.11607/prd.4138

[45] Binderman I, Halperin-Sternfeld M, Netanely E, Pohl S, Horowitz RA, Artzi Z. Biomaterials selection – Cellular interactions during regenerative and Remodeling phases – Chapter 3. In: Bone Augmentation by Anatomical Region: Techniques and Decision-Making. Wiley; 2020. pp. 43-60. DOI: 10.1002/9781119427926

[46] Garg V, Bhardwaj A, Chawla K. Treatment of periodontal infrabony defect using particulate dentin graft and recombinant human platelet-derived growth factor. Journal of Indian Society of Periodontology. 2024;**28**(4):489-493. DOI: 10.4103/jisp.jisp_449_23. Epub 2025 Jan 6

[47] Sánchez-Labrador L, Martín-Ares M, Cortés-Bretón Brinkmann J, López-Quiles J, Martínez-González JM. Assessment of changes in the outcome of autogenous tooth grafts over time: A clinical study evaluating periodontal healing in bone defects after lower third molar removal. Journal of Oral and Maxillofacial Surgery. 2024;**82**(9): 1121-1128. DOI: 10.1016/j.joms.2024.05.006. Epub 2024 May 22

[48] Mahajan S, Kaur RK, Grover V, Mehta M, Prashar S, Jain A. Efficacy of different sterilization protocols and its impact on osteogenic potential of autogenous tooth bone graft: A comparative in vitro study. Journal of Indian Society of Periodontology. 2024; **28**(6):673-679. DOI: 10.4103/jisp.jisp_19_24

[49] Imamura K, Hamada Y, Yoshida W, Murakami T, Nakane-Koyachi S,

Yoshikawa K, et al. Investigating the effects of dehydrated human amnion-chorion membrane on periodontal healing. Biomolecules. 2022;**12**(6):857. DOI: 10.3390/biom12060857

[50] Koob TJ, Lim JJ, Massee M, Zabek N, Rennert R, Gurtner G, et al. Angiogenic properties of dehydrated human amnion/chorion allografts: Therapeutic potential for soft tissue repair and regeneration. Vascular Cell. 2014;**6**:10. DOI: 10.1186/2045-824X-6-10

[51] Galvez P, Ahmed Omar N, Siadous R, Durand M, Comperat L, Lafarge X, et al. In vitro and in vivo assessment of a new acellular human amnion/chorion membrane device for guided bone regeneration. Scientific Reports. 2025;**15**(1):5483. DOI: 10.1038/s41598-025-88814-7

[52] Kim SG. Dehydrated human amnion–chorion membrane as a bioactive scaffold for dental pulp tissue regeneration. Biomimetics. 2024;**9**:771. DOI: 10.3390/biomimetics9120771

[53] Horowitz RA, Kurtzman GM. Improving the prognosis of periodontally involved teeth at the time of extraction of adjacent teeth with an amnion-chorion barrier and bioactive dentin graft. The Compendium of Continuing Education in Dentistry. 2024;**45**(7):e1-e4

[54] Nemati M, Nowrouzi M, Nemati F, Alizadeh A. The improving effects of the amnion and chorion membranes on tissue regeneration in periodontal disorders: A systematic review. Tissue & Cell. 2023;**83**:102147. DOI: 10.1016/j.tice.2023.102147. Epub 2023 Jun 27

[55] McCawley TK, McCawley MN, Rams TE. Immediate effect of Nd:YAG laser monotherapy on subgingival periodontal pathogens: A pilot clinical study. Journal of Periodontal & Implant Science. 2022;**52**(1):77-87. DOI: 10.5051/jpis.2100900045

[56] Zou Q, Zhang S, Jiang C, Xiao S, Wang Y, Wen B. Low-level laser therapy on soft tissue healing after implantation: A randomized controlled trial. BMC Oral Health. 2024;**24**(1):1477. DOI: 10.1186/s12903-024-05 a258-7

[57] Jha A, Gupta V, Adinarayan R. LANAP, periodontics and beyond: A review. Journal of Lasers in Medical Sciences. 2018;**9**(2):76-81. DOI: 10.15171/jlms.2018.16. Epub 2018 Mar 20

[58] Bechir ES. The clinical and microbiological effects of LANAP compared to scaling and root planing alone in the Management of Periodontal Conditions. Diagnostics (Basel). 2023;**13**(14):2450. DOI: 10.3390/diagnostics13142450

[59] Chhabrani A, Avinash BS, Bharadwaj RS, Gupta M. Laser light: Illuminating the path to enhanced periodontal care. Photodiagnosis and Photodynamic Therapy. 2024;**46**:104036. DOI: 10.1016/j.pdpdt.2024.104036. Epub 2024 Mar 2

[60] Berni M, Brancato AM, Torriani C, Bina V, Annunziata S, Cornella E, et al. The role of low-level laser therapy in bone healing: Systematic review. International Journal of Molecular Sciences. 2023;**24**(8):7094. DOI: 10.3390/ijms24087094

[61] Kurtzman GM, Horowitz RA, et al. Oral biofilms and its connection to diabetes, kidney disease and pancreatic cancer. Medical Research Archives, [S.l.]. 2025. ISSN 2375-1924;**13**(6):1-8. DOI: 10.18103/mra.v13i6.6700

[62] Kurtzman GM, Horowitz RA, et al. Oral biofilms and their connection to

cardiovascular health. Medical Research Archives, [S.l.]. 2025. ISSN 2375-1924;**13** (5):1-7. DOI: 10.18103/mra.v13i5.6585

[63] Huang N, Li Y, Li W, Zhao R, Ou Y, Chen J, et al. The clinical efficacy of laser in the nonsurgical treatment of peri-implantitis: A systematic review and meta-analysis. International Journal of Implant Dentistry. 2024;**10**(1):54. DOI: 10.1186/s40729-024-00570-x

[64] Shenoy A, Ganapathy D, Maiti S. Effectiveness of photobiomodulation with low-level laser therapy on the implant stability quotient at different time intervals: A randomized clinical trial. Cureus. 2024;**16**(1):e52160. DOI: 10.7759/cureus.52160

[65] Mellado-Valero A, Buitrago-Vera P, Solá-Ruiz MF, Ferrer-García JC. Decontamination of dental implant surface in peri-implantitis treatment: A literature review. Medicina Oral, Patología Oral y Cirugía Bucal. 2013; **18**(6):e869-e876. DOI: 10.4317/medoral.19420

[66] Gopal L, Palwankar P, Dhalla N. The efficacy of low-level laser therapy on the healing of oral wounds: A systematic review. Cureus. 2024;**16**(10):e70832. DOI: 10.7759/cureus.70832

[67] Wenzler JS, Wurzel SC, Falk W, Böcher S, Wurzel PP, Braun A. Bactericidal effect of different photochemical-based therapy options on implant surfaces-an In vitro study. Journal of Clinical Medicine. 2024; **13**(14):4212. DOI: 10.3390/jcm13144212

[68] Fiegler-Rudol J, Skaba D, Kawczyk-Krupka A, Wiench R. Antibacterial and bactericidal effects of the Er: YAG laser on oral bacteria: A systematic review of microbiological evidence. Journal of Functional Biomaterials. 2025;**16**(6):209. DOI: 10.3390/jfb16060209

[69] Yang H, Yang K. The biofilm removal and bactericidal effect of an 810-nm high-power laser on an orthodontic bracket surface: An in vitro study. Photobiomodulation, Photomedicine, and Laser Surgery. 2024; **42**(12):779-788. DOI: 10.1089/photob.2024.0088. Epub 2024 Oct 23

[70] Misischia WP, Xenoudi P, Yukna RA, Schurr MJ. Bacterial reduction effect of four different dental lasers on titanium surfaces in vitro. Lasers in Medical Science. 2021;**36**(8): 1759-1767. DOI: 10.1007/s10103-021-03349-3. Epub 2021 Jul 27. Erratum in: Lasers Med Sci. 2021 Oct;36(8):1769. doi: 10.1007/s10103-021-03403-0

[71] Mizutani K, Aoki A, Coluzzi D, Yukna R, Wang CY, Pavlic V, et al. Lasers in minimally invasive periodontal and peri-implant therapy. Periodontology 2000. 2016;**71**(1): 185-212. DOI: 10.1111/prd.12123

[72] Tavelli L, Barootchi S, Rodriguez MV, Mancini L, Majzoub J, Travan S, et al. Recombinant human platelet-derived growth factor improves root coverage of a collagen matrix for multiple adjacent gingival recessions: A triple-blinded, randomized, placebo-controlled trial. Journal of Clinical Periodontology. 2022;**49**(11): 1169-1184. DOI: 10.1111/jcpe.13706. Epub 2022 Jul 31

[73] Avila-Ortiz G, Ambruster J, Barootchi S, Chambrone L, Chen CY, Dixon DR, et al. American Academy of periodontology best evidence consensus statement on the use of biologics in clinical practice. Journal of Periodontology. 2022;**93**(12):1763-1770. DOI: 10.1002/JPER.22-0361. Epub 2022 Oct 24

[74] Tavelli L, Chen CJ, Barootchi S, Kim DM. Efficacy of biologics for the

treatment of periodontal infrabony defects: An American Academy of periodontology best evidence systematic review and network meta-analysis. Journal of Periodontology. 2022;**93**(12): 1803-1826. DOI: 10.1002/JPER.22-0120 Epub 2022 Oct 24

[75] Suárez-López Del Amo F, Monje A. Efficacy of biologics for alveolar ridge preservation/reconstruction and implant site development: An American Academy of Periodontology best evidence systematic review. Journal of Periodontology. 2022;**93**(12):1827-1847. DOI: 10.1002/JPER.22-0069. Epub 2022 Oct 24

[76] Misch MA. A Comparison of Growth Factor Release between Platelet Rich Fibrin and Recombinant Human Platelet Derived Growth Factor BB (RHPDGF-BB) and Beta-Tricalcium Phosphate: An In Vitro Analysis. All ETDs from UAB. University of Alabama at Birmingham; 2022. p. 571

[77] Khehra A, Shiba T, Chen CY, Kim DM. Latest update on the use of recombinant growth factors for periodontal regeneration: Existing evidence and clinical applications. Therapeutic Advances in Chronic Disease. 2024;**15**:20406223241302707. DOI: 10.1177/20406223241302707

[78] Nevins M, Giannobile WV, McGuire MK, Kao RT, Mellonig JT, Hinrichs JE, et al. Platelet-derived growth factor stimulates bone fill and rate of attachment level gain: Results of a large multicenter randomized controlled trial. Journal of Periodontology. 2005; **76**(12):2205-2215. DOI: 10.1902/jop.2005.76.12.2205

[79] Wallace SC, Snyder MB, Prasad H. Postextraction ridge preservation and augmentation with mineralized allograft with or without recombinant human platelet-derived growth factor BB (rhPDGF-BB): A consecutive case series. The International Journal of Periodontics & Restorative Dentistry. 2013;**33**(5):599-609. DOI: 10.11607/prd.1666

[80] Singh P, Suresh DK. Clinical evaluation of GEM 21S(®) and a collagen membrane with a coronally advanced flap as a root coverage procedure in the treatment of gingival recession defects: A comparative study. Journal of Indian Society of Periodontology. 2012;**16**(4): 577-583. DOI: 10.4103/0972-124X.106919

[81] Wright RF et al. Evaluation of GEM 21S for socket preservation after tooth extraction: A randomized controlled trial. Journal of Clinical Periodontology. 2010;**37**(11):999-1005

[82] Reis TG, Del Colletto AMS, Silva LAS, Koga BAA, Sogayar MC, Carreira ACO. Recombinant human peptide growth factors, bone morphogenetic Protein-7 (rhBMP7), and platelet-derived growth factor-BB (rhPDGF-BB) for osteoporosis treatment in an oophorectomized rat model. Biomolecules. 2024;**14**(3):317. DOI: 10.3390/biom14030317

[83] Li F, Yu F, Liao X, et al. Efficacy of recombinant human BMP2 and PDGF-BB in orofacial bone regeneration: A systematic review and meta-analysis. Scientific Reports. 2019;**9**:8073. DOI: 10.1038/s41598-019-44368-z

[84] Chantarawaratit P, Sangvanich P, Banlunara W, Soontornvipart K, Thunyakitpisal P. Acemannan sponges stimulate alveolar bone, cementum and periodontal ligament regeneration in a canine class II furcation defect model. Journal of Periodontal Research. 2014; **49**(2):164-178. DOI: 10.1111/jre.12090. Epub 2013 May 28

[85] Almutairi AS. Recombinant human PDGF-BB in combination with mineralized freeze-dried bone allograft in the treatment of Grade II furcation involvement: A case report. Asian Journal of Oral Health and Allied Sciences. 2021;**11**:4

[86] Monje A, Pons R, Barootchi S, Saleh MHA, Rosen PS, Sculean A. Recombinant human platelet-derived growth factor-BB-mediated reconstructive therapy of advanced peri-implantitis bone defects: A case series. International Journal of Oral Implantology (Berlin, Germany). 2025;**18**(1):47-57

[87] de Freitas LF, Hamblin MR. Proposed mechanisms of photobiomodulation or low-level light therapy. IEEE Journal of Selected Topics in Quantum Electronics. 2016;**22**(3):7000417. DOI: 10.1109/JSTQE.2016.2561201

[88] Woo K, Kim YS, Abueva C, Woo SH. Reprogramming macrophage phenotypes with photobiomodulation for improved inflammation control in ENT organ tissues. Clinical and Experimental Otorhinolaryngology. 2025;**18**(1):1-13. DOI: 10.21053/ceo.2024.00286. Epub 2024 Dec 19

[89] Leyane TS, Jere SW, Houreld NN. Cellular signalling and photobiomodulation in chronic wound repair. International Journal of Molecular Sciences. 2021;**22**(20):11223. DOI: 10.3390/ijms222011223

[90] Crous A, Abrahamse H. The signalling effects of photobiomodulation on osteoblast proliferation, maturation and differentiation: A review. Stem Cell Reviews and Reports. 2021;**17**(5):1570-1589. DOI: 10.1007/s12015-021-10142-w. Epub 2021 Mar 8

[91] Furtado GS, Martin V, Araújo R, Gomes PS, Lago ADN. Osteoinductive activity of photobiomodulation in an organotypic bone model. Photodiagnosis and Photodynamic Therapy. 2024;**45**:103936. DOI: 10.1016/j.pdpdt.2023.103936. Epub 2023 Dec 15

[92] Kim S, Park J, Choi Y, Jeon H, Lim N. Investigating the relevance of cyclic adenosine monophosphate response element-binding protein to the wound healing process: An in vivo study using photobiomodulation treatment. International Journal of Molecular Sciences. 2024;**25**(9):4838. DOI: 10.3390/ijms25094838

[93] Escudero JSB, Perez MGB, de Oliveira Rosso MP, Buchaim DV, Pomini KT, Campos LMG, et al. Photobiomodulation therapy (PBMT) in bone repair: A systematic review. Injury. 2019;**50**(11):1853-1867. DOI: 10.1016/j.injury.2019.09.031. Epub 2019 Sep 21

[94] Hamblin MR. Mechanisms and applications of the anti-inflammatory effects of photobiomodulation. AIMS Biophysics. 2017;**4**(3):337-361. DOI: 10.3934/biophy.2017.3.337. Epub 2017 May 19

[95] Serrage HJ, Cooper PR, Palin WM, Horstman P, Hadis M, Milward MR. Photobiomodulation of oral fibroblasts stimulated with periodontal pathogens. Lasers in Medical Science. 2021;**36**(9):1957-1969. DOI: 10.1007/s10103-021-03331-z. Epub 2021 May 15

[96] Zhong J, Zhang X, Ruan Y, Huang Y. Photobiomodulation therapy's impact on angiogenesis and osteogenesis in orthodontic tooth movement: In vitro and in vivo study. BMC Oral Health. 2024;**24**(1):147. DOI: 10.1186/s12903-023-03824-z

[97] Atarbashi-Moghadam F, Samadi-Rad A, Hakimiha N, Taghipour N, Mahmoudian A, Azadi A, et al. The impact of photobiomodulation on angiogenic differentiation of two different dental derived stem cells using two irradiation protocols: An in vitro investigation. BMC Oral Health. 2024; **24**(1):1090. DOI: 10.1186/s12903-024-04753-1

[98] Hosseinpour S, Tunér J, Fekrazad R. Photobiomodulation in oral surgery: A review. Photobiomodulation, Photomedicine, and Laser Surgery. 2019; **37**(12):814-825. DOI: 10.1089/photob.2019.4712. Epub 2019 Nov 21

[99] Ebrahimi P, Hadilou M, Naserneysari F, Dolatabadi A, Tarzemany R, Vahed N, et al. Effect of photobiomodulation in secondary intention gingival wound healing-A systematic review and meta-analysis. BMC Oral Health. 2021;**21**(1):258. DOI: 10.1186/s12903-021-01611-2

[100] Freitas NR, Guerrini LB, Esper LA, Sbrana MC, Dalben GDS, Soares S, et al. Evaluation of photobiomodulation therapy associated with guided bone regeneration in critical size defects. In vivo study. Journal of Applied Oral Science. 2018;**26**:e20170244. DOI: 10.1590/1678-7757-2017-0244. Epub 2018 May 7

[101] Marques MM, Diniz IM, de Cara SP, Pedroni AC, Abe GL, D'Almeida-Couto RS, et al. Photobiomodulation of dental derived mesenchymal stem cells: A systematic review. Photomedicine and Laser Surgery. 2016;**34**(11):500-508. DOI: 10.1089/pho.2015.4038. Epub 2016 Apr 8

[102] Rodriguez Salazar DY, Málaga Rivera JA, Laynes Effio JE, Valencia-Arias A. A systematic review of trends in photobiomodulation in dentistry between 2018 and 2022: Advances and investigative agenda. F1000Research. 2023;**12**:1415. DOI: 10.12688/f1000research.140950.2

[103] Joseph B, Janam P, Narayanan S, Anil S. Is antimicrobial photodynamic therapy effective as an adjunct to scaling and root planing in patients with chronic periodontitis? A systematic review. Biomolecules. 2017;**7**(4):79. DOI: 10.3390/biom7040079

[104] Maiti N, Benedicenti S, Appam S, Junaid I, Divyatammana, Kadam P, et al. Assessment of the efficacy of photobiomodulation (PBM) therapy in periodontal treatment: A longitudinal study. Journal of Pharmacy & Bioallied Sciences. 2024;**16**(Suppl. 3):S2449-S2451. DOI: 10.4103/jpbs.jpbs_286_24. Epub 2024 Jul 31

[105] Dalvi S, Benedicenti S, Hanna R. Effectiveness of photobiomodulation as an adjunct to nonsurgical periodontal therapy in the Management of Periodontitis - A systematic review of in vivo human studies. Photochemistry and Photobiology. 2021;**97**(2): 223-242. DOI: 10.1111/php.13348. Epub 2020 Nov 12

[106] Pawelczyk-Madalińska M, Benedicenti S, Sălăgean T, Bordea IR, Hanna R. Impact of adjunctive diode laser application to non-surgical periodontal therapy on clinical, microbiological and immunological outcomes in Management of Chronic Periodontitis: A systematic review of human randomized controlled clinical trials. Journal of Inflammation Research. 2021;**14**:2515-2545. DOI: 10.2147/JIR.S304946

[107] Sourvanos D, Lander B, Sarmiento H, Carroll J, Hall RD, Zhu TC, et al. Photobiomodulation in dental

extraction therapy: Postsurgical pain reduction and wound healing. Journal of the American Dental Association (1939). 2023;**154**(7):567-579. DOI: 10.1016/j.adaj.2023.03.004. Epub 2023 May 18

[108] Fekrazad S, Sohrabi M, Fekrazad R. Angiogenetic and anti-inflammatory effects of photobiomodulation on bone regeneration in rat: A histopathological, immunohistochemical, and molecular analysis. Journal of Photochemistry and Photobiology. B. 2023;**238**:112599. DOI: 10.1016/j.jphotobiol.2022.112599. Epub 2022 Nov 16

[109] Rosero KAV, Sampaio RMF, Deboni MCZ, Corrêa L, Marques MM, Ferraz EP, et al. Photobiomodulation as an adjunctive therapy for alveolar socket preservation: A preliminary study in humans. Lasers in Medical Science. 2020;**35**(8):1711-1720. DOI: 10.1007/s10103-020-02962-y. Epub 2020 Jan 22

[110] Abd-Elhaleem Othman MA, Zaky AA, Eltayeb EA, et al. A radiographic and histological study to compare red (650 nm) versus near infrared (810 nm) diode lasers photobiomodulation for alveolar socket preservation. Scientific Reports. 2024;**14**:6871. DOI: 10.1038/s41598-024-57114-x

[111] Doan N et al. Multidisciplinary approach to maximize angiogenesis and wound healing using piezoelectric surgery, concentrated growth factors and photobiomodulation for dental implant placement surgery involving lateral wall sinus lift: Two case reports. Vascular Cell, [S.l.]. 2020;**12**(1):2. ISSN 2045-824X

[112] Sahu N, Jalaluddin M, Kar SR, Swain SK, Brahma P, Nanda J. Effects of photo biomodulation on peri-implantitis. International Journal of Research in Medical Sciences. 2023;**11**:423-429

[113] Sahu N, Jalaluddin M, Kar SR, Swain SK, Brahma P, Nanda J. Effects of photo biomodulation on peri-implantitis. International Journal of Research in Medical Sciences. 2022;**11**(1):423-429. DOI: 10.18203/2320-6012.ijrms20223329

[114] Reza B, Soheil N, Ehsan B, Kourosh S, Reza F. Efficacy of photo biomodulation therapy for pain relief and soft tissue wound healing after dental implant surgery: A double-blind randomized clinical trial. Journal of Photochemistry and Photobiology. 2021; **8**:100062. ISSN 2666-4690. DOI: 10.1016/j.jpap.2021.100062

[115] Emecen-Huja P, Leblebicioglu B. Peri-implant wound healing and clinical outcomes. Current Oral Health Reports. 2024;**11**:215-225. DOI: 10.1007/s40496-024-00381-4

[116] Collado-Murcia Y, Parra-Perez F, López-Jornet P. Efficacy of photobiomodulation in the Management of Pain and Inflammation after dental implants: A randomized clinical trial. Journal of Clinical Medicine. 2024; **13**(19):5709. DOI: 10.3390/jcm13195709

[117] Rubin C, Xu G, Judex S. The anabolic activity of bone tissue, suppressed by disuse, is normalized by brief exposure to extremely low-magnitude mechanical stimuli. The FASEB Journal. 2001;**15**(12):2225-2229. DOI: 10.1096/fj.01-0166com

[118] Horowitz RA, Kurtzman GM. Utilization of low-magnitude high-frequency vibration (LMHFV) as an aid in treating peri-implantitis: Case presentations. The Journal of Oral Implantology. 2023;**49**(5):501-509. DOI: 10.1563/aaid-joi-D-21-00038

[119] Kurtzman GM, Horowitz R, Hallas M, El-Bialy T. Improving osseous conditions around teeth and implants

utilizing high frequency vibration. Journal of Osseointegration. 2021;**13**(1): 35-42. DOI: 10.23805/JO.2021.13.01.6

[120] Lau E, Al-Dujaili S, Guenther A, Liu D, Wang L, You L. Effect of low-magnitude, high-frequency vibration on osteocytes in the regulation of osteoclasts. Bone. 2010;**46**(6):1508-1515. DOI: 10.1016/j.bone.2010.02.031. Epub 2010 Mar 6

[121] Fu Z, Huang X, Zhou P, et al. Protective effects of low-magnitude high-frequency vibration on high glucose-induced osteoblast dysfunction and bone loss in diabetic rats. Journal of Orthopaedic Surgery and Research. 2021;**16**:650. DOI: 10.1186/s13018-021-02803-w

[122] Steppe L, Liedert A, Ignatius A, Haffner-Luntzer M. Influence of low-magnitude high-frequency vibration on bone cells and bone regeneration. Frontiers in Bioengineering and Biotechnology. 2020;**8**:595139. DOI: 10.3389/fbioe.2020.595139

[123] Ye X, Gu Y, Bai Y, Xia S, Zhang Y, Lou Y, et al. Does low-magnitude high-frequency vibration (LMHFV) worth for clinical trial on dental implant? A systematic review and meta-analysis on animal studies. Frontiers in Bioengineering and Biotechnology. 2021; **9**:626892. DOI: 10.3389/fbioe.2021.626892

[124] Chow DH, Leung KS, Qin L, Leung AH, Cheung WH. Low-magnitude high-frequency vibration (LMHFV) enhances bone remodeling in osteoporotic rat femoral fracture healing. Journal of Orthopaedic Research. 2011; **29**(5):746-752. DOI: 10.1002/jor.21303. Epub 2010 Dec 23

[125] Marędziak M, Lewandowski D, Tomaszewski KA, et al. The effect of low-magnitude low-frequency vibrations (LMLF) on osteogenic differentiation potential of human adipose derived mesenchymal stem cells. Cellular and Molecular Bioengineering. 2017;**10**:549-562. DOI: 10.1007/s12195-017-0501-z

[126] Mehta S, McClarren B, Aijaz A, Chalaby R, Cook-Chennault K, Olabisi RM. The effect of low-magnitude, high-frequency vibration on poly(ethylene glycol)-microencapsulated mesenchymal stem cells. Journal of Tissue Engineering. 2018;**9**. DOI: 10.1177/2041731418800101

[127] Nurrachman AS, Azhari A, Epsilawati L, Pramanik F. Temporal pattern of micro-CT angiography vascular parameters and VEGF mRNA expression in fracture healing: A radiograph and molecular comparison. European Journal of Dentistry. 2023; **17**(2):283-295. DOI: 10.1055/s-0042-1757466. Epub 2023 Jan 30

[128] Murphy J. The effect of mechanical vibration on alveolar bone following experimental periodontitis: A time course study [Master's theses] (2009). Marquette University; 2020. p. 603. Available from: https://epublications.marquette.edu/theses_open/603

[129] Qi Y, Zhang S, Zhang M, Zhou Z, Zhang X, Li W, et al. Effects of physical stimulation in the field of oral health. Scanning. 2021;**2021**:5517567. DOI: 10.1155/2021/5517567

[130] Wang S et al. The effect of low-magnitude high-frequency loading on peri-implant bone healing and implant osseointegration in beagle dogs. Journal of Prosthodontic Research. 2018;**62**(4): 497-502

Chapter 15

Perspective Chapter: The Impact of Electronic Cigarettes on the Oral Microenvironment

Giancarlo Cuadra, Alyssa Hanel, Nicole Christian, Sara Pecorelli, Vivian Ha, Sophie Tomov and Dominic Palazzolo

Abstract

The oral cavity is the first site in the human body affected by electronic cigarette aerosols, largely composed of humectants such as propylene glycol, glycerol, nicotine, and flavoring agents. Of these, flavoring agents have been shown to have notable detrimental effects on the oral microenvironment. This chapter focuses on the mucosal biology, immunology and the microbiology in the context of electronic cigarette use and (i) summarizes the current literature, (ii) indicates the gaps in knowledge, and (iii) proposes new directions of research in the topic. Considering the oral-systemic health connection and the increasing prevalence of electronic cigarette use, an understanding of the implications of vaping on oral tissues and the associated microbiome, especially as it relates to periodontitis, is paramount.

Keywords: electronic cigarettes, oral bacteria, oral epithelial cells, immune cells, inflammation

1. Introduction

Vaping is the act of inhaling aerosols generated from an electronic nicotine delivery system (ENDS) in a similar manner to which smokers inhale cigarette smoke. Originally, ENDS, or electronic cigarettes (ECIGs), were intended as a "harm-reduction" means for cessation of traditional smoking. However, it has now become a multimillion-dollar industry similar to that of "Big Tobacco" [1, 2]. The prevalence of vaping among young adults has increased exponentially, becoming a public health concern [3–8]. Although vaping is advertised as a safer alternative to smoking, the effects of inhaling ECIG-generated aerosols have not yet been fully explored [2, 9, 10].

In its simplest form, ECIGs are composed of a battery, a heating element, and a reservoir for the E-liquid (**Figure 1**). The battery powers the heating element typically integrated with the reservoir. When the battery is activated, the heating element vaporizes the E-liquid within the reservoir and generates an aerosol that the user

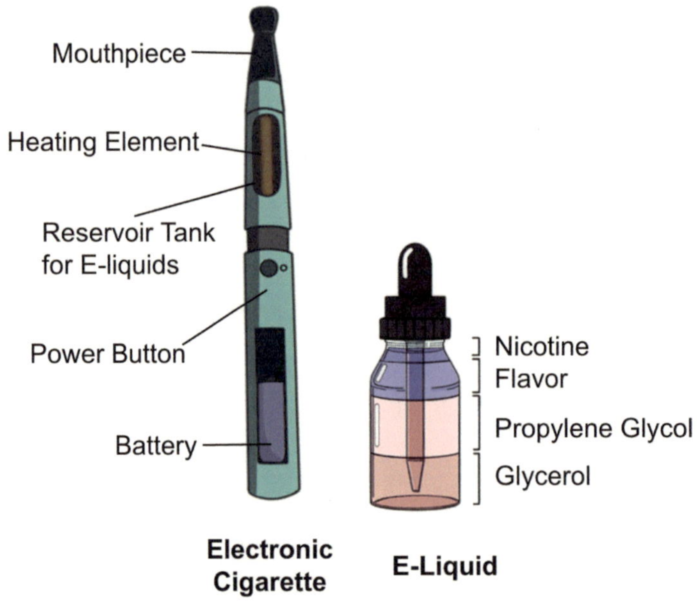

Figure 1.
Anatomy of a typical e-cigarette (ECIG) and the standard constituents of E-liquids.

inhales into the respiratory system [11]. **Figure 1** also shows the E-Liquid composition: the base humectants, propylene glycol (PG) and vegetable glycerol (VG); nicotine (ranging from 0 to 24 mg/mL); and flavoring agents which comprises up to 25% of the E-liquid [12, 13].

E-liquid aerosol particles range in size from <0.3 to >10 μm [14]. Biological effects of the particles depend largely on their deposition in the mouth and in the respiratory tract, being highly dependent on the manner of integration into biological fluids and tissues [15]. Vaping, its effects on the oral microenvironment, and the overall implications will be the focus of this chapter.

Consequently, this chapter covers three topics. First, the normal anatomy, physiology, and microflora of the oral cavity are presented. Next, we review the effects of vaping on the oral mucosa, particularly regarding oral epithelial cells, innate immune cells and saliva. Lastly, the effects of vaping on the oral microbiome and host-microbial interactions are outlined.

2. The oral cavity

As a dynamic, open biological system, the oral cavity serves as an interface between the internal and external environments where mechanical, chemical, and microbial components interact to maintain oral health and function. A description of the oral epithelium, the periodontium and the oral microbiota are briefly discussed.

Generally, the oral epithelium consists of squamous stratified epithelium and is classified according to variations in its thickness and extent of keratinization. Specific functions include protection of the underlying lamina propria and submucosal connective tissue layers as well as perception of temperature, touch, pain and taste [16].

The periodontium includes the alveolar bone, the junctional epithelium and the gingival tissues (**Figure 2**). The gingival sulcus is the space or periodontal pocket between the tooth and the surrounding gingival tissue and alveolar bone. The gingival crevicular fluid (GCF), as displayed in **Figure 2**, contains serum, inflammatory mediators, biomarkers, and antibodies [17].

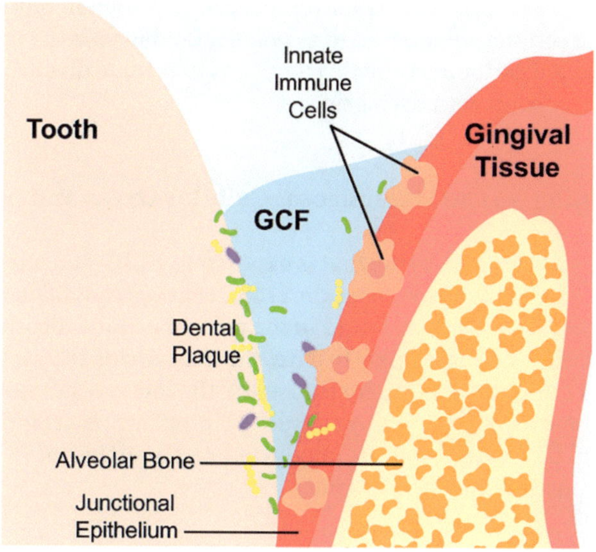

Figure 2.
The gingival sulcus includes the space between the tooth and the gum, and the main components are the gingival crevicular fluid (GCF), oral bacteria forming dental plaque, innate immune cells in the gingival tissue, the supporting alveolar bone and the connecting junctional epithelium adhered to the tooth.

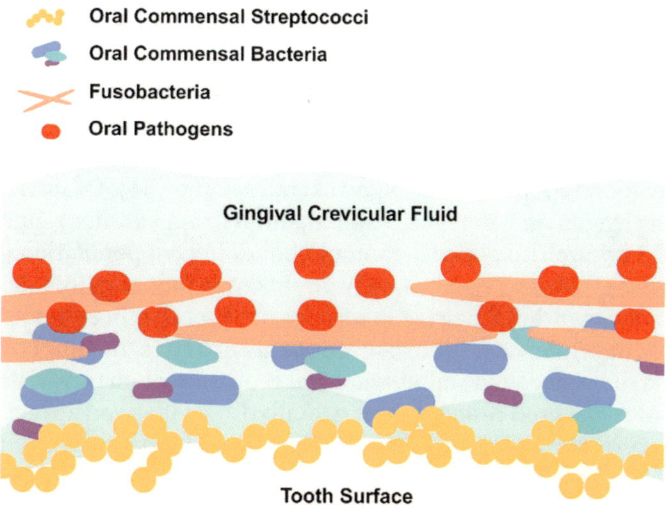

Figure 3.
Oral biofilm composed of various layers of bacteria. Oral biofilms begin with the attachment of oral commensal streptococci and other commensal bacteria. Fusobacteria can act as commensal bacteria but serve as a bridging taxa for oral pathogens. In the gingival sulcus, oral biofilms are bathed in gingival crevicular fluid (GCF).

The mucosal surface of the mouth is colonized with a natural microflora primarily in a commensal relationship with the host. These microbes include bacteria, fungi, viruses, and protozoa. The oral cavity has a vast and diverse microbiome with 834 taxa [18]. Oral streptococci are among the first to colonize the tooth surfaces (**Figure 3**) as they bind to the salivary pellicle, starting a biofilm [19]. As saliva and other nutrients flow across tooth surfaces, these early biofilms grow in number and diversity, as more species adhere to the streptococci, as shown in **Figure 3** [20]. These biofilms are commonly referred to as plaque. Dysbiosis is the imbalance in the microflora that may allow opportunistic pathogens to initiate disease. For example, periodontitis is associated with dysbiosis.

3. Effects of vaping on the oral mucosa: Cellular stress and inflammation

The oral mucosa is the first tissue that is exposed to ECIG-generated aerosols. Aerosol particles are dissolved into the saliva [15], coating and diffusing throughout the oral mucosal tissue. Substrates found in the aerosol include nicotine, propylene glycol, glycerol, and flavoring agents. To date, the majority of research *in vitro* and *in vivo* regarding E-liquid-related toxicity focuses on the lower respiratory tract [21, 22], with particular emphasis on respiratory tissues such as bronchial epithelia [23–27]. In contrast, minimal research has been conducted on the effects of ECIG-generated aerosols on oral epithelial tissues and saliva.

3.1 Effects of ECIGs on oral epithelial cells

3.1.1 Cytotoxicity

Nicotine concentrations in E-liquids range from 0 to 24 mg/mL, and depend on user preferences. With that said, nicotine doses less than 24 mg/mL do not usually reduce viability of different oral cell lines tested [28–32]. However, nicotine shows pathological effects on HaCaT keratinocytes at concentrations as low as 8 mg/mL [33].

E-liquids and their aerosols have been studied on oral cells and tissues and are found toxic. Typically, flavorless E-liquids are not cytotoxic, although flavorless aerosols composed of 30:70 PG/VG (v/v) were shown to induce cytotoxicity and Caspase 3 activation (apoptosis) in gingival keratinocytes [34]. Of interest, ECIGs utilize flavoring agents such as tobacco and menthol to appear more appealing for users. Other flavors are also prevalent among the adolescent population [29, 35–38]. Importantly, these flavoring agents have been shown to induce cytotoxic effects [39]. For example, menthol flavoring in tobacco products has been associated with greater nicotine dependence [40]. In conventional cigarettes, menthol reinforces smoking habits through cough suppression and reduction of airway irritation [41]. Fruit- and dessert-flavored E-liquids are particularly popular and attract adolescent users [36, 42], correlating with a higher number of inhalations per vaping session. Furthermore, a higher probability of vaping persistence after 6 months has been observed with fruit- and dessert-flavored E-liquids [43, 44].

As such, ECIG use is negatively implicated in the *in vitro* and *in vivo* wound healing capacity of mucosal cells (**Figure 4**), including complications in post-surgical oral wound healing [45, 46]. For example, cinnamaldehyde, the major component of cinnamon flavoring, is associated with cytotoxicity among other cellular responses

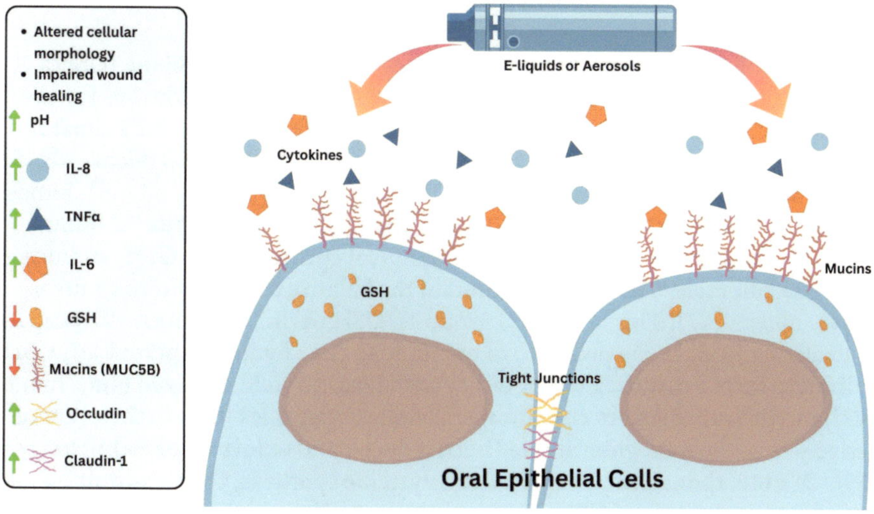

Figure 4.
Alterations in pro-inflammatory and oxidative stress biomarkers, including cytokines, glutathione, mucins and tight junctions of oral epithelial cells exposed to E-liquids and/or aerosols. Adapted from Shamim et al. [45].

[28, 39, 47–49]. In general, ECIG use is associated with observation of aberrant morphology (**Figure 4**) and cytotoxicity in epithelial cells located in the head and neck [50, 51]. ECIG-generated aerosols have also been shown to result in histological aberrations in the fungiform and circumvallate papillae of albino rats [52], indicating potential implications for taste and sensory deficits.

3.1.2 Gene expression and DNA damage

Oral epithelial cells play a critical role in wound closure post-injury. Wound closure curtails the invasion of microbes and microbial products into the lamina propria and bloodstream [53]. The production of salivary mucins is critical given their central role in the oral mucosa [54]. Along with tight junctions, mucins are responsible for maintaining the epithelial and mucosal barrier function [55]. A disruption in the ability of oral epithelial cells to recover from injury can pose a risk for infection and prolonged inflammation, in addition to systemic health risks [53]. Overall, as shown in **Figure 4**, physiological functions are altered on oral epithelial cells after exposure to flavoring agents in E-liquids, such as cinnamon, menthol, strawberry, and tobacco [45]. Additionally, gene expression profiles and critical molecular pathways may be affected by components in unflavored aerosolized E-liquid [56, 57]. Moreover, vaping leads to epigenetic DNA methylation of the tumor-suppressor HIC1 gene [58] and to DNA damage in oral epithelial cells [34, 50, 51, 59], making the tissues more susceptible to oral cancer. Noteworthy, traditional tobacco smokers who then became dual users, using both cigarettes and ECIGs, present with a significant reduction of DNA damage in the oral mucosa compared to smokers [60]. Presumably, this may be attributed to the fact that dual users smoke less conventional cigarettes. Nonetheless, smokers and vapers show a high prevalence for abnormal cells with increased risk to develop cancer (i.e., precancerous lesions) where the keratinized stratified squamous epithelium of the tongue is most commonly affected [61].

3.1.3 Oxidative stress and inflammation

Pathophysiological indicators in the oral mucosa include glutathione (GSH), cytokines, mucins, and tight junctions, among others (**Figure 4**). Various flavoring agents, particularly cinnamaldehyde, induce production of pro-inflammatory cytokines [48, 49], reactive oxygen species (ROS) and cytochrome c release [49, 62], leading to epithelial barrier dysfunction [63] and apoptosis [49, 62, 64–66]. Exposure to flavored E-liquids result in oxidative stress and cytokine production in human periodontal ligament fibroblasts and in the gingival epithelia [66]. GSH, an intracellular antioxidant molecule, helps to maintain the balance of ROS and to combat oxidative injuries [67]. The sulfhydryl group on GSH permits its antioxidant capacity by neutralizing ROS. In the presence of excess ROS (i.e., hydrogen peroxide), GSH is oxidized to form a disulfide bond, either with itself to yield oxidized glutathione (GSSG), or with other sulfur-containing proteins or peptides [68]. In the event of oxidative stress, the total glutathione (both reduced and oxidized forms) increases [67, 69]. Of note, the activity of γ-glutamyl cysteine synthase, the rate-limiting enzyme for the synthesis of GSH, has been shown to increase in response to oxidative stressors [70, 71]. Conversely, the amount of GSH may decrease as it is oxidized by exposure to oxidative stress [68]. This depletion of intracellular GSH, due to its conversion to GSSG or reacted with other sulfhydryl-containing molecules, typically signals apoptosis [72]. For example, unflavored aerosols [73] or E-liquids [45] may decrease intracellular GSH levels in human oral keratinocytes (**Figure 4**), suggesting heightened cytotoxicity and oxidative stress [74].

The inflammatory response of epithelial cells can be monitored by measuring the release of a number of pro-inflammatory cytokines such as tumor necrosis factor (TNF)α, interleukin (IL)-6, and IL-8. Expression of these signaling cytokines are under the control of transcriptional and post-transcriptional mechanisms in response to tissue injury [75] and thus are responsible for stimulating the large-scale host defense through acute phase responses, hematopoiesis, and a number of other immune processes [75].

Elevated total glutathione represents a localized cellular oxidative challenge, whereas an increase in pro-inflammatory cytokine expression suggests the initiation of inflammation. The immune and oxidative responses of oral epithelial cells induced by ECIG flavoring agents must be further examined to contribute to knowledge concerning their acute effects in the oral cavity [50, 51].

The specific correlation between ECIG usage and periodontal disease has recently been evaluated. ECIG use imposes an inflammatory burden *in vivo*, where pro-inflammatory cytokines, including interferon (IFN)γ, IL-2, IL-4, IL-6, IL-8, IL-10, granulocyte-monocyte colony stimulating factor, and TNFα are upregulated suggesting that ECIG use is associated with greater inflammation [76]. In addition, an *in vitro* study by Ramenzoni et al. using reverse transcription quantitative polymerase chain reaction, revealed an increase in pro-inflammatory cytokines (IL-1α, IL-1β, and IL-6) from oral epithelial cells exposed to ECIG aerosol [77], thus supporting the *in vivo* data by Ganesan et al. [76]. In addition, exposure of the 3D engineered human oral mucosal cells to ECIG aerosols reveal tissue structural damage including a decrease in type IV collagen and laminin as well as increased levels of matrix metalloproteinase (MMP)-2, MMP-3, MMP-9, lactate dehydrogenase activity and pro-inflammatory cytokines [78]. Similarly, gingival epithelial cells exposed to flavored and unflavored ECIG aerosols with varying ratios of PG/VG [79] increase production of similar biomarkers, however, at a lower extent than when cells are exposed to cigarette smoke [80].

Therefore, cigarette smoke appears to be more harmful than ECIG aerosols on mucosal immunity.

3.1.4 Immune response on macrophages and neutrophils

Macrophages are involved in phagocytosis of pathogenic bacteria and pro-inflammatory cytokine secretion. Polarization of naïve macrophage to the M1 pro-inflammatory subtype is hindered when these cells are exposed to E-liquids, specifically altered morphology, gene expression of inflammatory markers and cytokines [81]. Alveolar macrophages exposed to E-liquids die of necrosis and/or apoptosis, whereas exposure to ECIG aerosols is less cytotoxic [82]. In addition, these authors report that phagocytosis is significantly hindered, whereas ROS, IL-6, TNFα, and MMP-9 production is elevated, concluding that aerosol exposure is detrimental to macrophage immunobiology [49, 83]. Impaired functions were observed in alveolar macrophages after exposure to flavored E-liquids containing cinnamaldehyde [84]. Additionally, ECIG flavorings induce a proinflammatory state in macrophages, with cinnamon and menthol flavorings causing the most detrimental effects [85]. Moreover, neutrophils exposed to E-liquids with flavors display altered morphology and decreased formation of neutrophil extracellular traps, indicating impaired immune function [84].

3.2 Effects of ECIG on saliva and sputum

The assimilation of recondensed E-liquid in saliva results in a wide range of physiological effects [86, 87]. Saliva of ECIG users contains decreased levels of antimicrobial lysozyme and IgA in comparison to non-ECIG users [88]. Additionally, salivary flow rate and pH are significantly lower in individuals who vape [89]. This decrease in flow rate and pH may be attributed to the effects of nicotine and the generated aldehyde levels within the aerosol [90–92], as well as other E-liquid constituents. A decrease in salivary flow and pH, as well as reduced levels of mucin (MUC) 5B [45], may result in xerostomia [93], dental caries, [94, 95] and other pathologies such as periodontitis [96]. Interestingly, analysis of saliva can help evaluate the effects of vaping on oral health because it is easily attainable and contains various cellular secretions. Saliva of ECIG users has higher protein, phosphate and calcium concentrations as well as lower pH [90]. Although still under study, high calcium content in the saliva of ECIG users could serve as a biomarker for periodontal disease, as salivary calcium is positively correlated with bone resorption and weakened tooth attachment [97]. Excess salivary calcium may lead to faster mineralization of plaque.

Increased levels of inflammatory MMP-9, cytokines IL-6, TNFα and IL-1β, IL-8, IL-17, IL-4, and IFNγ are found in saliva of ECIG users [98]. In addition, GCF analysis, although limited, shows increased concentrations of TNFα and IL-1β [99]. A significant correlation between ECIG-generated aerosol and oxidative damage indicators such as malondialdehyde, superoxide dismutase and 8-hydroxy-2′-deoxyguanosine has also been observed, indicating metabolic alterations in the saliva of ECIG users [100]. Increasing prevalence of E-liquids and ECIGs necessitates further research regarding their physiologic effects in the oral cavity.

Sputum collected from vapers contains significantly higher amounts of bronchial epithelial cells, indicating an airway injury [101]. Analysis of sputum from ECIG users also reveals overall immunosuppression, with low levels of soluble intercellular adhesion molecule 1, soluble vascular cell adhesion molecule 1, C-reactive protein, IFNγ, monocyte chemoattractant protein-1, MMP-2, anti-inflammatory uteroglobin, and vascular endothelial growth factor. If the oropharyngeal mucosal immune system is suppressed due to vaping, there is a higher risk for infection as the mucosa between the oral cavity and airway is always exposed to the external environment [101].

4. Effects of vaping on the oral microbiota

ECIG-generated aerosols have the potential to disturb the homeostasis of the oral microbiota, leading to dysbiosis. Therefore, it is critical that the effect of ECIGs on the oral cavity, oral microbiome, and host-bacteria interactions are further explored. Perturbation of the oral microbiota are implicated in oral diseases such as periodontitis [102].

4.1 Commensal bacteria

Existing studies on the effects of ECIG components include comparisons between ECIG-generated aerosols, conventional cigarette smoke, E-liquids, nicotine, and flavors. In regards to the effects of nicotine by itself, commensal *Streptococcus gordonii* planktonic growth (i.e., free flowing bacteria in a suspension), biofilm formation, aggregation, and gene expression of binding proteins is increased after exposure from 0 to 4 mg/mL of nicotine [103]. Studies comparing the effects of flavorless E-liquids and cigarette smoke show that the latter has a strong cytotoxic effect [104, 105]. While flavorless E-liquids do not show any significant effect, Fischman et al. [12] found that flavored E-liquids—such as tobacco, menthol, cinnamon, strawberry, blueberry—tend to have an inhibitory effect in a dose-dependent manner on the planktonic growth of several oral commensal streptococci, including *S. gordonii*, *Streptococcus intermedius*, *Streptococcus mitis*, and *Streptococcus oralis* [12]. It is worth noting that in that study, the nicotine concentration was as high as 1 mg/mL, resulting in no change in planktonic growth [12]. Similarly, the effects of flavored E-liquids on single and multispecies commensal biofilm formation using oral commensal streptococci also reveals a dose-dependent inhibitory effect [106]. Others show that ECIG generated aerosols further inhibit the growth of commensals *S. gordonii* and *Streptococcus sanguinis* while enhancing biofilm formation [107]. Thus, the smoke from combusted tobacco and E-liquid flavors elicit a significant harmful effect on oral streptococci while nicotine concentrations in ECIGs do not appear toxic.

Hydrophobic interactions facilitate bacterial cell adherence to each other and to oral surfaces [108]. An increase in hydrophobicity allows for better adherence and biofilm formation [109]. Therefore, it is important to investigate the effects of ECIG aerosols and E-liquids on bacterial cell hydrophobicity. To this end, Catala-Valentin et al. [107] investigated the effects of ECIG aerosols on the hydrophobicity of the commensal bacteria *S. sanguinis* and *S. gordonii*, and the opportunistic pathogen *Streptococcus mutans*. Authors observe relatively little change in the hydrophobicity of the commensal organisms, while the hydrophobicity of *S. mutans* significantly increased. This also correlates with a significant increase in the adherence of *S. mutans* to oral epithelial cells [107]. Cinnamon and menthol stock ECIG flavors has been observed to increase the hydrophobicity of oral streptococci including *S. gordonii*, *S. mitis* and *S. oralis* [110]. Additionally, exposure of oral commensal population to cinnamon- and menthol-flavored E-liquids induce a bactericidal effect, which is supported by a decrease in the viability of multispecies communities composed of the same bacteria treated with cinnamon aerosol [110]. Overall, E-liquids and their aerosols appear to alter the hydrophobicity of oral commensal streptococci, and it is speculated that such alterations may contribute to microbial dysbiosis. While some of the effects of ECIG aerosols and E-liquids on the growth and biofilm formation of oral streptococci have been documented, more research is needed to elucidate multi-species interactions between oral commensals, pathogens and the host.

4.2 Pathogenic bacteria

The effects of nicotine on oral pathogenic bacteria and periodontitis are well documented [111]. For example, single exposure to nicotine inhibits the growth of oral pathogen *Porphyromonas gingivalis* in a dose-dependent manner; however, multiple exposures to nicotine result in increased bacterial growth indicating development of resistance [112]. This suggests that chronic nicotine exposure may lead to pathogenicity. In addition, after exposure to nicotine *Lactobacillus casei*, *Actinomyces viscosus*, *Actinomyces naeslundii*, *Rothia dentocariosa*, *Enterococcus faecalis*, and *S. mutans* show inconsistent effects on planktonic growth, but most species exhibit an upward trend in biofilm formation [113, 114]. The effects of flavored E-liquids on individual oral pathogen species are limited. For example, an increase in biofilm biomass and expression of virulent carbohydrate metabolic genes in *S. mutans* is observed after exposure to ECIG aerosols [107, 115]. Overall, these studies lead to the following observation: E-liquids and their aerosols affect the survival of oral pathogenic bacteria and promote biofilm formation *in vitro*, suggesting plaque formation may occur on tooth surfaces *in vivo,* thus increasing the risk of oral diseases. While few studies focus on the effects of vaping on individual pathogens, most studies are observational in nature. For the most part, studies on the effects of vaping on the oral microbiome *in vivo* lack mechanistic data which would help elucidate this observation. This gap in knowledge begs for further research (**Figure 5**).

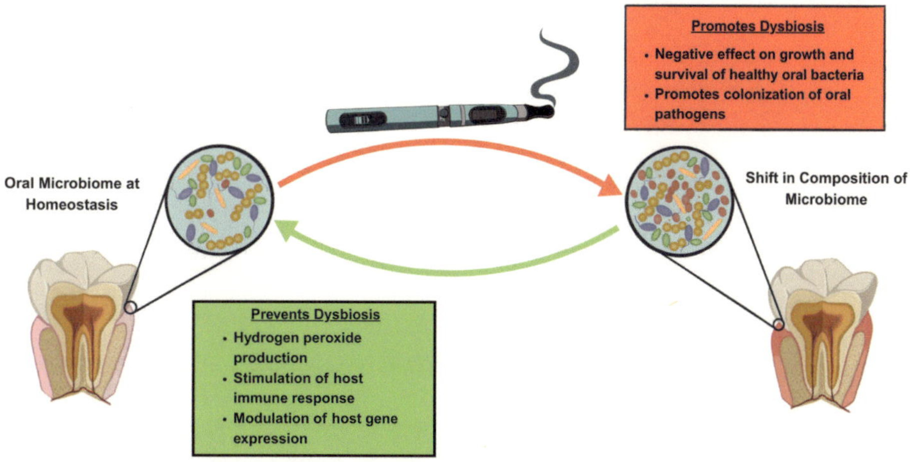

Figure 5.
Effect of vaping on oral microbiome and, by extension, the status of health and disease in the oral cavity. Under homeostasis, some oral commensal bacteria produce hydrogen peroxide, which prevents the growth and colonization of oral pathogens. Exposure to ECIG aerosols has no effect on the growth of oral commensal bacteria while having a positive effect on that of oral pathogens. The resulting dysbiosis, as a consequence of vaping, is implicated in oral diseases. Cessation of vaping may reverse oral dysbiosis.

4.3 Microbial diversity

Considering the wide microbial diversity in the oral cavity, maintaining a balanced species composition is important to the host health status. For example, as depicted in **Figure 6**, commensal bacteria produce bacteriocins, such as hydrogen peroxide, which prevent excess growth of pathogenic species [116, 117]. Dysbiosis could offset the healthy host-bacteria interactions and lead to oral, and therefore systemic, pathogenesis [118]. Therefore, it is critical to understand the effects of ECIGs on the composition of the oral microbiome *in vivo*. Pushalkar et al. [119] found a significant shift in the relative composition of microbial species between ECIG users and non-users, where *Porphyromonas* and *Veillonella* are in higher abundance among vapers [119] (**Figure 6**). *Porphyromonas* is known to have a pathogenic role and has been implicated in gingivitis and periodontitis [120]. *Veillonella* is mainly commensal, although it may support the colonization of pathogenic bacteria [121]. Other observational

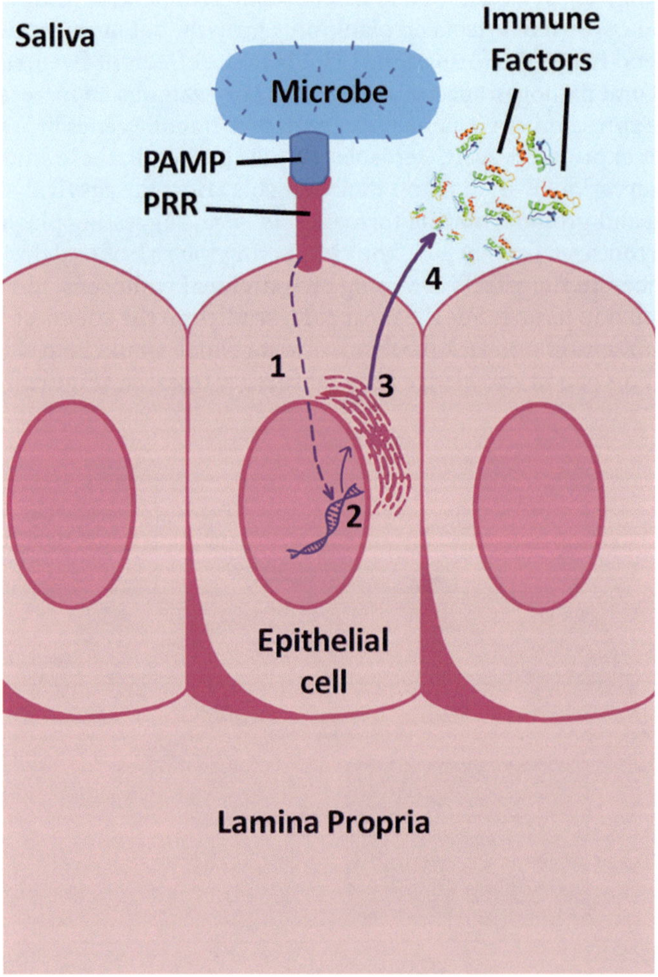

Figure 6.
Host-microbe interaction between microbe and oral epithelial cell. Microbial pathogen associated molecular patterns (PAMP) and pattern recognition receptors (PRR) bind, leading to a signal transduction pathways (1), inducing gene expression (2), and production/secretion (3) of inflammatory mediators (4).

studies have also found similar results, in that there was a difference in the microbial diversity of ECIG users (**Figure 6**) when compared to cigarette smokers and non-users [76, 122]. Furthermore, vaping may be associated with increased periodontal tissue destruction, leading to the development of periodontitis [123]. To emphasize, the overall compositional shift towards dysbiosis is a multifactorial deviation from the optimal that includes changes in oral microbial diversity, metabolic processes, bacteria-bacteria interactions, and responses to external stimuli [102, 124–126]. *In vitro* studies demonstrate that exposure to ECIG aerosols favors the growth and colonization of oral pathogens over commensals [107, 115], supporting the shift in the microbial community (**Figure 5**). However, blanket statements indicating that vaping increases or decreases a specific species may not provide an accurate holistic depiction of the oral microbiota as it relates to health status.

4.4 Oral epithelial cells and oral microbe interactions

The oral cavity serves as an entryway for microbial pathogens and environmental insults, and therefore has developed an advanced innate and adaptive immune system. **Figure 6** portrays pattern recognition receptors (PRRs) on host cells detecting microbial threats and initiate innate immune responses that mobilize immune cells including neutrophils, macrophages, dendritic cells, and lymphocytes, typically found in the mucosal tissues, lamina propria, and saliva [127]. Through PRRs, immune cells detect pathogen-associated molecular patterns (PAMPs) (**Figure 6**), such as lipopolysaccharides, flagella, peptidoglycan, and carbohydrates [128–130], which activate immune cells to produce cytokines, chemokines, ROS (**Figure 6**) and ultimately mount an immune response [23]. In addition antibodies, mucin glycoproteins, lysozyme, lactoferrin and antimicrobial peptides also help regulate the microbial burden and keep the oral cavity at homeostasis [131, 132].

Pathogenic oral bacteria, such as *P. gingivalis*, are known to invade host oral epithelial cells [133]. This process is associated with inflammation and oral diseases, such as gingivitis and periodontitis [134]. However, oral commensal streptococci, such as *S. gordonii* and *S. intermedius*, are protective against *P. gingivalis* invasion [135]. These interactions between microbes and host cells play an important role in determining the status of health or disease in the oral cavity. Thus, it is important to investigate how exposure to ECIG aerosols might affect such interactions. Opportunistic *S. mutans* has a higher capacity to adhere to oral epithelial cells than the oral commensals *S. sanguinis* and *S. gordonii*, and exposure to E-liquids increases the adherence of *S. mutans* [107]. Unfortunately, studies examining opportunistic invasive microbes, such as *P. gingivalis*, interacting with oral epithelial cells while exposed to E-liquids or their aerosols are insufficient. In addition, exposure of *Candida albicans*—an opportunistic pathogenic yeast—to ECIG aerosol increases growth, chitin production, and adherence to gingival epithelial cells, which may enhance pathogenesis and risk of oral candidiasis [136]. Furthermore, ECIG use is positively correlated with the presence of Human Papillomavirus-16 infections [137, 138]. Overall, these studies indicate that exposure to ECIG aerosols and E-liquids has the potential to modulate host-microbe interactions, which could affect the health of the oral cavity, but further research is still required.

Based on the current evidence in the primary literature, conflicting results exist regarding the impact of ECIG on oral health. Microbiological evidence overwhelmingly suggests that ECIG use prompts dysbiosis, which is supported by clinical studies [50, 119, 123, 139, 140]. Other clinical studies investigating vaping-induced periodontal destruction have not shown such correlation, yet other studies have observed higher plaque scores [123, 141]. Further research will clarify these conflicting results.

5. Chapter summary

This chapter reviews the current literature regarding the effects of ECIG use on the oral microenvironment with an emphasis on oral immunology and microbiology. The available primary literature indicates that vaping, the inhalation of ECIG aerosols, induces alterations in both the oral mucosa and associated microbiota. Specifically, aerosols promote inflammation and oxidative stress, are cytotoxic to the oral epithelium and cause alterations in the genetic makeup which could lead to various pathologies, such as precancerous lesions. Also, many E-liquids lead to pro-inflammatory cytokine production and changes in glutathione, an indicator of oxidative stress. In addition, cinnamon flavor E-liquids and their aerosols induce cell death on many cell models, presumably via apoptosis. Moreover, E-liquids and their aerosols disrupt the balance of the oral microbiota, killing some species while promoting growth of others, which leads to dysbiosis. For instance, E-liquids are cytotoxic as displayed in many studies testing the planktonic growth of oral commensal bacteria as well as biofilm formation. However, not much research focuses on pathogens, including bacteria, fungi and viruses.

Over the past decade, paramount and elegant investigations have increased our knowledge on the effects of vaping within the oral cavity. Nevertheless, there are still major gaps in our current understanding, especially in regards to host-bacteria interactions and the accompanying immune response. Furthermore, the majority of studies are observational in nature and do not explore in-depth mechanisms of action. Therefore, this area of research would benefit from mechanistic studies on the effects of vaping compounds on host cells, microbes and their interactions. For example, an investigation on the effects of vaping compounds on the adherence of commensal bacteria as well as the invasion of *P. gingivalis* into oral epithelial cells in the presence or absence of commensal bacteria would provide insights into the mechanistic host-bacteria interactions in the context of vaping. In addition, well-designed studies that explore changes in gene expression of oral epithelial cells, oral commensal and pathogenic bacteria might include exposure to E-liquids or their aerosol followed by RNA extraction and sequencing. Such investigations would further elucidate the effects of vaping on the molecular biology of microbes and the host in within the oral cavity. More importantly, these studies will expand our understanding of how vaping may relate to periodontal inflammation.

Author details

Giancarlo Cuadra[1*], Alyssa Hanel[2], Nicole Christian[3], Sara Pecorelli[4], Vivian Ha[5], Sophie Tomov[1] and Dominic Palazzolo[6]

1 Department of Biology, Muhlenberg College, Allentown, PA, USA

2 Dental Department, Robert Wood Johnson University Hospital, New Brunswick, NJ, USA

3 School of Dentistry, University of Michigan, Ann Arbor, MI, USA

4 School of Dental Medicine, Rutgers, The State University of New Jersey, Newark, NJ, USA

5 College of Dentistry, University of Illinois – Chicago, Chicago, IL, USA

6 DeBusk College of Osteopathic Medicine, Lincoln Memorial University, Harrogate, TN, USA

*Address all correspondence to: giancarlocuadra@muhlenberg.edu

References

[1] Cahn Z, Siegel M. Electronic cigarettes as a harm reduction strategy for tobacco control: A step forward or a repeat of past mistakes? Journal of Public Health Policy. 2011;**32**(1):16-31. DOI: 10.1057/jphp.2010.41

[2] Palazzolo DL. Electronic cigarettes and vaping: A new challenge in clinical medicine and public health. A literature review. Frontiers in Public Health. 2013;**1**:56. DOI: 10.3389/fpubh.2013.00056

[3] Agaku IT, King BA, Husten CG, Bunnell R, Ambrose BK, Sean Hu S, et al. Tobacco product use among adults--United States, 2012-2013. MMWR: Morbidity and Mortality Weekly Report. 2014;**63**(25):542-547

[4] Bunnell RE, Agaku IT, Arrazola RA, Apelberg BJ, Caraballo RS, Corey CG, et al. Intentions to smoke cigarettes among never-smoking US middle and high school electronic cigarette users: National Youth Tobacco Survey, 2011-2013. Nicotine & Tobacco Research: Official Journal of the Society for Research on Nicotine and Tobacco. 2015;**17**(2):228-235. DOI: 10.1093/ntr/ntu166

[5] King BA, Alam S, Promoff G, Arrazola R, Dube SR. Awareness and ever-use of electronic cigarettes among U.S. adults, 2010-2011. Nicotine & Tobacco Research: Official Journal of the Society for Research on Nicotine and Tobacco. 2013;**15**(9):1623-1627. DOI: 10.1093/ntr/ntt013

[6] Li J, Newcombe R, Walton D. The prevalence, correlates and reasons for using electronic cigarettes among New Zealand adults. Addictive Behaviors. 2015;**45**(June):245-251. DOI: 10.1016/j.addbeh.2015.02.006

[7] McMillen RC, Gottlieb MA, Whitmore Shaefer RM, Winickoff JP, Klein JD. Trends in electronic cigarette use among U.S. adults: Use is increasing in both smokers and nonsmokers. Nicotine & Tobacco Research: Official Journal of the Society for Research on Nicotine and Tobacco. 2015;**17**(10):1195-1202. DOI: 10.1093/ntr/ntu213

[8] Regan AK, Promoff G, Dube SR, Arrazola R. Electronic nicotine delivery systems: Adult use and awareness of the 'e-cigarette' in the USA. Tobacco Control. 2013;**22**(1):19-23. DOI: 10.1136/tobaccocontrol-2011-050044

[9] Foulds J, Veldheer S, Berg A. Electronic cigarettes (e-cigs): Views of aficionados and clinical/public health perspectives. International Journal of Clinical Practice. 2011;**65**(10):1037-1042. DOI: 10.1111/j.1742-1241.2011.02751.x

[10] Foulds J, Veldheer S. Commentary on Etter & Bullen (2011): Could e-cigs become the ultimate nicotine maintenance device? Addiction (Abingdon, England). 2011;**106**(11):2029-2030. DOI: 10.1111/j.1360-0443.2011.03532.x

[11] Palazzolo DL, Nelson JM, Ely EA, Crow AP, Distin J, Kunigelis SC. The effects of electronic cigarette (ECIG)-generated aerosol and conventional cigarette smoke on the mucociliary transport velocity (MTV) using the bullfrog (R. Catesbiana) palate paradigm. Frontiers in Physiology. 2017;**8**:1023. DOI: 10.3389/fphys.2017.01023

[12] Fischman JS, Sista S, Lee DK, Cuadra GA, Palazzolo DL. Flavorless vs. flavored electronic cigarette-generated aerosol and e-liquid on the growth of common oral commensal streptococci.

Frontiers in Physiology. 2020;**11**:585416. DOI: 10.3389/fphys.2020.585416

[13] Krüsemann EJZ, Boesveldt S, de Graaf K, Talhout R. An e-liquid flavor wheel: A shared vocabulary based on systematically reviewing e-liquid flavor classifications in literature. Nicotine & Tobacco Research: Official Journal of the Society for Research on Nicotine and Tobacco. 2019;**21**(10):1310-1319. DOI: 10.1093/ntr/nty101

[14] Palazzolo DL, Caudill J, Baron J, Cooper K. Fabrication and validation of an economical, programmable, dual-channel, electronic cigarette aerosol generator. International Journal of Environmental Research and Public Health. 2021;**18**(24):13190. DOI: 10.3390/ijerph182413190

[15] Sosnowski TR, Odziomek M. Particle size dynamics: Toward a better understanding of electronic cigarette aerosol interactions with the respiratory system. Frontiers in Physiology. 2018;**9**:74-81. Available from: https://www.frontiersin.org/article/10.3389/fphys.2018.00853:74-81

[16] Squier CA, Kremer MJ. Biology of oral mucosa and esophagus. JNCI Monographs. 2001;**2001**(29):7-15. DOI: 10.1093/oxfordjournals.jncimonographs.a003443

[17] Subbarao KC, Nattuthurai GS, Sundararajan SK, Sujith I, Joseph J, Syedshah YP. Gingival crevicular fluid: An overview. Journal of Pharmacy and Bioallied Sciences. 2019;**11**(Suppl 2):S135-S139

[18] HOMD:: Human Oral Microbiome Database. n.d. Available from: https://www.homd.org/# [Accessed: May 28, 2025]

[19] Abranches J, Zeng L, Kajfasz JK, Palmer SR, Chakraborty B, Wen ZT, et al. Biology of oral streptococci. Microbiology Spectrum. 2018;**6**(5):10-1128. DOI: 10.1128/microbiolspec.gpp3-0042-2018

[20] Dieckow S, Szafrański SP, Grischke J, Qu T, Doll-Nikutta K, Steglich M, et al. Structure and composition of early biofilms formed on dental implants are complex, diverse, subject-specific and dynamic. npj Biofilms and Microbiomes. 2024;**10**(1):1-16. DOI: 10.1038/s41522-024-00624-3

[21] Chun LF, Moazed F, Calfee CS, Matthay MA, Gotts JE. Pulmonary toxicity of e-cigarettes. American Journal of Physiology-Lung Cellular and Molecular Physiology. 2017;**313**(2):L193-L206. DOI: 10.1152/ajplung.00071.2017

[22] Merecz-Sadowska A, Sitarek P, Zielinska-Blizniewska H, Malinowska K, Zajdel K, Zakonnik L, et al. A summary of in vitro and in vivo studies evaluating the impact of e-cigarette exposure on living organisms and the environment. International Journal of Molecular Sciences. 2020;**21**(2):652. DOI: 10.3390/ijms21020652

[23] Chen L, Deng H, Cui H, Fang J, Zuo Z, Deng J, et al. Inflammatory responses and inflammation-associated diseases in organs. Oncotarget. 2017;**9**(6):7204-7218. DOI: 10.18632/oncotarget.23208

[24] Ghosh A, Coakley RC, Mascenik T, Rowell TR, Davis ES, Rogers K, et al. Chronic e-cigarette exposure alters the human bronchial epithelial proteome. American Journal of Respiratory and Critical Care Medicine. 2018;**198**(1):67-76. DOI: 10.1164/rccm.201710-2033OC

[25] Ghosh A, Coakley RD, Ghio AJ, Muhlebach MS, Esther CR, Alexis NE, et al. Chronic e-cigarette

use increases neutrophil elastase and matrix metalloprotease levels in the lung. American Journal of Respiratory and Critical Care Medicine. 2019;**200**(11):1392-1401. DOI: 10.1164/rccm.201903-0615OC

[26] Higham A, Bostock D, Booth G, Dungwa JV, Singh D. The effect of electronic cigarette and tobacco smoke exposure on COPD bronchial epithelial cell inflammatory responses. International Journal of Chronic Obstructive Pulmonary Disease. 2018;**13**(March):989-1000. DOI: 10.2147/COPD.S157728

[27] Reidel B, Radicioni G, Clapp PW, Ford AA, Abdelwahab S, Rebuli ME, et al. E-cigarette use causes a unique innate immune response in the lung, involving increased neutrophilic activation and altered mucin secretion. American Journal of Respiratory and Critical Care Medicine. 2018;**197**(4):492-501. DOI: 10.1164/rccm.201708-1590OC

[28] Bahl V, Lin S, Xu N, Davis B, Wang Y-h, Talbot P. Comparison of electronic cigarette refill fluid cytotoxicity using embryonic and adult models. Reproductive Toxicology (Elmsford, N.Y.). 2012;**34**(4):529-537. DOI: 10.1016/j.reprotox.2012.08.001

[29] Farsalinos KE, Romagna G, Allifranchini E, Ripamonti E, Bocchietto E, Todeschi S, et al. Comparison of the cytotoxic potential of cigarette smoke and electronic cigarette vapour extract on cultured myocardial cells. International Journal of Environmental Research and Public Health. 2013;**10**(10):5146-5162. DOI: 10.3390/ijerph10105146

[30] Misra M, Leverette RD, Cooper BT, Bennett MB, Brown SE. Comparative in vitro toxicity profile of electronic and tobacco cigarettes, smokeless tobacco and nicotine replacement therapy products: E-liquids, extracts and collected aerosols. International Journal of Environmental Research and Public Health. 2014;**11**(11):11325-11347. DOI: 10.3390/ijerph111111325

[31] Sancilio S, Gallorini M, Cataldi A, di Giacomo V. Cytotoxicity and apoptosis induction by e-cigarette fluids in human gingival fibroblasts. Clinical Oral Investigations. 2016;**20**(3):477-483. DOI: 10.1007/s00784-015-1537-x

[32] Scheffler S, Dieken H, Krischenowski O, Förster C, Branscheid D, Aufderheide M. Evaluation of e-cigarette liquid vapor and mainstream cigarette smoke after direct exposure of primary human bronchial epithelial cells. International Journal of Environmental Research and Public Health. 2015;**12**(4):3915-3925. DOI: 10.3390/ijerph120403915

[33] Hwang JH, Lyes M, Sladewski K, Enany S, McEachern E, Mathew DP, et al. Electronic cigarette inhalation alters innate immunity and airway cytokines while increasing the virulence of colonizing bacteria. Journal of Molecular Medicine (Berlin, Germany). 2016;**94**(6):667-679. DOI: 10.1007/s00109-016-1378-3

[34] Ma T, Lee A, Eng B, Patel V, Michel SLJ, Kane MA, et al. Aerosolized e-liquid base constituents induce cytotoxicity and genotoxicity in oral keratinocytes. Oral Diseases. 2025;**31**(2):482-491. DOI: 10.1111/odi.15104

[35] Czoli CD, Goniewicz M, Islam T, Kotnowski K, Hammond D. Consumer preferences for electronic cigarettes: Results from a discrete choice experiment. Tobacco Control. 2016;**25**(e1):e30-e36. DOI: 10.1136/tobaccocontrol-2015-052422

[36] Kreslake JM, Wayne GF, Alpert HR, Koh HK, Connolly GN. Tobacco industry control of menthol in cigarettes and targeting of adolescents and young adults. American Journal of Public Health. 2008;**98**(9):1685-1692. DOI: 10.2105/AJPH.2007.125542

[37] Morean ME, Butler ER, Bold KW, Kong G, Camenga DR, Cavallo DA, et al. Preferring more e-cigarette flavors is associated with e-cigarette use frequency among adolescents but not adults. PLoS One. 2018;**13**(1):e0189015. DOI: 10.1371/journal.pone.0189015

[38] Tackett AP, Lechner WV, Meier E, Grant DMM, Driskill LM, Tahirkheli NN, et al. Biochemically verified smoking cessation and vaping beliefs among vape store customers. Addiction. 2015;**110**(5):868-874. DOI: 10.1111/add.12878

[39] Cuadra GA, Shamim A, Shah R, Morgan J, Palazzolo DL. Comparison of culture media for in vitro expansion of oral epithelial keratinocytes. Applied Biosciences. 2023;**2**(2):308-327. DOI: 10.3390/applbiosci2020021

[40] Yerger VB. Menthol's potential effects on nicotine dependence: A tobacco industry perspective. Tobacco Control. 2011;**20**(Suppl 2):ii29-ii36. DOI: 10.1136/tc.2010.041970

[41] McCarthy WJ, Caskey NH, Jarvik ME, Gross TM, Rosenblatt MR, Carpenter C. Menthol vs nonmenthol cigarettes: Effects on smoking behavior. American Journal of Public Health. 1995;**85**(1):67-72. DOI: 10.2105/AJPH.85.1.67

[42] Lewis MJ, Wackowski O. Dealing with an innovative industry: A look at flavored cigarettes promoted by mainstream brands. American Journal of Public Health. 2006;**96**(2):244-251. DOI: 10.2105/AJPH.2004.061200

[43] Leventhal AM, Goldenson NI, Cho J, Kirkpatrick MG, McConnell RS, Stone MD, et al. Flavored e-cigarette use and progression of vaping in adolescents. Pediatrics. 2019;**144**(5):e20190789. DOI: 10.1542/peds.2019-0789

[44] Soneji S, Barrington-Trimis JL, Wills TA, Leventhal AM, Unger JB, Gibson LA, et al. Association between initial use of e-cigarettes and subsequent cigarette smoking among adolescents and young adults: A systematic review and meta-analysis. JAMA Pediatrics. 2017;**171**(8):788-797. DOI: 10.1001/jamapediatrics.2017.1488

[45] Shamim A, Herzog H, Shah R, Pecorelli S, Nisbet V, George A, et al. Pathophysiological responses of oral keratinocytes after exposure to flavored e-cigarette liquids. Dentistry Journal. 2025;**13**(2):60. DOI: 10.3390/dj13020060

[46] Majid OW. Preliminary evidence of impaired oral wound healing in e-cigarette users: A call for perioperative vaping cessation. Evidence-Based Dentistry. 2024;**25**(January):63-64. DOI: 10.1038/s41432-024-00982-z

[47] Behar RZ, Davis B, Wang Y, Bahl V, Lin S, Talbot P. Identification of toxicants in cinnamon-flavored electronic cigarette refill fluids. Toxicology In Vitro. 2014;**28**(2):198-208. DOI: 10.1016/j.tiv.2013.10.006

[48] Lerner CA, Sundar IK, Yao H, Gerloff J, Ossip DJ, McIntosh S, et al. Vapors produced by electronic cigarettes and e-juices with flavorings induce toxicity, oxidative stress, and inflammatory response in lung epithelial cells and in mouse lung. PLoS One. 2015;**10**(2):e0116732. DOI: 10.1371/journal.pone.0116732

[49] Muthumalage T, Prinz M, Ansah KO, Gerloff J, Sundar IK, Rahman I. Inflammatory and oxidative responses induced by exposure to commonly used e-cigarette flavoring chemicals and flavored e-liquids without nicotine. Frontiers in Physiology. 2018;**8**:1130. DOI: 10.3389/fphys.2017.01130

[50] Szumilas P, Wilk A, Szumilas K, Karakiewicz B. The effects of e-cigarette aerosol on oral cavity cells and tissues: A narrative review. Toxics. 2022;**10**(2):74. DOI: 10.3390/toxics10020074

[51] Wilson C, Tellez Freitas CM, Awan KH, Ajdaharian J, Geiler J, Thirucenthilvelan P. Adverse effects of e-cigarettes on head, neck, and oral cells: A systematic review. Journal of Oral Pathology & Medicine. 2022;**51**(2):113-125. DOI: 10.1111/jop.13273

[52] Tolba YM, Omar SS, El Hak AR, Nagui DA. Electronic cigarettes can damage lingual papillae and taste buds. Can vitamins C and E supplementation reverse this damage? Life Sciences. 2023;**329**(September):121955. DOI: 10.1016/j.lfs.2023.121955

[53] Groeger S, Meyle J. Oral mucosal epithelial cells. Frontiers in Immunology. 2019;**10**(February):1-22. DOI: 10.3389/fimmu.2019.00208

[54] King MW. Glycoproteins: Roles in cellular homeostasis and disease. In: Reviews in Cell Biology and Molecular Medicine. Hoboken, NJ, USA: John Wiley & Sons, Ltd., Wiley-Blackwell; 2006. DOI: 10.1002/3527600906.mcb.200300040

[55] Wang S-S, Tang Y-L, Pang X, Zheng M, Tang Y-J, Liang X-H. The maintenance of an oral epithelial barrier. Life Sciences. 2019;**227**(June):129-136. DOI: 10.1016/j.lfs.2019.04.029

[56] Ji EH, Elzakra N, Chen W, Cui L, Lee ES, Sun B, et al. E-cigarette aerosols induce unfolded protein response in normal human oral keratinocytes. Journal of Cancer. 2019;**10**(27):6915-6924. DOI: 10.7150/jca.31319

[57] Tommasi S, Caliri AW, Caceres A, Moreno DE, Li M, Chen Y, et al. Deregulation of biologically significant genes and associated molecular pathways in the oral epithelium of electronic cigarette users. International Journal of Molecular Sciences. 2019;**20**(3):738. DOI: 10.3390/ijms20030738

[58] Tommasi S, Brocchieri L, Tornaletti S, Besaratinia A. Epigenomic dysregulation in youth vapers: Implications for disease risk assessment. American Journal of Respiratory Cell and Molecular Biology. 2025;**72**(2):206-218. DOI: 10.1165/rcmb.2024-0207OC

[59] Guo J, Hecht SS. DNA damage in human oral cells induced by use of e-cigarettes. Drug Testing and Analysis. 2023;**15**(10):1189-1197. DOI: 10.1002/dta.3375

[60] Ganapathy V, Chinnaiyan M, Brobst D, Sadhasivam B, Nshimiyimana JD, Zhao Y, et al. Abstract LB086: Measuring oral DNA damage to evaluate electronic cigarette use as a tobacco harmreduction strategy. Cancer Research. 2024;**84**(7_Supplement):LB086. DOI: 10.1158/1538-7445.AM2024-LB086

[61] Pérez-Leal M, El Helou B, Roger I. Electronic cigarettes versus combustible cigarettes in oral squamous cell cancer patients: A systematic review. Journal of Oral Pathology & Medicine: Official Publication of the International Association of Oral Pathologists and the American Academy of Oral Pathology. 2025;**54**(4):199-206. DOI: 10.1111/jop.13618

[62] Ka H, Park H-J, Jung H-J, Choi J-W, Cho K-S, Ha J, et al. Cinnamaldehyde induces apoptosis by ROS-mediated mitochondrial permeability transition in human promyelocytic leukemia HL-60 cells. Cancer Letters. 2003;**196**(2):143-152. DOI: 10.1016/S0304-3835(03)00238-6

[63] Gerloff J, Sundar IK, Freter R, Sekera ER, Friedman AE, Robinson R, et al. Inflammatory response and barrier dysfunction by different e-cigarette flavoring chemicals identified by gas chromatography-mass spectrometry in e-liquids and e-vapors on human lung epithelial cells and fibroblasts. Applied In Vitro Toxicology. 2017;**3**(1):28-40. DOI: 10.1089/aivt.2016.0030

[64] Javed F, Kellesarian SV, Sundar IK, Romanos GE, Rahman I. Recent updates on electronic cigarette aerosol and inhaled nicotine effects on periodontal and pulmonary tissues. Oral Diseases. 2017;**23**(8):1052-1057. DOI: 10.1111/odi.12652

[65] Leigh NJ, Lawton RI, Hershberger PA, Goniewicz ML. Flavourings significantly affect inhalation toxicity of aerosol generated from electronic nicotine delivery systems (ENDS). Tobacco Control. 2016;**25**(Suppl 2):ii81-ii87. DOI: 10.1136/tobaccocontrol-2016-053205

[66] Sundar IK, Javed F, Romanos GE, Rahman I. E-cigarettes and flavorings induce inflammatory and pro-senescence responses in oral epithelial cells and periodontal fibroblasts. Oncotarget. 2016;**7**(47):77196-77204. DOI: 10.18632/oncotarget.12857

[67] Adeoye O, Olawumi J, Opeyemi A, Christiania O. Review on the role of glutathione on oxidative stress and infertility. JBRA Assisted Reproduction. 2018;**22**(1):61-66. DOI: 10.5935/1518-0557.20180003

[68] Lushchak VI. Glutathione homeostasis and functions: Potential targets for medical interventions. Journal of Amino Acids. 2012;**2012**:736837. DOI: 10.1155/2012/736837

[69] Owen JB, Butterfield DA. Measurement of oxidized/reduced glutathione ratio. Methods in Molecular Biology (Clifton, N.J.). 2010;**648**:269-277. DOI: 10.1007/978-1-60761-756-3_18

[70] Rahman I, Bel A, Mulier B, Donaldson K, MacNee W. Differential regulation of glutathione by oxidants and dexamethasone in alveolar epithelial cells. American Journal of Physiology-Lung Cellular and Molecular Physiology. 1998;**275**(1):L80-L86. DOI: 10.1152/ajplung.1998.275.1.L80

[71] Seo YJ, Lee JW, Lee EH, Lee HK, Kim HW, Kim Y-H. Role of glutathione in the adaptive tolerance to H_2O_2. Free Radical Biology & Medicine. 2004;**37**(8):1272-1281. DOI: 10.1016/j.freeradbiomed.2004.07.012

[72] Franco R, Bortner CD, Schmitz I, Cidlowski JA. Glutathione depletion regulates both extrinsic and intrinsic apoptotic signaling cascades independent from multidrug resistance protein 1. Apoptosis. 2014;**19**(1):117-134. DOI: 10.1007/s10495-013-0900-0

[73] Ji EH, Sun B, Zhao T, Shu S, Chang CH, Messadi D, et al. Characterization of electronic cigarette aerosol and its induction of oxidative stress response in oral keratinocytes. PLoS One. 2016;**11**(5):e0154447. DOI: 10.1371/journal.pone.0154447

[74] Franco R, DeHaven WI, Sifre MI, Bortner CD, Cidlowski JA. Glutathione depletion and disruption of intracellular ionic homeostasis regulate lymphoid cell apoptosis. The Journal of Biological

Chemistry. 2008;**283**(52):36071-36087. DOI: 10.1074/jbc.M807061200

[75] Tanaka T, Narazaki M, Kishimoto T. IL-6 in inflammation, immunity, and disease. Cold Spring Harbor Perspectives in Biology. 2014;**6**(10):a016295. DOI: 10.1101/cshperspect.a016295

[76] Ganesan SM, Dabdoub SM, Nagaraja HN, Scott ML, Pamulapati S, Berman ML, et al. Adverse effects of electronic cigarettes on the disease-naive oral microbiome. Science Advances. 2020;**6**(22):eaaz0108. DOI: 10.1126/sciadv.aaz0108

[77] Ramenzoni LL, Schneider A, Fox SC, Meyer M, Meboldt M, Attin T, et al. Cytotoxic and inflammatory effects of electronic and traditional cigarettes on oral gingival cells using a novel automated smoking instrument: An in vitro study. Toxics. 2022;**10**(4):179. DOI: 10.3390/toxics10040179

[78] Alanazi H, Rouabhia M. Effect of e-cigarette aerosol on gingival mucosa structure and proinflammatory cytokine response. Toxicology Reports. 2022;**9**(August):1624-1631. DOI: 10.1016/j.toxrep.2022.08.003

[79] Beklen A, Uckan D. Electronic cigarette liquid substances propylene glycol and vegetable glycerin induce an inflammatory response in gingival epithelial cells. Human & Experimental Toxicology. 2021;**40**(1):25-34. DOI: 10.1177/0960327120943934

[80] Su L, Liu J, Yue Q, Zhang S, Zhao C, Sun X, et al. Evaluation of the effects of e-cigarette aerosol extracts and tobacco cigarette smoke extracts on human gingival epithelial cells. ACS Omega. 2023;**8**(12):10919-10929. DOI: 10.1021/acsomega.2c07324

[81] Shah R, Luo ED, Shaffer CA, Tabakha M, Tomov S, Minton SH, et al. Polarization of THP-1-derived human M0 to M1 macrophages exposed to flavored e-liquids. Toxics. 2025;**13**(6):451. DOI: 10.3390/toxics13060451

[82] Scott A, Lugg ST, Aldridge K, Lewis KE, Bowden A, Mahida RY, et al. Pro-inflammatory effects of e-cigarette vapour condensate on human alveolar macrophages. Thorax. 2018;**73**(12):1161-1169. DOI: 10.1136/thoraxjnl-2018-211663

[83] Lamb T, Rahman I. Pro-inflammatory effects of aerosols from e-cigarette-derived flavoring chemicals on murine macrophages. Toxicology Reports. 2023;**10**:431-435. DOI: 10.1016/j.toxrep.2023.04.003

[84] Clapp PW, Pawlak EA, Lackey JT, Keating JE, Reeber SL, Glish GL, et al. Flavored e-cigarette liquids and cinnamaldehyde impair respiratory innate immune cell function. American Journal of Physiology-Lung Cellular and Molecular Physiology. 2017;**313**(2):L278-L292. DOI: 10.1152/ajplung.00452.2016

[85] Lee WH, Ong S-G, Zhou Y, Tian L, Bae HR, Baker N, et al. Modeling cardiovascular risks of e-cigarettes with human-induced pluripotent stem cell-derived endothelial cells. Journal of the American College of Cardiology. 2019;**73**(21):2722-2737. DOI: 10.1016/j.jacc.2019.03.476

[86] Effah F, Taiwo B, Baines D, Bailey A, Marczylo T. Pulmonary effects of e-liquid flavors: A systematic review. Journal of Toxicology and Environmental Health, Part B. 2022;**25**(7):343-371. DOI: 10.1080/10937404.2022.2124563

[87] Iacob AM, Escobedo Martínez MF, Barbeito Castro E, Junquera Olay S, Olay García S, Junquera Gutiérrez LM. Effects of vape use on oral health: A review of

the literature. Medicina. 2024;**60**(3):365. DOI: 10.3390/medicina60030365

[88] Cichońska D, Kusiak A, Kochańska B, Ochocińska J, Świetlik D. Influence of electronic cigarettes on selected antibacterial properties of saliva. International Journal of Environmental Research and Public Health. 2019;**16**(22):1-7. DOI: 10.3390/ijerph16224433

[89] Kurniawan AV, Amtha R, Gunardi I, Heriandi A, Sari EF. The impact of electronic and conventional cigarette use towards saliva profile and oral microbiota in adolescents. Asian Pacific Journal of Cancer Prevention: APJCP. 2025;**26**(1):309-318. DOI: 10.31557/APJCP.2025.26.1.309

[90] Cichońska D, Kusiak A, Kochańska B, Ochocińska J, Świetlik D. Influence of electronic cigarettes on selected physicochemical properties of saliva. International Journal of Environmental Research and Public Health. 2022;**19**(6):3314. DOI: 10.3390/ijerph19063314

[91] Marques P, Piqueras L, Sanz M-J. An updated overview of e-cigarette impact on human health. Respiratory Research. 2021;**22**(1):151. DOI: 10.1186/s12931-021-01737-5

[92] Saputri D, Nasution AI, Surbakti MRW, Gani BA. The correlation between pH and flow rate of salivary smokers related to nicotine levels labelled on cigarettes. Dental Journal. 2017;**50**(2):61-65. DOI: 10.20473/j.djmkg.v50.i2.p61-65

[93] Guo X, Hou L, Peng X, Tang F. The prevalence of xerostomia among e-cigarette or combustible tobacco users: A systematic review and meta-analysis. Tobacco Induced Diseases. 2023;**21**:22. DOI: 10.18332/tid/156676

[94] Jawed M, Shahid SM, Qader SA, Azhar A. Dental caries in diabetes mellitus: Role of salivary flow rate and minerals. Journal of Diabetes and its Complications. 2011;**25**(3):183-186. DOI: 10.1016/j.jdiacomp.2010.07.001

[95] Modéer T, Blomberg CC, Wondimu B, Julihn A, Marcus C. Association between obesity, flow rate of whole saliva, and dental caries in adolescents. Obesity. 2010;**18**(12):2367-2373. DOI: 10.1038/oby.2010.63

[96] Vallabhan CG, Sivarajan S, Shivkumar AD, Narayanan V, Vijayakumar S, Indhuja RS. Assessment of salivary flow rate in patients with chronic periodontitis. Journal of Pharmacy and Bioallied Sciences. 2020;**12**(Suppl 1):S308. DOI: 10.4103/jpbs.JPBS_92_20

[97] Kumar V, Na A, Pratap M, Rawat G, Verma A, Kumar G. Estimation of salivary level of calcium in chronic periodontitis patients: A biochemical study. International Journal of Dentistry Research. 2018;**3**(3):47-49. DOI: 10.31254/dentistry.2018.3204

[98] Śniadach J, Kicman A, Michalska-Falkowska A, Jończyk K, Waszkiewicz N. Changes in concentration of selected biomarkers of exposure in users of classic cigarettes, e-cigarettes, and heated tobacco products—A narrative review. International Journal of Molecular Sciences. 2025;**26**(5):1796. DOI: 10.3390/ijms26051796

[99] Tabnjh AK, Alizadehgharib S, Campus G, Lingström P. The effects of electronic smoking on dental caries and proinflammatory markers: A systematic review and meta-analysis. Frontiers in Oral Health. 2025;**6**(April):1569806. DOI: 10.3389/froh.2025.1569806

[100] He X, Meister M, Jeon J, Shinde A, Zhang Q, Chepaitis P, et al. Multi-omics

assessment of puff volume-mediated salivary biomarkers of metal exposure and oxidative injury associated with electronic nicotine delivery systems. Environmental Health Perspectives. 2025;**133**(1):017005. DOI: 10.1289/EHP14321

[101] Hickman E, Payton A, Duffney P, Wells H, Ceppe AS, Brocke S, et al. Biomarkers of airway immune homeostasis differ significantly with generation of e-cigarettes. American Journal of Respiratory and Critical Care Medicine. 2022;**206**(10):1248-1258. DOI: 10.1164/rccm.202202-0373OC

[102] Radaic A, Kapila YL. The oralome and its dysbiosis: New insights into oral microbiome-host interactions. Computational and Structural Biotechnology Journal. 2021;**19**:1335-1360. DOI: 10.1016/j.csbj.2021.02.010

[103] Huang R, Li M, Ye M, Yang K, Xu X, Gregory RL. Effects of nicotine on *Streptococcus gordonii* growth, biofilm formation, and cell aggregation. Applied and Environmental Microbiology. 2014;**80**(23):7212-7218. DOI: 10.1128/AEM.02395-14

[104] Cuadra GA, Smith MT, Nelson JM, Loh EK, Palazzolo DL. A comparison of flavorless electronic cigarette-generated aerosol and conventional cigarette smoke on the survival and growth of common oral commensal streptococci. International Journal of Environmental Research and Public Health. 2019;**16**(10):e1669. DOI: 10.3390/ijerph16101669

[105] Nelson JM, Cuadra GA, Palazzolo DL. A comparison of flavorless electronic cigarette-generated aerosol and conventional cigarette smoke on the planktonic growth of common oral commensal streptococci. International Journal of Environmental Research and Public Health. 2019;**16**(24):5004. DOI: 10.3390/ijerph16245004

[106] Xu CP, Palazzolo DL, Cuadra GA. Mechanistic effects of e-liquids on biofilm formation and growth of oral commensal streptococcal communities: Effect of flavoring agents. Dentistry Journal. 2022;**10**(5):85. DOI: 10.3390/dj10050085

[107] Catala-Valentin A, Bernard JN, Caldwell M, Maxson J, Moore SD, Andl CD. E-cigarette aerosol exposure favors the growth and colonization of oral *Streptococcus mutans* compared to commensal streptococci. Microbiology Spectrum. 2022;**10**(2):e02421-e02421. DOI: 10.1128/spectrum.02421-21

[108] Sharma S, Mohler J, Mahajan SD, Schwartz SA, Bruggemann L, Aalinkeel R. Microbial biofilm: A review on formation, infection, antibiotic resistance, control measures, and innovative treatment. Microorganisms. 2023;**11**(6):1614. DOI: 10.3390/microorganisms11061614

[109] Mirani ZA, Fatima A, Urooj S, Aziz M, Khan MN, Abbas T. Relationship of cell surface hydrophobicity with biofilm formation and growth rate: A study on *Pseudomonas aeruginosa*, *Staphylococcus aureus*, and *Escherichia coli*. Iranian Journal of Basic Medical Sciences. 2018;**21**(7):760-769. DOI: 10.22038/IJBMS.2018.28525.6917

[110] Christian N, Burden D, Emam A, Brenk A, Sperber S, Kalu M, et al. Effects of e-liquids and their aerosols on biofilm formation and growth of oral commensal streptococcal communities: Effect of cinnamon and menthol flavors. Dentistry Journal. 2024;**12**(8):232. DOI: 10.3390/dj12080232

[111] Trybek G, Aniko-Wlodarczyk M, Preuss O, Kuligowski P,

Gabrysz-Trybek E, Suchanecka A, et al. The effect of nicotine on oral health. Baltic Journal of Health and Physical Activity. 2022;**10**(2):1. DOI: 10.29359/BJHPA.10.2.1

[112] Baek O, Zhu W, Kim HC, Lee S-W. Effects of nicotine on the growth and protein expression of *Porphyromonas gingivalis*. The Journal of Microbiology. 2012;**50**(1):143-148. DOI: 10.1007/s12275-012-1212-8

[113] DuBois AE, Bennett ZC, Khalid U, Khalid A, Meece RA, Difiore GJ, et al. Nicotine: Its stimulating and inhibitory effects on oral microorganisms. Fine Focus. 2014;**1**(1):63-75. DOI: 10.33043/FF.1.1.63-75

[114] Huang R, Li M, Gregory RL. Effect of nicotine on growth and metabolism of *Streptococcus mutans*. European Journal of Oral Sciences. 2012;**120**(4):319-325. DOI: 10.1111/j.1600-0722.2012.00971.x

[115] Rouabhia M, Semlali A. Electronic cigarette vapor increases *Streptococcus mutans* growth, adhesion, biofilm formation, and expression of the biofilm-associated genes. Oral Diseases. 2021;**27**(3):639-647. DOI: 10.1111/odi.13564

[116] Kreth J, Merritt J, Shi W, Qi F. Competition and coexistence between *Streptococcus mutans* and *Streptococcus sanguinis* in the dental biofilm. Journal of Bacteriology. 2005;**187**(21):7193-7203. DOI: 10.1128/jb.187.21.7193-7203.2005

[117] Herrero ER, Slomka V, Boon N, Bernaerts K, Hernandez-Sanabria E, Quirynen M, et al. Dysbiosis by neutralizing commensal mediated inhibition of pathobionts. Scientific Reports. 2016;**6**(1):38179. DOI: 10.1038/srep38179

[118] Giordano-Kelhoffer B, Lorca C, Llanes JM, Rábano A, del Ser T, Serra A, et al. Oral microbiota, its equilibrium and implications in the pathophysiology of human diseases: A systematic review. Biomedicine. 2022;**10**(8):1803. DOI: 10.3390/biomedicines10081803

[119] Pushalkar S, Paul B, Li Q, Yang J, Vasconcelos R, Makwana S, et al. Electronic cigarette aerosol modulates the oral microbiome and increases risk of infection. iScience. 2020;**23**(3):1-14. DOI: 10.1016/j.isci.2020.100884

[120] Bostanci N, Belibasakis GN. *Porphyromonas gingivalis*: An invasive and evasive opportunistic oral pathogen. FEMS Microbiology Letters. 2012;**333**(1):1-9. DOI: 10.1111/j.1574-6968.2012.02579.x

[121] Zhou P, Manoil D, Belibasakis GN, Kotsakis GA. Veillonellae: Beyond bridging species in oral biofilm ecology. Frontiers in Oral Health. 2021;**2**(October):774115. DOI: 10.3389/froh.2021.774115

[122] Chopyk J, Bojanowski CM, Shin J, Moshensky A, Fuentes AL, Bonde SS, et al. Compositional differences in the oral microbiome of e-cigarette users. Frontiers in Microbiology. 2021;**12**(May):1-12. DOI: 10.3389/fmicb.2021.599664

[123] Figueredo CA, Abdelhay N, Figueredo CM, Catunda R, Gibson MP. The impact of vaping on periodontitis: A systematic review. Clinical and Experimental Dental Research. 2021;7(3):376-384. DOI: 10.1002/cre2.360

[124] Cugini C, Ramasubbu N, Tsiagbe VK, Fine DH. Dysbiosis from a microbial and host perspective relative to oral health and disease. Frontiers in Microbiology. 2021;**12**(March):617485. DOI: 10.3389/fmicb.2021.617485

[125] Hrncir T. Gut microbiota dysbiosis: Triggers, consequences, diagnostic and therapeutic options. Microorganisms. 2022;**10**(3):578. DOI: 10.3390/microorganisms10030578

[126] Kriss M, Hazleton KZ, Nusbacher NM, Martin CG, Lozupone CA. Low diversity gut microbiota dysbiosis: Drivers, functional implications and recovery. Current Opinion in Microbiology. 2018;**44**(August):34-40. DOI: 10.1016/j.mib.2018.07.003

[127] Chaplin DD. Overview of the immune response. The Journal of Allergy and Clinical Immunology. 2010;**125**(2 Suppl 2):S3-S23. DOI: 10.1016/j.jaci.2009.12.980

[128] Kieser KJ, Kagan JC. Multi-receptor detection of individual bacterial products by the innate immune system. Nature Reviews. Immunology. 2017;**17**(6):376-390. DOI: 10.1038/nri.2017.25

[129] Li D, Wu M. Pattern recognition receptors in health and diseases. Signal Transduction and Targeted Therapy. 2021;**6**(1):1-24. DOI: 10.1038/s41392-021-00687-0

[130] Uehara A, Sugawara Y, Kurata S, Fujimoto Y, Fukase K, Kusumoto S, et al. Chemically synthesized pathogen-associated molecular patterns increase the expression of peptidoglycan recognition proteins via toll-like receptors, NOD1 and NOD2 in human oral epithelial cells. Cellular Microbiology. 2005;**7**(5):675-686. DOI: 10.1111/j.1462-5822.2004.00500.x

[131] Mallapragada S, Wadhwa A, Agrawal P. Antimicrobial peptides: The miraculous biological molecules. Journal of Indian Society of Periodontology. 2017;**21**(6):434-438. DOI: 10.4103/jisp.jisp_325_16

[132] Ptasiewicz M, Grywalska E, Mertowska P, Korona-Głowniak I, Poniewierska-Baran A, Niedźwiedzka-Rystwej P, et al. Armed to the teeth—The oral mucosa immunity system and microbiota. International Journal of Molecular Sciences. 2022;**23**(2):882. DOI: 10.3390/ijms23020882

[133] Dickinson BC, Moffatt CE, Hagerty D, Whitmore SE, Brown TA, Graves DT, et al. Interaction of oral bacteria with gingival epithelial cell multilayers. Molecular Oral Microbiology. 2011;**26**(3):210-220. DOI: 10.1111/j.2041-1014.2011.00609.x

[134] How KY, Song KP, Chan KG. Porphyromonas gingivalis: An overview of periodontopathic pathogen below the gum line. Frontiers in Microbiology. 2016;**7**(February):53. DOI: 10.3389/fmicb.2016.00053

[135] Hanel AN, Herzog HM, James MG, Cuadra GA. Effects of oral commensal streptococci on *Porphyromonas gingivalis* invasion into oral epithelial cells. Dentistry Journal. 2020;**8**(2):39

[136] Alanazi H, Semlali A, Chmielewski W, Rouabhia M. E-cigarettes increase *Candida albicans* growth and modulate its interaction with gingival epithelial cells. International Journal of Environmental Research and Public Health. 2019;**16**(2):294. DOI: 10.3390/ijerph16020294

[137] Herndon P, Jassal JS, Cramer JD. Association between e-cigarette use and oral HPV-16 infection. Oral Oncology. 2022;**125**(February):105676. DOI: 10.1016/j.oraloncology.2021.105676

[138] Hong Y-R, Mainous AG. Electronic cigarette use and oral human papillomavirus infection among US adult population: Analysis of 2013-2016 NHANES. Journal of General Internal

Medicine. 2021;**36**(5):1454-1456. DOI: 10.1007/s11606-020-05874-3

[139] Charde P, Ali K, Hamdan N. Effects of e-cigarette smoking on periodontal health: A scoping review. PLOS Global Public Health. 2024;**4**(3):e0002311. DOI: 10.1371/journal.pgph.0002311

[140] Cichońska D, Kusiak A, Goniewicz ML. The impact of e-cigarettes on oral health—A narrative review. Dentistry Journal. 2024;**12**(12):404. DOI: 10.3390/dj12120404

[141] Tattar R, Jackson J, Holliday R. The impact of e-cigarette use on periodontal health: A systematic review and meta-analysis. Evidence-Based Dentistry. 2025;**26**(February):1-7. DOI: 10.1038/s41432-025-01119-6